DATE DUE			
Apr 25 '80			

Physiological Adaptation to the Environment

Physiological Adaptation to the Environment

Proceedings of a symposium
held at the 1973 meeting
of the American Institute
of Biological Sciences

Edited by

F. John Vernberg
Belle W. Baruch Institute for Marine Biology and Coastal Research
University of South Carolina

Intext Educational Publishers
New York

Library of Congress Cataloging in Publication Data

Main entry under title:

Physiological adaptation to the environment.

 Proceedings of a symposium held at the AIBS meeting, June 20–22, 1973.

  Bibliography: p.
  Includes index.
  1. Adaptation (Physiology)—Congresses.
I. Vernberg, F. John, 1925–   ed. II. American Institute of Biological Sciences.
QP82.P46 1975   574.1   74-30177
ISBN 0-7002-2465-3

Intext Educational Publishers
666 Fifth Avenue
New York, New York 10019

Typography by Robert Sugar

Manufactured in the United States of America

Contents

PART IV: Adaptations of Aquatic Organisms

Part V: Adaptive Value of Biological Time Measurements

Part VI: Synergisms, Models, and What Next

List of Contributors

Numbers in parentheses indicate the pages on which the authors' contributions begin.

U. Buschbom (111)
Botanisches Institut II, Botanische Anstalter der Universität Würzburg

G. M. Courtin (201)
Laurentian University

E. B. Edney (77)
University of California, Los Angeles

J. T. Enright (465)
Scripps Institution of Oceanography, University of California, La Jolla

M. Evenari (111)
The Hebrew University of Jerusalem

Raymond A. Galloway (365)
University of Maryland

E. Gwinner (417)
Max Planck Institut für Verhaltensphysiologie, Seewiesen und Erling-Andechs/Obbs.

K. C. Hamner (477)
University of California, Los Angeles

Klaus Hoffmann (435)
Max Planck Institut für Verhaltensphysiologie, Erling-Andechs

T. Hoshizaki (477)
University of California, Los Angeles

L. Kappen (111)
Botanisches Institut II, Botanische Anstalten der Universität Würzburg

H. Kleerekoper (383)
Texas A&M University

O. L. Lange (111)
Botanisches Institut II, Botanische Anstalten der Universität Würzburg

Brent H. McCown (225)
The University of Wisconsin

Stephen F. MacLean, Jr. (269)
Institute of Arctic Biology, University of Alaska

J. M. Mayo (201)
University of Alberta

H. A. Mooney (19)
Stanford University

Dietrich Neumann (451)
University of Cologne

David W. Norton (301)
Institute of Arctic Biology, University of Alaska

William R. A. Osborne (37)
University of Michigan Medical School

Olga v. H. Owens (355)
The Johns Hopkins University

C. Ladd Prosser (3)
University of Illinois

John L. Roberts (395)
University of Massachusetts

Frank B. Salisbury (501)
Utah State University

E. D. Schulze (111)
Botanisches Institut II, Botanische Anstalten der Universität Würzburg

H. H. Seliger (355)
The Johns Hopkins University

Vaughan H. Shoemaker (143)
University of California, Riverside

Constantine Sorokin (333)
University of Maryland

Richard E. Tashian (37)
University of Michigan Medical School

C. Richard Taylor (131)
Museum of Comparative Zoology and Harvard University

Larry L. Tieszen (157)
Augustana College

Irwin P. Ting (99)
University of California, Riverside

W. B. Vernberg (521)
University of South Carolina

Paul E. Waggoner (547)
The Connecticut Agricultural Experiment Station, New Haven

F. W. Went (67)
Desert Research Institute, University of Nevada System, Reno

George C. West (301)
Institute of Arctic Biology, University of Alaska

Robert G. White (239)
University of Alaska

Nancy K. Wieland (157)
Augustana College

G. M. Woodwell (51)
Brookhaven National Laboratory

F. Eugene Yates (539)
University of Southern California

Preface

In recent years there has been increasing research emphasis on the nature of the physiological mechanisms that enable organisms to meet the stress of environmental fluctuation. This trend has been the result of a number of developments. Perhaps one of the more important of these has been the increasing awareness of environmental problems. Questions have been raised about the ability of organisms to survive in an environment which is being insulted at an alarming rate, and there is much societal interest in how organisms are adapted to live where they do. Many of these questions cannot now be answered on a scientific basis because of the lack of information. But emotionalism is giving way to rational approaches. An increasing number of scientists are studying and analyzing the impact of the environment on the functional capacity of organisms, and powerful scientific techniques have become available.

Because growth in our knowledge of physiological adaptation has been rapid, and because the work has involved scientists working in different disciplines and on different levels of biological organization, the need for a major symposium, cosponsored by divergent scientific societies, to deal with the topic of "Physiological Adaptation to the Environment" was evident. This symposium was held at the AIBS meetings at the University of Massachusetts June 20–22, 1973.

A primary objective of this symposium was to examine newly acquired information on the mechanisms of physiological adaptation of plants and animals as they relate to cellular and subcellular, organ system, whole organism, and ecosystem levels of organization. By bringing together investigators who do not normally have contact with each other, it was hoped that new insights and useful evaluation of lines of research would be possible.

To completely resolve environmental adaptation problems at one symposium was impossible. Hence, another objective of this symposium was to serve as a catalyst to bring together at future meetings those scientists representing diverse disciplines to discuss in greater detail those problems which they share.

Lastly the need to publish was strongly felt; and this volume, comprising six parts, includes most of the papers presented at this interdisciplinary symposium. Part I deals with the general nature of physiological adaptation as seen at the whole organism, tissue-organ system, cellular, biochemical, and the ecosystem level of biological organization. Parts II–IV emphasize adaptations by plants and animals from three major habitat types—the desert, polar-alpine, and aquatic. The fifth part focuses on the adaptive nature of biological time measurements, and the volume concludes with papers on the positive and negative aspects of modeling and on the interaction of multiple factors on plants and animals.

Special praise is due the following individuals who organized and chaired specific sections:

Section II.   The Desert Organisms. *E. Edney and F. Went*
Section III.   Polar-Alpine Organisms. *L. Bliss*
Section IV.   Aquatic Organisms. *R. Krauss and F. J. Vernberg*
Section V.   Biological Time Measurements. *E. Gwinner and C. Pittendrigh*

The general program was planned by an appointed committee representing various societies:

Dr. F. John Vernberg, Chairman
University of South Carolina
Physiological Ecology Section
Ecological Society of America

Dr. Bert Drake
Smithsonian Institution
American Society of Plant
Physiologists

Dr. Henry Hellmers
Duke University
Physiological Ecology Section
Ecological Society of America

Dr. Frank Salisbury
Utah State University
American Society of Plant
Physiologists

Dr. Bodil Schmidt-Nielsen
Mount Desert Island
Biological Laboratory
American Physiological Society

Dr. George Bartholomew
University of California,
Los Angeles
Division of Comparative Physiology
and Biochemistry, American Society
of Zoologists

Dr. G. Edgar Folk
University of Iowa
Physiological Ecology Section
Ecological Society of America

Dr. William Hoar
University of British Columbia
Division of Comparative Physiology
and Biochemistry, American Society
of Zoologists

The many colleagues who refereed the individual papers are to be thanked for their invaluable contribution of their skill and time. Drs. Bliss, DeCoursey, and W. Vernberg are to be singled out for their extensive editorial duties. The Ms. H. Merritt, S. Counts, and B. Dudley prepared the final copy while tolerating both authors and me.

A grant from the National Science Foundation (GB-37353) provided travel funds for some of the participants.

Finally, the encouragement and vital assistance of the late Dr. John R. Olive, AIBS, in bringing this symposium to fruition is gratefully acknowledged. This volume is dedicated to his memory in honor of his long continuing efforts to serve the biological community.

This volume is dedicated to
the memory of
John R. Olive
who
dedicated his life to
the biological community

Part I
The Nature of Physiological Adaptation to the Environment

Physiological Adaptations in Animals

C. Ladd Prosser

Physiology Department
University of Illinois
Urbana, Illinois

One purpose of this volume is to seek a general terminology for organism—environment interactions which may be common to animals, plants, and microorganisms. Table 1 lists a number of definitions. Most examples will be for poikilothermic aquatic animals, mainly fish; but many of these definitions can equally well be used for other organisms and for environmental parameters other than temperature.

The word adaptation has so many meanings as to be of questionable value, but I shall use physiological adaptation to refer to any state or rate function which favors normal biological activity in a specific, but often stressful environment. Physiological variation refers to diversity in adaptive properties. Such variations may have two bases: (1) they may be genetically determined, or (2) they may be environmentally induced. The genotype sets the limits within which individuals in a population respond to environmental pressure. Genetically determined variations can be separated from those environmentally induced by breeding or transplantation experiments, or by laboratory acclimation with respect to a single factor or by acclimatization in nature where multiple factors vary.

Genetic variations provide the basis for speciation. A physiological species is a population of similar individuals occupying throughout their

3

Table 1 Some Definitions for Environmental Physiology

Physiological adaptation: Any functional adjustment (state or rate function) which favors normal biological activity in an altered, often a stressful, environment.

Physiological variations: Differences in physiological properties which are adaptive with respect to some stressful environmental factor. These may be either:
1. Genetically determined as in physiological races, subspecies, etc., or
2. Environmentally induced as in populations in different environments—either laboratory or nature.

Resistance adaptations: Adaptations which favor survival at environmental extremes.

Capacity adaptations: Adaptations which favor normal rate functions within a mid- or "normal" environmental range.

Measures of lethality, for:
enzymes—denaturation, inactivation, conformational changes.
lipids—change in physical state, melting.
cells—change in leakiness of membranes; loss of ATP synthesis.
organs and organ systems—loss of coordinated and integrative functions.
organisms—loss of integration in nervous and other systems which, with continued stress, could lead to death.
populations—failure of reproduction.
The limits of tolerance are widest for molecules, narrower for tissues and very narrow for organisms and populations.

Homeostasis: Maintenance of relative constancy of an internal state. Feedback control mechanisms are activated when environment changes; for example, constancy of body temperature, or of intracellular potassium concentration.

Homeokinesis: Maintenance of relative constancy of energy output, hence of capacity for biological activity irrespective of whether internal state varies, e.g., ATP production in osmoconforming animals.

Conformity: Change in some parameter of internal state in proportion to change in this parameter of environment. Internal state may equal that in the environment (e.g., temperature in poikilotherms) or may increase or decrease with the environment but at a constant difference (e.g., osmoconcentration in many osmoconformers).

Regulation of state: Maintenance of relative constancy of some internal parameter in face of environmental stress; control mechanisms insufficient at limits; essentially similar to homeostasis, e.g., homeotherms. Regulation may occur in some body regions, not in others, as in heterotherms.

Ectotherms: Animals dependent on external sources of heat.

Endotherms: Animals that generate most body heat internally.
The terms poikilothermy and homeothermy refer to conformity and regulation; ectothermy and endothermy refer to processes, outside or within the animal, for gaining heat. Many combinations of these characters occur.

Time course of adaptations: (1) direct responses, (2) acclimatory compensations, (3) selection of genetic variants.

Direct responses: Changes in state or rate function occurring immediately after exposure to an altered environment, e.g. rates used to calculate Q_{10}'s; also homeostatic alterations which eliminate variation of a regulated function, e.g., homeothermy.

Table 1 (continued)

Compensatory acclimation or acclimatization: Long-term changes in an organism after exposure to an altered environment so that rate function (e.g., energy output) is similar for two groups at different environments of acclimation and measurement but different for the two groups if both are measured at an intermediate environment, e.g., metabolic rate of cold-acclimated poikilotherms is greater than that of warm-acclimated when measured at intermediate temperature. Also homeostatic changes which conserve energy or shift from a direct response to a more permanent one, e.g., changes in insulation or shift to nonshivering thermogenesis in a homeotherm.

Acclimation: Compensatory changes in a morphological, biochemical, or biophysical function permitting constancy in rate functions after prolonged change in a single environmental variable, e.g., with controlled laboratory parameters.

Acclimatization: Compensatory changes permitting constancy of rate functions after prolonged exposures to altered multiple environmental factors in nature, e.g., seasonal, geographic effects.

Euryhaline, eurythermal: Tolerant of wide ranges of salinity, temperature.

Stenohaline, stenothermal: Limited in range of tolerable salinity, temperature.

---

life cycles the same ecological niche and geographic range. That is, a physiological species is uniquely adapted, and, if the mechanisms of such adaptation could be described in detail, the species would be truly described in terms of natural selection.

Physiological adaptations are of two sorts and these may, but need not, be related as to underlying mechanisms. Resistance adaptations are those which permit survival at environmental extremes, e.g., in heat or cold. Capacity adaptations are those which permit relative constancy of biological activity over a "normal" or tolerable environmental range; these may refer to internal states, such as temperature, or to rate functions, such as energy output.

Resistance adaptations can be considered in terms of survival, the limits and mechanisms of which differ according to the level of biological organization being studied. In general, entire integrated organisms have narrower limits of survival than the limits of their enzyme proteins. We may think of environmental limits for enzymes in terms of denaturation, inactivation, or block of synthesis, and for lipids in terms of melting point or change in physical state. Survival limits of cells are shown by leakiness of cell membranes for ions, particularly potassium and sodium, and by reduction of synthesis of adequate amounts of ATP. Approach of death with respect to organs and whole organisms is shown by loss of coordinated function; in animals the most sensitive part is usually the nervous system, loss of coordination of which may lead to organismic death. At the level of populations, survival fails when reproduction is no longer effective. Thus resistance adaptation may be observed and its mechanisms analyzed in terms of molecules, organisms, and populations.

Capacity adaptations may provide for homeostasis or relative constancy of internal state in the face of environmental change. As internal deviation occurs, feedback mechanisms are activated and these bring about regulation of the internal state, e.g., constancy of body temperature in homeotherms, and maintenance of high intracellular concentrations of potassium in excitable cells. Thus we may separate organismic and cellular homeostasis.

A more general form of capacity adaptation is homeokinesis or maintenance of constancy of energy output, hence of capacity for biological activity irrespective of internal state variations. Another form of homeokinesis, largely nonmetabolic, is behavioral; in many animal tropisms and kineses keep the animal in an "optimal" environment.

In contrast to regulation of internal state, there may be conformity, or internal change in proportion to change in a given parameter of the environment. Internal state may equal that of the environment (e.g., body temperature in strict poikilotherms) or may increase or decrease by a constant difference with respect to the environment (e.g., many osmoconforming invertebrates). An animal may be a conformer in internal state (varying with the environment) yet show homeokinesis as to energy production. For some states, e.g., osmoconcentration, regulation may occur for deviation in one direction and not in the opposite direction. Also some tissues may conform with the environment, whereas regulation occurs in other body regions, as in heterothermic animals.

In an analysis of adaptations to an environmental stress we may recognize three time periods. First are direct responses which may be homeostatic or homeokinetic. They may consist of increases or decreases in metabolic rates. One measure of enzyme response at different conditions is the maximum velocity (V_{max}) measured at saturating levels of substrate; this is a measure of total enzyme activity. Another measure is the concentration of substrate required for 50% activity of the enzyme; this is often given as K_m for hyperbolic activity – substrate concentration curves, or it may be given as S_{50} of substrate as in reactions with sigmoid curves. K_m in its strict definition for a simple Michaelis–Menton reaction scheme is a ratio of velocity constants $(K_2 + K_3)/K_1$. When K_m equals the enzyme–substrate dissociation constant $(K_s = K_2/K_1)$ and only under this condition is $1/K_m$ a true measure of enzyme–substrate affinity. Generally the K_m for one substrate depends on the concentrations of other substrates and cofactors, hence the designation: apparent K_m. Although apparent K_m or S_{50} are imprecise as measures of true affinity, they do characterize velocity – substrate curves, particularly in physiological ranges. V_{max} indicates activity when enzyme is rate-limiting and gives information regarding amount of enzyme. Both apparent K_m and V_{max} are useful kinetic measures and they vary directly in response to environmental change.

Another type of direct response involves activation of peripheral (or central) sensors followed by direct behavioral responses. Such direct responses may initiate chains of hormonal and nervous reactions which maintain internal constancy, e.g., body temperature in homeotherms.

After the environmental alteration has been in effect for some time — usually days or weeks — a second major kind of response takes place, compensatory acclimation or acclimatization. In individuals, biochemical changes occur which result in constancy of energy output or of internal state in the altered environment. Some poikilothermic animals, such as fish, undergo metabolic compensation over several weeks in an altered environment; other poikilotherms, e.g., some snails and amphibians, become lethargic at temperature extremes and remain dormant or noncompensating. Homeotherms may alter their insulation and hormonal state over periods of weeks at changed temperatures. Cold-hardening of some plants is a compensatory acclimatization. Evidence is accumulating that animals which live in a constant as opposed to a cycling environment may lose capacity for compensatory acclimation. Fish living in Antarctic waters have very limited acclimatory capacity (Somero et al., 1968). Species of rockfish living below the thermocline show less acclimation than a shallow-water species (Wilson et al., 1974).

The third major time period is of many generations duration and permits selection of genetic variants which are adaptive (Somero, 1969a). These provide the basis for races and subspecies, and, under conditions of isolation, they lead to speciation. Analysis of physiological variation in related populations reveals selected differences in primary structure of proteins and innate behavior patterns. In organisms with short life cycles, as bacteria and yeast, selection of mutants may be a more evident adaptation to environmental alteration than are acclimatory changes. An example of the selection of primary structure of a protein in animals is the increasing content of proline-hydroxyproline in collagen, correlated with higher melting point in animals which live in the tropics (or at 37°C) as compared with those in colder environments (Josse and Harrington, 1964). Species of the fish *Catastomus* from fast mountain streams have 20% of their hemoglobin molecules with terminal amino acid groups so modified that they show no Bohr effect, an advantage for O_2 loading under exercise (Powers, 1972). An example of a selected innate behavior is that of the characteristic song patterns which function in reproductive isolation of different species of sparrows.

Natural selection acts on phenotypes; and the genotype usually contains much more genetic potential than is realized in a given environment. An organism must be adapted in its entirety to a particular environmental parameter. However, specific mechanisms may differ in different tissues and enzymes as well as for a given organism at different stages in its life cycle. Thus, adaptational physiology bridges molecular or reductionistic biology and organismic or holistic biology. Our objective is to describe in cellular and molecular terms both the metabolic and behavioral adaptations which occur in intact animals. Unfortunately many ecological and eco-engineering decisions are based on short-term observations at one biological level.

Adaptations of Direct Responses

The following specific examples of direct responses were selected because they exhibit adaptive value. Generally, in temperature-conforming animals, metabolism and behavioral activity rise and fall with temperature. Those species which become lethargic or dormant at temperature extremes follow the typical Q_{10} relation only over a limited thermal range. In many active species the body temperature rises or falls with that of the environment, but there is some independence of temperature in that the metabolic Q_{10} approaches unity over the "optimal" thermal range (Newell, 1966).

One mechanism of instantaneous temperature compensation relates to enzyme kinetics, specifically to enzyme–substrate affinity. Measurements of apparent K_m or of S_{50}, while not measuring affinity directly are related to it qualitatively, are much used experimentally. As the temperature falls, the K_m decreases for all enzymes, i.e., the apparent affinity increases. The position of the curve on the temperature axis for given enzymes is such that for warm-water species it is far to the right of curves for cold-water species. The same enzyme differs in its primary structure such that the form which is used in polar species would be useless in the tropics. At lower temperatures the K_m curves sometimes plateau or even pass through a minimum; these temperatures of maximum apparent enzyme–substrate affinity correspond to optimal environmental ranges. Many enzymes occur in multiple forms of isozymes in one tissue, and these may differ in their temperature ranges. In a cold-climate snake one isozyme of liver s-malic dehydrogenase is more active at 5°, another form at 35° (Hoskins and Aleksiuk, 1973). An isozyme of LDH from a Manitoba, Canada, population of the snake *Thamnophis* has a lower K_m value (higher apparent affinity) at low temperatures than isozymes from a Florida population (Aleksiuk, 1971). Kinetic curves of pyruvate kinase of the Alaskan king crab show one state with minimal

K_m at 12°, another below 5° (Somero, 1969b). Populations of *Fundulus* from 20 localities on the Atlantic coast with mean annual temperature ranging from 5° to 22° show a gradual increase from one homozygote for one LDH locus, BB, to another, B'B', with heterozygotes in intermediate localities. It is evident from data on K_m's and activation energies that the B'B' homozygote is selected in warm regions (Powers, 1973).

A second kinetic parameter relates to how activation energies for given reactions are related to temperature. Temperature coefficients (Q_{10} or Arrhenius μ) are maximal at saturating substrate concentrations, i.e., V_{max}, but decline with decreasing substrate concentrations which approach those which probably occur physiologically. Thus Q_{10}'s obtained for V_{max}'s give a misleading picture of what may happen physiologically. The decreasing K_m with cooling combined with decreased temperature coefficient at physiological substrate concentrations provide some direct independence of metabolism with temperature alteration (Hochachka and Somero, 1973). Q_{10} is not constant over a wide temperature range. For many intertidal and subtidal invertebrates, standard metabolism is independent of temperature over a range corresponding to the normal (Newell, 1966; Newell and Pye, 1971).

A third physical consideration which is difficult to apply physiologically is the effect of temperature on conformation of proteins. The third and fourth order conformations depend on weak bonds within a protein in particular thermal ranges and folding can result (Hochachka and Somero, 1973). Many enzyme systems show breaks in their Arrhenius plots at critical temperatures; usually the activation energy is greater in the tolerable low temperature range than at higher temperatures. Some 20 mammalian enzymes have been shown to be cold labile and to break into subunits at temperatures below 7°–15°C. Their quaternary structure, which depends on hydrogen bonding, and hence their enzymatic activity are temperature sensitive. At these low temperatures the corresponding enzymes from poikilotherms are unaffected (Beyer, 1972).

A different type of direct response which is adaptive is behavioral. Many poikilothermic animals in a thermal gradient go to a particular temperature—the so-called preferred temperature. Desert lizards bask in the sun at low air temperatures and rest in the shade on hot days. When temperature is suddenly reduced or raised, many animals become hyperactive. The net effect of hyperactivity is to bring the animals into "preferred" temperatures (Prosser, 1973).

In general, axonal conduction continues down to lower temperatures than synaptic transmission and block occurs with less cooling in highly integrating parts of the brain, such as optic tectum and cerebellum, than in lower distributive centers. In the optic tectum of goldfish, conditioned-evoked potentials block with less cooling than do direct visual responses. Also, in goldfish a series of behavioral responses — hyperactivity, disorientation, loss of equilibrium and finally coma — occur during cooling. Similarly at critical degrees of cooling these functions in the cerebellum fail in the following sequence: inhibitory synapses, climbing fiber excitatory synapses, spontaneity of Purkinje neurons, and responses of these neurons to antidromic stimulation (Kotchabakdi and Prosser, in preparation; Prosser and Nagai, 1968).

Poikilotherms, such as large flying insects, must raise the temperature of the nervous system to some critical level before they can fly. They produce heat by movement of thoracic muscles or absorb radiant heat by body positioning. Thus they continue to thermoregulate during locomotor activity (Kammer, 1970; McCrea and Heath, 1971).

At temperature extremes, some poikilotherms go into a behavioral coma and there is much evidence that this results from failure of neural integration rather than of muscle activity. For example, tropical marine snails which live in the subtidal zone succumb to heat coma more readily than those which live high in the intertidal zone. The nervous system of Arctic beetles continues to show spontaneous electrical activity at temperatures below 0°C. This thermal range would cause death in temperate zone beetles (Baust and Miller, 1970). The nature of the synaptic membranes which have been selected for differences in thermal tolerance is unknown.

Compensatory Acclimations

Several patterns of acclimation or long-term adaptation of individual animals have been identified with respect to temperature. When a poikilotherm is transferred from an intermediate temperature to a higher or lower one, a rate function may change according to temperature and may be maintained at the new level. Or, the rate may change to a compensating increase in the cold and decrease in the warm; compensation may be partial or complete. A few functions overcompensate, and a few change in reverse direction, i.e., become reduced with time in cold or increased with time in warm. The transition to the acclimated state is not smooth, and, for goldfish, we have recently found initial oscillations or instability before a new steady state is reached in 3 – 4 weeks (Sidell *et al.*, 1973).

Both compensatory acclimations (Precht types 1 – 3) and no or inverse acclimations (types 4, 5) have been observed for different classes of enzymes (Precht, 1958; Prosser, 1967). The best known of those which compensate positively are involved in oxidative metabolism (enzymes of pentose shunt, TCA cycle and the electron transport cytochrome system) (Freed, 1965) and some synthetic enzymes (Prosser, 1967). Those enzymes which compensate negatively or fail to compensate are concerned with degradation of metabolic intermediates and with nitrogen excretion (Hazel and Prosser, 1970). Also glycolytic enzymes in fishes may fail to show positive compensation; this relates to the predominantly aerobic metabolism of active fish and the greater supply of oxygen in the cold, and conversely to the reduced availability of O_2 in the warm. Thus it would be nonadaptive for glycolysis to increase in the cold if it can already provide sufficient two-carbon fragments to the Krebs cycle, or to decrease in the warm where anaerobiosis is more important. Ion transport enzymes vary with the species and ionic conditions; sometimes they are compensating, sometimes not. Compensation varies in organs of the same animal and with stage in the life cycle. Also, as mentioned previously, neither compensatory nor noncompensatory acclimations occur in animals which become dormant in cold or warm. A temperate zone frog (Holzman and McManus, 1973) and also a salamander (Fitzpatrick, 1973) show little or no thermal acclimation of O_2 consumption. However the frog does show changes in high critical temperature (resistance acclimation).

The molecular mechanisms of compensatory acclimation are multiple. Changes in the primary structure of enzymes may be excluded on the grounds that amino acid sequences are coded by RNA and ultimately by DNA and that genetic coding cannot change within an individual. This is supported by identical K_m's and kinetic curves for nonisozymal enzymes such as succinic dehydrogenase from cold- and warm-acclimated fish (Hazel, 1970).

Greater incorporation of labeled amino acids into proteins of cold-acclimated than into those of warm-acclimated goldfish indicates increased protein turnover (Das and Prosser, 1966). Whether this enhanced turnover applies to particular enzyme proteins has been examined by my student, F. R. Wilson, by use of immunological methods (Wilson, 1973). Antibodies to cytochrome oxidase were used to inactivate quantitatively the cytochrome oxidase in mitochondrial extracts from cold- and warm-acclimated goldfish. Results showed unequivocally that the cold fish have more cytochrome oxidase per milligram mitochondrial protein than the warm-acclimated fish. Since total protein content apparently does not change, it is evident that specific proteins do change in amount; whether this is due to increased synthesis or to decreased degradation is under study now. One of the early events in cold-acclimation is increased activity of aminoacyl transferase of liver (Haschmeyer, 1969).

It has been suggested that for enzymes which are isozymal, more of one form may be synthesized in the cold and more of another in the

warm. Such selective synthesis has been found in rainbow trout for enzymes such as acetylcholine esterase (Baldwin, 1971), isocitrate dehydrogenase (Moon and Hochachka, 1972), pyruvate kinase and phosphofructokinase (Somero, 1972), and liver citrate synthase (Hochachka and
Lewis, 1970). In goldfish and green sunfish, no differences were found in
relative band patterns of LDH and m-MDH from several tissues
(Wilson et al., 1973). The polymorphism of goldfish can lead to misinter-
pretation of isozyme patterns unless sufficient numbers of fish are examined. Also we have found that the quantitative change in LDH is one of
decreased activity in the cold. Thus, at least for goldfish and green sunfish, no qualitative selective synthesis of particular isozymes of LDH
occurs and the total activity shows inverse acclimation. Also s-MDH in
snake liver, which consists of two adaptively different isozymes, shows
no acclimation effect on synthesis of relative amounts of the two isozymes (Hoskins and Aleksiuk, 1973). In poikilotherms in general there
is unquestionably genetic selection of isozymes corresponding to minimal K_m's in optimal temperature ranges.

   Another suggested mechanism of compensatory acclimation is that
concontrations of modifying ions may be changed. The reported alterations in tissue ions such as sodium are relatively small and unlikely to be
significant. However, the activity of enzymes such as PFK changes with
pH so that they go from essentially zero to full activity over 0.2 pH unit
(Freed, 1971; Trivedi and Danforth, 1966). It is established that the pH
of body fluids of most poikilotherms decreases by 0.016 pH unit per
degree rise in temperature. A recent contention (Houston, 1971) that
this relation between pH and blood temperature does not hold for fishes
is invalidated by the extreme sensitivity of fish to handling. Hence pH
values are different according to the method of blood removal and it is
not useful to compare data from different investigators. Thus it is possible that changes in intracellular pH with temperature may modify enzyme kinetics. However, the changes, in blood pH which involve acid –
base adjustments are relatively fast ($\frac{1}{2}$ hour to less than 3 days) and
seem unlikely to be responsible for acclimation which requires a month
to develop.

   Important modulation of many membrane-bound oxidative enzymes
is provided by phospholipids. It is established for many sorts of organisms that lipids which are deposited at low temperatures are more unsaturated than those deposited at high temperatures (Johnston and
Roots, 1964). Also, there tend to be more long-chain acids. My student,
Anderson (1970), showed by use of labeled acetate and phosphate that
there is increased turnover of phospholipids in cold-acclimated goldfish.
When mitochondrial phospholipid (PL) from cold-acclimated fish is ad-

ded to succinic dehydrogenase protein from either cold or warm fish the enzyme activation is much greater than when the activating PL comes from mitochondria of warm-acclimated fish. Hazel (1970) has some evidence that the amount of activation may depend on the degree of unsaturation but that the threshold concentration for activation may depend on the specific bases of the PL.

It is concluded that metabolic acclimation of poikilotherms results from changes in the following: turnover or amount of specific proteins, limited selective isozyme synthesis (at least in trout), and marked changes in unsaturation of lipid cofactors.

Acclimatory changes in fish nervous systems occur faster than metabolic changes and compensations are noted within a day or two at an altered temperature. Conduction in peripheral nerves is relatively unaffected by thermal acclimation, spinal reflexes show cold-block at slightly higher temperature than nerves and show some effect of acclimation, whereas conditioned visual responses are blocked at still higher temperatures. Blocking temperatures are directly proportional to the acclimation temperature. Also the minimum temperature at which conditioning can occur is modified by thermal acclimation (Prosser and Nagai, 1968). Lethal temperature for several freshwater fish changes by 1° for each 3° difference in acclimation temperature. Evidence from measurements on neuromuscular junctions and brain indicates that synapses are more sensitive to temperature and are more modifiable by acclimation than axons. Since synaptic function depends on lipoproteins in membranes which are selective for particular ion conductances, it is possible that the clue to central nervous acclimation is, like that of metabolic acclimation, in the synthesis of lipoproteins.

Birds and mammals show metabolic, behavioral, and morphological acclimation to temperature extremes. Seasonal changes occur in thermoneutral limits, metabolic response to cooling, insulation, and vascular sensitivity to cooling of appendages. Some species enter a state of hibernation during which the set-point of their thermoregulating center is shifted to a few degrees above zero. Discussion of the cellular mechanisms of acclimation in homeotherms is beyond the scope of this summary.

Osmotic Adaptation

It may be useful to cite examples of some of the preceding generalizations for another environmental parameter, salinity. All living organisms regulate intracellular ion concentrations and virtually all animal cells are isosmotic with the extracellular fluid. Some animals, cnidarians and echinoderms, show very little ionic regulation of extracellular body fluids, others, some bivalve mollusks and annelids, show moderate regulation, and still others, many crustaceans and vertebrates, show considerable ionic regulation of body fluids. Osmotic regulation is much more limited and many regulators of body volume and of ion concentrations are osmoconformers. Some intertidal worms, mollusks and crustaceans, especially those in estuaries, may live subject to extreme fluctuations in salinity with each change of the tide. When certain of these animals are transferred in the laboratory from one salinity to another they show initial volume change corresponding to the osmotic gradient. As excretory processes for ions become active, volume is gradually restored. With prolonged change in internal osmoconcentration, a series of compensatory reactions takes over (Prosser, 1973). The concentrations of amino acids and of such nitrogenous bases as taurine decrease in dilute animals and increase in more concentrated ones. These changes in organic solutes, particularly amino acids, are marked in cells such as muscle but they also occur in hemolymph. For example, in a euryhaline crab *Carcinus* the free amino acid concentration in hemolymph and muscle was some 80% higher in seawater than in freshwater acclimated animals. Similar changes in taurine occur in *Mytilus*. The net effect is to minimize changes in concentrations of inorganic ions while permitting considerable change in osmotic concentrations. The acclimatory compensations can occur only within certain limits for a given animal and they involve either binding and release or synthesis and degradation of amino acids.

Another mechanism of long-term alteration with salinity is in euryhaline fish and crustaceans which can either migrate between fresh water and seawater (salmon, eels, estuarine blue crabs) or can tolerate extreme salinity shifts *(Fundulus)*. In fresh water, certain cells of the gills of these animals develop the capacity actively to absorb ions. When the crab *Callinectes* is exposed to fresh or very dilute seawater, patches of specialized secretory cells appear on the gills. At a concentration of external sodium lower than in sea water active absorption is initiated (Copeland, 1968). In freshwater fish the gills have a sodium exchange pump which seems to be coupled with excretion of H^+ or NH_4^+. Conversely when fishes such as eels become acclimatized to seawater the activity of a gill ATPase associated with active Na extrusion is doubled.

The result of biochemical acclimatory changes is maintenance of some constancy of osmoconcentration and of ion concentrations in the face of a reversed gradient between the organism and the milieu. The location and nature of the receptors which trigger changes in concentrations of organic solutes and in activity of ion pumps are not known.

Conclusions

The preceding kinds of examples of immediate compensations in direct responses and long-term acclimations can be observed for other environmental parameters. Specific biochemical characters have been selected over many generations so that ecologically separated populations, species and related genera differ for specific properties of enzymes in an adaptive fashion. Similar selection of behavior patterns has occurred. The net effect is to provide some independence of the environment, with varying degrees of homeostasis and homeokinesis.

The next step in the analysis of physiological adaptation is to investigate the feedback to the genetic control of protein and lipid synthesis. Haschmeyer (1969) has shown enhancement of activity of aminoacyl transferase in liver of cold-acclimated toadfish, and one of the first steps in thermal acclimation may be stimulation of the transfer enzymes of RNA associated with protein synthesis. To what extent are the biochemical changes due to direct action of temperature (or osmoconcentration or P_{O_2}) at the cellular level and to what extent is there endocrine and nervous system mediation? Since compensatory acclimations to physical parameters can occur in microorganisms and since changes have been found in isolated gill tissues, direct cellular compensations seem probable. Hormones may play a mediating role, particularly in ionic acclimation in fishes. Possibly hormones are especially important in resistance adaptations. Turnover rates for enzyme proteins are faster than formerly believed and both synthesis and degradation may be involved (Shimke, 1970; Shimke and Doyle, 1970).

A most difficult question concerns the sensing mechanisms. We really have no reasonable ideas concerning the cellular detectors of changes in temperature and can only postulate that mass action kinetics is involved. Evidence from effects of Na and K gradients across cells of excitable tissues provide suggestions for ionic detectors in general. Specific detectors of temperature which result in constancy of OH/H ratio appear to be the imidazole groups (principally histidine) of buffer proteins (Reeves, 1972). Different parts of the brain and different cell types in the cerebellum of goldfish show different sensitivities to cooling, and specific neurons in the mammalian hypothalamus detect thermal change, others detect osmotic and ionic alterations.

In conclusion, analysis of environment–organism interactions bridges between molecular and holistic biology for all kinds of organisms. Investigations are required at all levels of organization from protein synthesis to animal behavior.

References

Aleksiuk, M. (1971). An isoenzymic basis for instantaneous cold compensation in reptiles: lactate dehydrogenase kinetics in *Thamnophis sirtalis*. *Comp. Biochem. Physiol* **40B,** 671–681.

Anderson, T. R. (1970). Temperature adaptation and the phospholipids of membranes in goldfish *(Carassius auratus). Comp. Biochem. Physiol.* 33, 663–687.

Baldwin, J. (1971). Adaptation of enzymes to temperature: acetylcholinesterases in the central nervous system of fishes. *Comp. Biochem. Physiol.* 40, 181–187.

Baust, J. G., and Miller, L. K. (1970). Variations in glycerol content and its influence on cold hardiness of the Alaskan carabid beetle, *Pterostichus brevicornis. Inst. Physiol.* 16, 979–990.

Beyer, R. E. (1972). *In* "Hibernation and Hypothermia," (F. E. South *et al.,* eds.), pp. 17–54. Elsevier, New York.

Copeland, D. E. (1968). Ultrastructure of salt absorbing cells in gills of *Callinectes. Z. Zellforsch.* 92, 1–22.

Das, A. B., and Prosser, C. L. (1966). Biochemical changes in tissues of goldfish acclimated to high and low temperatures. I. Protein synthesis. *Comp. Biochem. Physiol.* 21, 447–467.

Fitzpatrick, L. C. (1973). Effect of seasonal temperatures on energy budget and metabolic rates of northern salamander, *Eurycea bislineata. Comp. Biochem. Physiol.* 14, 651–659.

Freed, J. M. (1965). Temperature acclimation of cytochrome oxidase in goldfish. *Comp. Biochem. Physiol.* 14, 651–659.

Freed, J. M. (1971). Phosphofructokinase in temperature adaptation of goldfish. *Comp. Biochem. Physiol.* **39B,** 747–764, 765–774.

Haschmeyer, A. E. V. (1969). Synthesis of polypeptide chains in temperature acclimation of *Opsanus. Proc. Nat. Acad. Sci.* 62, 128–135.

Hazel, J. R. (1970). The effect of temperature acclimation upon succinic dehydrogenase activity from the epaxial muscle of the common goldfish (*Carassius auratus* L.): lipid reactivation of the soluble enzyme. *Comp. Biochem. Physiol.* **43B,** 837–861, 863–882.

Hazel, J., and Prosser, C. L. (1970). Interpretation of inverse acclimation to temperature. *Z. Vergl. Physiol.* 67, 217–228.

Hochachka, P. W., and Lewis, J. K. (1970). Enzyme variants in thermal acclimation: trout liver citrate synthases. *Biol. Chem.* 245, 6567–6573.

Hochachka, P. W., and Somero, G. N. (1973). "Strategies of Biochemical Adaptation." Saunders, Philadelphia.

Holzman, N., and McManus, J. J. (1973). Acclimation effects on metabolism and thermal tolerance in frog, *Rana vegatipes. Comp. Biochem. Physiol.* **45A,** 833–842.

Hoskins, M. A. H., and Aleksiuk, M. (1973). Temperature effects on MDH of cold climate snake, *Thamnophis sirtalis. Comp. Biochem. Physiol.* **45B,** 343–353.

Houston, A. H. (1971). Some comments upon acid–base balance in teleost fishes and its relationship to environmental temperature. *Comp. Biochem. Physiol.* **40A,** 535–542.

Johnston, P. V., and Roots, B. J. (1964). Brain lipid fatty acids and temperature acclimation. *Comp. Biochem. Physiol.* **11,** 303–310.

Josse, J., and Harrington, W. F. (1964). Composition of collagen as a function of temperature. *J. Mol. Biol.* **9,** 269–287.

Kammer, A. E. (1970). Thoracic temperature and flight in monarch butterfly. *Z. Vergl. Physiol.* **68,** 334–344.

Kotchabakdi, N., and Prosser, C. L. (in preparation). Effects of cooling on behavior and on electrical activity in goldfish cerebellum.

McCrea, M., and Heath, J. E. (1971). Dependence of flight on temperature regulation in moth *Munduca. J. Exp. Biol.* **54,** 415–535.

Moon, T. W., and Hochachka, P. W. (1972). Temperature and the kinetic analysis of trout isocitrate dehydrogenase. *Comp. Biochem. Physiol.* **42B,** 725–730.

Newell, R. C. (1966). Metabolic independence of temperature over limited ranges in poikilotherms. *Nature London* **212,** 426–428; *J. Zool. London* **151,** 299–311, 1967; *also* Newell, R. C., and Northcraft, H. R. (1967). *J. Zool. London* **151,** 277–298.

Newell, R. C., and Pye, V. I. (1971). Quantitative aspects of the relationship between metabolism and temperature in the winkle *Littorina littorea* (L.). *Comp. Biochem. Physiol.* **38B,** 635–650.

Powers, D. A. (1972). Hemoglobin adaptation for fast and slow water habitats in sympatric catostomid fishes. *Science* **177,** 360–362.

Powers, D. A. (1973). Ecological meaning of specific LDH alleles in *Fundulus.* (Personal communication.)

Precht, H. (1958). *In* "Physiological Adaptation," (C. L. Prosser, ed.) pp. 50–78. Amer. Phys. Soc., Washington, D.C.

Prosser, C. L. (1967). *In* "Molecular Mechanisms of Temperature Adaptation," (C. L. Prosser, ed.) pp. 351–376. Amer. Ass. Advan. Sci., Washington, D.C.

Prosser, C. L. (1973). Chapter 1. Water. Chapter 9. Temperature. *In* "Comparative Animal Physiology," (C. L. Prosser, ed.), Chaps. 1 and 9, pp. 1–78, 362–428. Saunders, Philadelphia, Pennsylvania.

Prosser, C. L., and Farhi, E. (1965). Effects of temperature on conditioned reflexes. *Z. Vergl. Physiol.* **50,** 91–101.

Prosser, C. L., and Nagai, T. (1968). *In* "The Central Nervous System and Fish Behavior," (D. Ingle, ed.), pp. 171–180, University of Chicago Press, Chicago, Illinois.

Reeves, R. B. (1972). An imidazole alphastat hypothesis for vertebrate acid–

base regulation: tissue carbon dioxide content and body temperature in bull-frogs. *Resp. Physiol.* **14,** 219–236.

Shimke, R. T. (1970). Regulation of protein degradation in mammalian tissues. *In* "Mammalian Protein Metabolism," Vol. IV, (H. N. Monro, ed.), pp. 1–7, 228, Academic Press, New York.

Shimke, R. T., and Doyle, D. (1970). Control of enzyme levels in animal tissues. *Annu. Rev. Biochem.* **39,** 929–976.

Sidell, B., Wilson, F. R., Hazel, J., and Prosser, C. L. (1973). Time course of thermal acclimation in goldfish. *J. Comp. Phys.* **84**(2), 119–127.

Somero, G. N. (1969a). Enzymic mechanisms of temperature compensation: immediate and evolutionary effects of temperature on enzymes of aquatic poikilotherms. *Amer. Natur.* **103,** 517–530.

Somero, G. N. (1969b). Pyruvate kinase variants of the Alaskan king crab: evidence for a temperature-dependent interconversion between two forms having distinct and adaptive kinetic properties. *Biochem. J.* **114,** 237–241.

Somero, G. N. (1972). *In* "Hibernation–Hypothermia," (F. South *et al.,* eds. by), pp. 55–80. Elsevier, New York.

Somero, G. N., Giese, A. C., and Wohlschlag, D. E. (1968). Cold adaptation of the Antractic fish, *Trematomus bernacchii. Comp. Biochem. Physiol.* **26,** 223–233.

Trivedi, B., and Danforth, W. H. (1966). Effect of pH on the kinetics of frog muscle phosphofructokinase. *J. Biol. Chem.* **241,** 4110–4114.

Wilson, F. R. (1973). Quantitative changes of enzymes of the goldfish (*Carassius auratus* L.) in response to temperature acclimation: an immunological approach. Ph.D. Thesis, University of Illinois.

Wilson, F. R., Whitt, G., and Prosser, C. L. (1973). Lactate dehydrogenase and malate dehydrogenase isozyme patterns in tissues of temperature acclimated goldfish (*Carassius auratus* L.). *Comp. Biochem. Physiol.* **46B,** 105–116.

Wilson, F. R., Somero, G., and Prosser, C. L. (1974). Temperature-metabolism relations of two species of *Sebastes* from different thermal environments. *Comp. Biochem. Physiol.* **47B,** 485–491.

Plant Physiological Ecology — A Synthetic View

H. A. Mooney

Department of Biological Sciences
Stanford University
Stanford, California

The objective of this chapter is to present a brief overview of the physiological ecology of plants. I have taken a very broad approach and have focused on vascular plants, and on whole plant processes. No attempt was made to cover the field entirely, for obvious reasons, or to present all of the various approaches possible. Rather, I have concentrated on processes, plants, systems, and approaches of particular interest to me, and which hopefully illustrate the general adaptive pathways of plants. Particular emphasis is placed on the ecological significance of a particular adaptive mechanism rather than on the nature of the mechanism itself, since examples of the latter are discussed in detail elsewhere in this volume. I further emphasize that in order to understand the adaptations of plants to their environment one must consider not only the physiological possibilities but also how morphological means can in some cases accomplish the same end. There are apparently certain morphological–physiological combinations which represent the optimal type for a given environment since analogs occur in unrelated stock in climatically similar, but disjunct regions. Finally, I consider the plant as having a set amount of capital to expend to meet the demands of any given environment. Since it may not be able to meet all of these demands simultaneously, a plant must make a developmental "choice" which has competitive implications. To start this discussion let us examine the distribution of certain plants in nature.

Life Form Gradients and Plant Adaptation

As one progresses along gradients of increasing climatic severity, either in the high mountains, or at high latitudes, there is a comparable change in the dominant life forms. Trees give way to shrubs, then herbs, and finally, in the severest climates, only lichens will be evident. In the southern hemisphere, for example, there is a latitudinal treeline at 54° S on the shores of the Beagle Channel, 700 miles north of the tip of Antarctica (Llano, 1962). Here the mean annual temperature is near 6°C (Taylor, 1955). In Antarctica proper there are but two herbaceous plants found, and they do not extend beyond 68° S. Lichens are found, however, at latitudes higher than 85° S (Greene *et al.*, 1967).

It is within the interior Antarctic Plateau that the lowest temperatures thus far recorded on earth have been noted (−88.3°C; Vostok, 78°27′ S). However, it is apparently not temperature but water which is the primary limiting factor for plant life in Antarctica (Ugolini, 1970). For example, some Antarctic lichens can withstand rapid cooling to −196°C and, furthermore, they can assimilate carbon while frozen. Lange and Kappen (1970) have measured positive carbon fixation in Antarctic lichens at temperatures as low as −18°C. It is such characteristics as these − plus their capacity to survive long periods in a semihydrated state and to quickly absorb moisture when it becomes available (Greene and Longton, 1970) − which enables these plants to cope with one of the earth's most hostile environments. The same life-form gradients exist at high elevations and here, too, the upper absolute limit of plant growth is principally due to the lack of free water (Billings and Mooney, 1968).

The factors which limit the other growth forms, such as trees or shrubs, at lower elevations and latitudes, in environments less severe in temperature and moisture availability, are more complex and involve factors such as the economy of wood production in relation to temperature (Billings and Mooney, 1968). With increasing elevation, for example, thermal conditions for metabolism become restricted to levels closer and closer to the earth's surface, which places restrictions on the growth form possibilities.

If one looks to the other extremes of the earth's habitats, the deserts, it can be seen that higher plants can adapt to the highest air temperatures found on earth, such as those found on the floor of Death Valley,

California. Here, there are herbs and shrubs in water-limited habitats and even trees where water is unlimited. It is interesting that some of the plants which inhabit these extremely hot habitats do not avoid these conditions by dormancy, but rather they have their optimal metabolism at these temperatures. For example, *Tidestromia oblongifolia* (Wats.) Standl. has its optimal temperature of photosynthesis at 47°C (Figure 1) Björkman *et al.*, 1972) which is presumably close to its lethal thermal

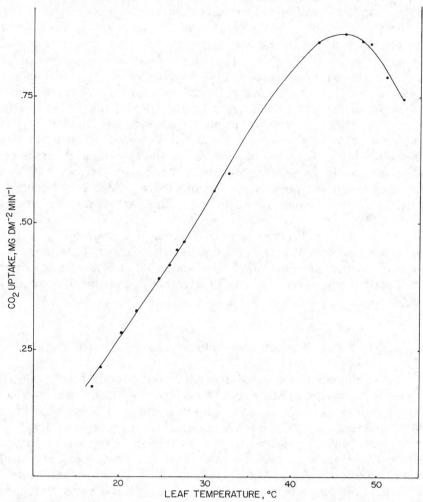

Figure 1 Temperature-related net photosynthesis of *Tidestromia oblongifolia* as measured *in situ* in Death Valley, California (from Björkman *et al.*, 1972).

limit. Levitt (1972) has noted that desert plants have thermal limits in the range of 44°–59°C, a range which is not too different from many plants originating from considerably cooler environments. It is only in those deserts where water is essentially absent, such as the Atacama Desert of Chile and Peru, that higher plants are totally lacking.

There are two themes which I would like to derive from these observations and to develop further. One is that adaptation to a limited water supply has been more difficult to accomplish through evolution by higher plants than has been thermal adaptation. Secondly, it appears that there are only a limited number of successful adaptive combinations which inhabit the earth's diverse environments and that whenever these habitats occur you will find these plant forms. Thus, we have areas of the world which may be quite disjunct but which have comparable dominant life forms, be they evergreen conifers of cold temperate climates, cushion plants of the alpine, or evergreen sclerophyll shrubs of Mediterranean climates. A given environment selects for such functional types, and phylogeny may have only a small influence on the outcome (Parsons, 1973). Thus, we may have coexisting similar morphotypes which are totally unrelated in any given climate. Further, we may have unrelated unique adaptive types in disjunct areas such as the giant rosette plants of the Andean Paramo and of the East African high mountains.

The relationship between form, physiology, and environmental adaptation will subsequently be pursued somewhat further. First, however, let us examine plant distributions at a somewhat finer level, that of species distributions, to see what sort of inferences can be made about plant adaptation.

Widespread Species-Adaptive Inferences

One of the most widespread angiosperms in the world is *Phragmites communis* Trin., the common reed. It occurs on all of the continents and from latitudes extending from equatorial regions to the low arctic at 70°29′ N (Haslam, 1972). Further, it occurs from sea level to elevations over 3000 m in Tibet (Ridley, 1923). In all of these regions it occurs in wet, open habitats in either fresh or brackish water (vigorous growth occurs up to a salinity of 1.2%) (Haslam, 1972). Between these various habitats, these plants may be exposed to quite diverse thermal regimes. For example, in Death Valley, California, the plants actively grow in water which reaches temperatures of at least 37°C and where air temperatures can exceed 48°C (Deacon *et al.*, 1972). Leaf temperatures under these extreme conditions may, however, be as much as 9° under ambient (Pearcy *et al.,* 1972).

Almost equally as widespread is another aquatic macrophyte, *Typha latifolia* L. It, too, grows in open wet habitats of differing salinities and is found across a wide range of latitudes from the subarctic to the tropics (Smith, 1967). An indication of the thermal diversity in the habitats in which a closely related species, *Typha domingensis,* is found is shown for two populations, one from a markedly cool maritime climate in Bodega Bay, California, and the other for Death Valley, California (Figure 2). During the midgrowing season, plants of these populations scarcely experience the same range of temperatures. The Bodega plants are often operating at air temperatures in the 10°–15°C range, and those of Death Valley at temperatures between 30° and 50°C.

Another group of plants which has an unusually wide latitudinal distribution is that which is found in arctic-alpine habitats. An example of this type is *Oxyria digyna* (L.) Hill. It covers a vast range encompassing 50 degrees of latitude from the high arctic to the mountains of southern California and Arizona (Mooney and Billings, 1961). Over this range during the summer growing season, there can be considerable differences in the quality, intensity, and duration of incoming radiation and in the amplitude of thermal fluctuation (Billings and Mooney, 1968).

All of these examples indicate that there can be wide limits in the adaptation of a single genetic system. This appears to be particularly true for plants which span a range of thermal environments. There are

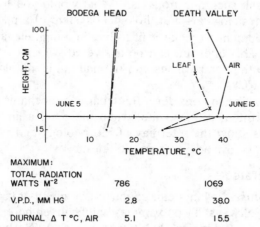

Figure 2 The microclimate of a *Typha* stand in June 1973, in contrasting coastal (Bodega Bay, California) and desert (Furnace Creek, Death Valley, California) environments.

also indications that many of the examples of the seemingly widely adapted species are those which grow in habitats where there is *apparently* a low degree of competition from other species. Thus, we see that these plants include not only those of the marshes and arctic-alpine habitats cited above, but also those of the strand, salt deserts, as well as weeds of disturbed habitats (Good, 1964).

A single generalized genetic system appears to adapt to an exceptionally wide range of thermal environments as well as to habitats differing in a number of radiation parameters. Further, there seems to be a relationship between the range of adaptability of a species and the degree of competition it encounters in the community.

In many instances it has been amply documented that these widespread species are actually composed of populations of differing ecological fitness for dissimilar thermal, radiation, or nutrient levels (Heslop-Harrison, 1964). Thus, in most instances, a single genetic system is of course not adapted to the whole gamut of environmental conditions of the species, but rather there is a series of adaptively finely tuned populations spanning the entire range. However, plants with these wide distributions are indicative of the adaptability limits of a single generalized genetic system.

Ecotypes have been intensively utilized, particularly by the Plant Biology Department of the Carnegie Institute of Washington, as experimental material to understand the origin of adaptations. Many plants can be easily cloned and comparisons can be made of the behavior of an ecotype in its own environment as well as in that of a contrasting ecotype. Thus, one can ask such questions as, "What would you have to modify in a genetic–physiological–morphological system of a plant adapted to a coastal environment to make it fit to live in a high elevation or desert environment?" This question can be answered with a certain degree of precision, since the comparisons can be made utilizing plants with very similar genetic stock.

I would now like to consider a few adaptive mechanisms that plants utilize to capture minerals or water when these are a limiting resource. These examples show the interplay of morphology and physiology and of short- and long-term adaptive possibilities.

Adaptive Strategies

Mineral Uptake.   Plants can adapt to any given environmental factor in a number of ways. Two examples will be given here. One is mineral uptake in mineral-deficient habitats. Chapin (1973) has shown that plants which grow in arctic soils have a potentially reduced mineral absorption due to both the physiological effects of cold temperature and the low nutrient status of the substrate. Arctic marsh plants differ from more temperate origin genetic counterparts both morphologically and physiologically in a manner which enhances their nutrient gathering capacity. Roots of arctic plants were concentrated in the upper, warmer soil levels (alternatively, they were concentrated in mineral-rich regions). Also they had relatively higher root/shoot ratios and a greater root surface-to-volume ratio than temperate zone specimens. Further, these northern plant populations differed from temperate counterparts in having both a higher capacity of phosphorous uptake, and a lower temperature optimum for root production at any given temperature when grown under comparable conditions. Temperate counterparts from thermally more unstable environments, however, had a greater capacity to adjust to temporal temperature changes (Figure 3). That is, they have a greater capacity to adjust their mineral uptake potential according to the prevailing temperature which changes through the season.

Northern plants thus divert a greater proportion of their capital into structural and biochemical machinery to gain nutrients. Although these adjustments have been made on an evolutionary time scale, they can also be made on shorter time scales of days or weeks by the adjustment of apportionment of carbon to greater enzyme and root production. In an analogous fashion, plants can enhance their carbon-gaining capacity through a variety of biochemical and morphological means.

Carbon-Gaining Capacity. Higher plants have evolved only a few biochemical photosynthetic pathways in response to the earth's many diverse environments. For example, certain plants of bright habitats

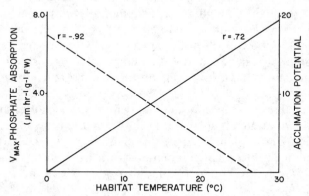

Figure 3 Influence of soil thermal regime of origin upon V_{max} and acclimation potential of phosphate absorption in marsh plants. V_{max} was determined on roots of nine species grown and measured at 5°C root temperature. Acclimation potential (ratio of V_{max} of 5° and 20°C acclimated individuals) was measured at 20°C on the same species (from Chapin, 1973).

where water is often limiting have a C_4-dicarboxylic acid cycle type of photosynthesis. Plants of this type, which occur in a variety of dicotyledonous and monocotyledonous families, usually have exceptionally high photosynthetic rates, high temperature optima of photosynthesis, high light-saturation values, and are relatively efficient at producing dry matter per unit of water loss. All of these features are a consequence of the greater capacity of C_4 plants to utilize intercellular CO_2.

Another photosynthetic type, crassulacean acid metabolism, or CAM, is restricted to succulent plants of a number of different families. CAM plants are also restricted to bright habitats where water is limiting. In contrast to C_4 plants, they generally have quite low rate of CO_2 uptake; however, they are even more efficient at the production of dry matter per unit of water lost. Their water-use efficiency is accomplished in quite a different manner. These plants have the capacity to open their stomata at night, when evaporative stress is low, and to store CO_2 temporarily in organic acids. During the day, while the stomates remain closed and hence evaporative water loss is minimal, the CO_2 is released within the plant and refixed via the C_3 pathway into carbohydrate utilizing light energy. Not all succulents have crassulacean acid metabolism, nor do all CAM plants open their stomates only at night; however, all CAM plants are succulents. Many CAM plants will fix carbon directly through the C_3-type (Calvin cycle) of metabolism during the light periods when significant soil moisture is available, and shift to a greater proportion of CAM as water becomes limiting (Bartholomew, 1973). Thus, the source of CO_2 in the light for these plants may be either endogenous or exogenous, or both, depending on environmental conditions.

Most of the world's higher plants apparently carry out their photosynthesis utilizing the unmodified Calvin cycle. These plants are found in virtually all of the world's environments, including the extremes of hot and cold, bright and shady, and wet and dry. In comparison to C_4 plants, C_3 plants generally have low temperature optima and lower water-use efficiencies.

It is clear that in open, hot habitats where water is often limiting, C_4 plants would be at an advantage at least during the growing season. The slow-growing CAM plants can be competitive only where there is no light limitation due to plant interaction, such as in deserts or in rocky sites. Also they can be productive in those sites where there is very low water availability.

In certain habitats, plants having all three photosynthetic pathways coexist. In these habitats, the C_3 plants are generally active in the cool periods of the year, and the C_4 plants in the hot periods. In a sense, then, they are dividing the available resources.

CAM plants are quite specialized, but to a lesser degree than C_4 species. It is the C_3 plants which have the widest ecological tolerances. How has niche separation been accomplished through the use of a single metabolic strategy? Apparently, both morphological and physiological features have been used. One example of differing physiological traits can be seen in the comparisons of sun and shade plants. Shade plants have lower light saturated rates of photosynthesis than do sun plants. This trait is to a large degree genetically fixed and is related to a low level of the carboxylating enzyme, carboxydismutase, maintained in their leaves (Björkman, 1968). Sun leaves, in contrast, divert considerably more protein into this enzyme for a greater return, since more light energy for photosynthesis is available. Some plants when grown in shade can modify their photosynthetic response to a certain degree by enzyme adjustment.

Plants of the same genotype, when grown under dissimilar thermal regimes, may not only have different light saturated maximum rates of photosynthesis, but also differing temperatures of optimum photosynthesis. Furthermore, changes in physiological states can occur in time spans in the order of a day (Mooney and Shropshire, 1967). Plants thus appear to have the potential to respond to the environment in a plastic and adaptive manner within certain limits. There is some evidence that genotypes from thermally unstable environments are more plastic than those from stable environments (Billings *et al.*, 1971).

Plants can employ a variety of morphological strategies in order to enhance their carbon gain. However, the benefits of the potential additional carbon gain must be greater than the cost of employing these strategies. A simple example can be utilized to illustrate this concept (Figure 4). Photosynthesis in plants is limited by water. Thus, in drought envi-

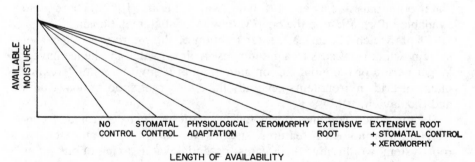

Figure 4 Physiological and morphological strategies to prolong water availability in a water-limited habitat. The various slopes are diagrammatic only and do not imply exact quantitative relationships.

ronments, anything a plant can do to capture more water or to prolong the availability of water will result in greater carbon fixation.

Drought evaders usually have mesophytic leaves with minimal morphological features, in addition to stomatal control, to prevent water loss (and hence to block carbon dioxide diffusion). Thus, these leaves have high photosynthetic capacities when water is available (Mooney and Dunn, 1970).

During periods of excessive evaporative demands, such as during midday, stomatal closure can result in considerable water saving. This closure can enhance water-use efficiency in two ways. First, when stomates close, water loss is affected to a proportionally greater extent than is carbon gain, since water vapor has a shorter diffusional pathway than carbon dioxide. Secondly, the stomatal closure results in a water savings which can be used during periods of lower evaporative demands.

Although water saving may be accomplished by stomatal closure, this may result in leaf over-temperature if there is a high radiation load and if the leaves are large and thus have a low convection coefficient (Gates, 1968). It is probably significant that in arid environments large-leaved plants are generally drought deciduous (Mooney and Harrison, 1972).

Plants can also conserve water by having a leaf anatomy which is so constructed as to impede water loss (xeromorphy). However, the consequence of this strategy is also to impede carbon influx and thus may be of a positive benefit only in certain environments (Mooney and Dunn, 1970).

A plant can prolong its water availability for carbon gain by simply being more efficient at extracting it against low water potentials and utilizing it. For example, certain desert xerophytes can photosynthesize at water potentials as low as −118 bars (Kappen et al., 1972). There is no available information on the energy "costs" of such metabolism.

Plants which allocate a greater fraction of their carbon to their root system will have access to a greater reservoir of water and hence have a longer period of potential carbon gain in an arid environment. Perennial plants of arid environments generally have high root/shoot ratios (Rodin and Bazilevich, 1967).

Plants which combine physiological features, such as stomatal control, and morphological features, such as xeromorphy and an extensive root system, would have the greatest potential water saving of our series of adaptive strategies (Figure 4).

All of these water-saving features do not have equal metabolic "costs" and some may not even repay the plant's carbon investment in

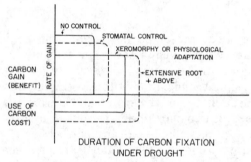

Figure 5 A carbon balance cost/benefit analysis.

them in all environments. An illustration of their relationships is given in Figure 5. The height above the horizontal line indicates the amount of carbon gained by the given strategy and the extent below the line is the estimated relative carbon cost, or loss in carbon-gaining potential, of this strategy. The width of the bars along the horizontal indicates the time duration of carbon fixation that would be possible in a drought environment employing the given strategy.

As described above, a mesophytic leaf has a high rate of carbon gain. It invests nothing into xerophytism and thus can maintain this rate only when water is available. By controlling stomata, an unknown cost, it extends its carbon-gaining period somewhat. A xerophytic leaf has invested carbon into water conservation, at the same time it has restricted carbon gain. Extensive roots do not decrease carbon gain directly, but they have a cost which may be compensated for by the greater period of potential carbon gain.

The cost of certain of these strategies is fixed. Although under some conditions, as in our drought examples, they may repay the plant's investment, in others they may not. For example, it can be seen in Figure 5 that if water were not limiting, there would be no time dimension. The "winning" strategy under these conditions would be the plant with the mesophytic leaf, where there is no fixed cost, and a high carbon-gaining capacity. Intermediate drought environments would lead to those strategy combinations midway along the time axis.

Similar analyses can be made for the cost and benefits of enhancing nutrient and light capture or optimizing thermal relationships in varied environments. Such analyses would have to take into consideration leaf display, leaf duration, leaf area index, enzyme level, and acclimation, among other parameters. There have already been attempts to predict optimal leaf sizes on the basis of water-use efficiency for any given environment (Parkhurst and Loucks, 1972).

Apportionment Theory

The case has been presented that plants can employ a variety of strategies to adapt to any given factor in short supply. A similar case can be made for adaptation to factors in excess. I would now like to build further on this theme to indicate that these strategies are primarily ones of resource allocation within the plant; and, further, that allocation of resources to meet the demands of one particular environment will necessarily make the plant less adaptive in another.

In any given environment, plants must produce, maintain, and protect systems for gaining carbon, water, and minerals. Further, they must produce, maintain, and protect a reproductive system (Figure 6).

These demands, of course, vary with time. An example of seasonal carbon apportionment is given for the Mediterranean-climate evergreen sclerophyll, *Heteromeles arbutifolia* (Figure 7). Although this Californian native shrub photosynthesizes year round, it produces stem growth mainly during the spring. Root growth is principally in fall and winter. It is also during the period of low demand for carbon by the shoot that the plant synthesizes such compounds as phenolics, which are possibly involved in predator protection.

In *Heteromeles*, reproduction occurs after stem growth, presumably not on reserves but on current photosynthate. These events indicate a seasonal partitioning of the plant's carbon to meet best the internal as well as external demands.

This sort of information has been synthesized along with data for similar species to produce a preliminary model of the limitations on the timing of apportionment in evergreens in Mediterranean climates (Table 1). It can be seen that there may be very different environmental and

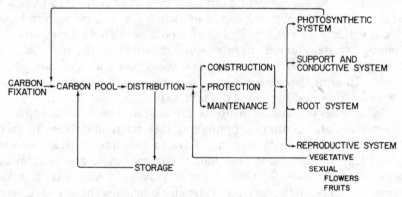

Figure 6   The uses of carbon by plants (from Mooney *et al.*, 1973).

biological elements which are selective for the timing of appointment, or in other terms, the plant phenology. A few of these elements will be explored here.

In Mediterranean environments there are sufficient resources to produce a closed canopy of vegetation. Thus, there is presumably competition for light. Hence, any species which produces its new canopy first would be at a competitive advantage. However, if a plant starts building its canopy too soon, it will be subject to a late freeze and it will lose its entire investment and any competitive gain. These constraints are probably responsible for the synchronous growth of the dominants in most light-limited habitats.

As already stated, during the period of high demand for carbon for canopy development, there may be little diversion to other vital functions such as root development, construction of protection systems, and

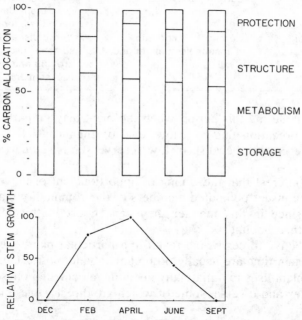

Figure 7 Seasonal carbon apportionment in the evergreen shrub, *Heteromeles arbutifolia.* The values given are the amount of ^{14}C found in the various categories one month after fixation as $^{14}CO_2$. The compounds were assigned to the functional categories in the following manner: storage, sugar and starch; metabolism, amino acids, organic acids, and proteins; structure, cell wall material; protection, phenolics, terpenes, resin acids, etc. (Mooney and Chu, in press).

Table 1 The Environmental Limitations on Carbon Appointment and Their Physiological Consequences in Mediterranean-Climate Evergreen Sclerophylls

Process	Environmental limitations	Physiological or evolutionary result
Carbon gain	Summer drought, winter cold	Rate reduction during winter and summer
Carbon allocation		
Canopy	Competition for light, winter freeze, carbon limitations	Synchronous growth initiation in spring
Roots	Carbon limitation	Regulation of activity to noncanopy development period (winter – fall)
Flowers	Competition for pollinators	Asynchrony of flowering
Protection	Carbon limitation	Regulation of activity to noncanopy development period (winter – fall)
Fruit dispersal	Germination conditions unsuitable summer and fall	Fall fruit dispersal or summer dispersal with drought and predator escape mechanisms

storage. It is during this period when the plant may be particularly vulnerable to predation due to a low level of chemical defense (Feeney, 1970), or to grazing because of low reserve status (Donart and Cook, 1970).

It is of interest that the timing of apportionment of flower development for the insect pollinated members of the community may be asynchronous, since in this manner they can apportion the pollinator resources of their habitat.

The selective forces which result in a particular plant event happening at a certain time are usually both climatic and biotic. Thus, the cues which the plant uses to initiate any given developmental phase are probably complex and diverse, some of which are direct while others are indirect.

Although timing of apportionment is of great competitive importance so is the form and amount of the allocation. A scheme linking these elements and the factors selecting for them is given in Figure 8. This figure is illustrative only and is directed toward carbon apportionment. It does not consider all of the possible selective forces.

As was indicated earlier, we should be able to predict the optimal photosynthetic system for a given climatic region. This system has been evolutionarily selected to have the greatest net carbon gain for these general conditions. The actual amount of carbon gained is of course regulated by the weather. The amount of carbon apportioned to root versus shoots is genetically programmed by past selective events in the environment, such as soil moisture regions, nutrient level, etc; and further, any plant is plastic to a certain degree and can modify apportionments to optimally adjust to the extant conditions.

The actual form the leaf or stem takes may be determined by those climatic and competitive forces which lead to the optimal productive

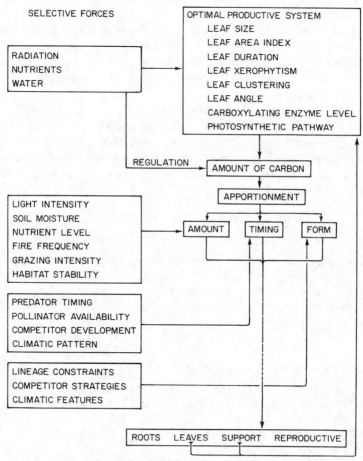

Figure 8 Environmental features which select for the timing, form, and amount of carbon apportionment.

system but built within heritage restraints. Some taxa are apparently more genetically fixed than others, e.g., pines versus oaks. Also, the form of apportionment can be modified greatly depending on the extant environment and to differing degrees depending on the average nature of the habitat, e.g., sun versus shade leaves, submerged versus aerial leaves.

There are few examples which have evaluated the significance of apportionment strategy in the survival of plants in a natural community, However, Gulmon (1973) has shown that plants which have virtually identical forms and generalized phenologies (annual, Mediterranean climate, grasses) coexist by keying their apportionment of synthetic or structural material to root or shoots to environmental cues which differ slightly. They in a sense are betting on winning (greater reproductive output) by strongly linking to a given climatic sequence. Since the climate fluctuates greatly from day to day and between weeks, the winning combination is constantly changing, resulting in a relatively stable but diverse community.

A very broad view of the adaptive possibilities of plants has been presented. They are diverse and involve complex morphological and physiological responses of both a long- and short-term nature and yet there are only a finite number of "winning" combinations for any environmental type. These are the forms which are repeated wherever similar environments exist.

Acknowledgments

This paper grew out of studies supported by the National Science Foundation (GB 27151 and GB 35854). Olle Björkman, F. C. Chapin, S. L. Gulmon, and J. Troughton made valuable comments on the manuscript for which I express sincere appreciation. Jim Ehleringer and Barbara Rice provided important information.

References

Bartholomew, B. (1973). Drought response in the gas exchange of *Dudleya farinosa* (Crassulaceae) grown under natural conditions. *Photosynthetica* **7**, 114–120.

Billings, W. D., and Mooney, H. A. (1968). The ecology of Arctic and Alpine plants. *Biol. Rev.* **43**, 481–529.

Billings, W. D., Godfrey, P. J., Chabot, B. F., and Bourgue, D. (1971). Metabolic acclimation to temperature in Arctic and Alpine ecotypes of *Oxyria digyna*. *Arctic Alpine Res.* **3**, 277–289.

Björkman, O. (1968). Carboxydismutase activity in shade-adapted species of higher plants. *Physiol. Plant* **21**, 1 – 10.

Björkman, O., Pearcy, R., Harrison, A., and Mooney, H. (1972). Photosynthetic adaptation to high temperatures: a field study in Death Valley, California. *Science* **175**, 786 – 789.

Chapin, F. S. (1973). Morphological and physiological mechanisms of temperature compensation in phosphate absorption along a latitudinal gradient. Ph.D. Thesis, Stanford University.

Deacon, J., Bradley, W., and Moor, K. (1972). Saratoga Springs Validation Site U. S. International Biological Program. *Desert Biome Res. Memorandum*, pp. 72 – 50.

Donart, G. B., and Cook, C. W. (1970). Carbohydrate reserve content of mountain range plants following defoliation and growth. *J. Range Manage.* **23**, 15 – 19.

Feeney, P. (1970). Seasonal changes in oak leaf tannins and nutrients as a cause of spring feeding by winter moth caterpillars. *Ecology* **51**, 565 – 581.

Gates, D. M. (1968). Transpiration and leaf temperature. *Annu. Rev. Plant Physiol.* **19**, 211 – 238.

Good, R. 1964. "The Geography of the Flowering Plants," 3rd Ed. John Wiley, New York.

Greene, S., and Longton, R. (1970). The effects of climate on Antarctic plants. *In* "Antarctic Ecology," Vol. 2. Academic Press, New York.

Greene, S. W., Gressitt, J., Koob, D., Llano, G., Rudolph, E., Singer, R., Steere, W., and Ugolini, F. (1967). Terrestrial life in Antarctica. Antarctic map folio series. Amer. Georgr. Soc., New York.

Gulmon, S. L. (1973). Maintenance of diversity in California grasslands. *Bull. Ecol. Soc. Amer.* **54**, 31.

Haslam, S. (1972). *Phragmites communis* Trin. *J. Ecol.* **60**, 585 – 610.

Heslop-Harrison, J. (1964). Forty years in genecology. *Advan. Ecol. Res.* **2**, 159 – 247.

Kappen, L., Lange, O. L., Schulze, E. D., Evenari, M., and Buschbom, U. (1972). Extreme water stress and photosynthetic activity of the desert plant *Artemisia herbaalba* Asso. *Oecologia* **10**, 177 – 182.

Lange, O., and Kappen, L. (1970). Photosynthesis of lichens from Antarctica. *In* "Antarctic Terrestrial Biology," G. Llano, ed., pp. 23 – 95. Ed. Amer. Geophysical Union, Washington, D. C.

Levitt, J. (1972). "Responses of Plants to Environmental Stresses." Academic Press, New York.

Llano, G. A. (1962). The terrestrial life of the Antarctic. *Sci. Amer.* **207**, 212 – 230.

Mooney, H. A., and Billings, W. D. (1961). Comparative physiological ecology of Arctic and Alpine populations of *Oxyria digyna. Ecol. Monogr.* **31**, 1 – 29.

Mooney, H. A., and Chu, C. (in press). Carbon allocation in *Heteromeles arbutifolia,* a California evergreen shrub. *Oecologia.*

Mooney, H. A., and Dunn, E. L. (1970). Photosynthetic systems of Mediterranean-climate shrubs and trees of California and Chile. *Amer. Natur.* **104,** 447–453.

Mooney, H. A., and Harrison, A. T. (1972). The vegetational gradient on the lower slopes of the Sierra San Pedro Martir in northwest Baja California. *Madroño* **21,** 439–445.

Mooney, H. A., and Shropshire, F. (1967). Population variability in temperature-related photosynthetic acclimation. *Oecol. Plantarum* **2,** 1–13.

Mooney, H. A., Parsons, D., and Kummerow, J. (1973). Plant development in Mediterranean climates. *In* "Phenology and Seasonality Modeling," (H. Lieth, ed.). Springer Verlag, Heidelberg.

Parkhurst, D., and Loucks, O. (1972). Optimal leaf size in relation to environment. *J. Ecol.* **60,** 505–537.

Parsons, D. (1973). A comparative study of vegetation structure of Mediterranean shrub communities of California and Chile. Ph.D. Thesis, Stanford University.

Pearcy, R., Berry, J., and Bartholomew, B. (1972). Field measurements of the gas exchange capacities of *Phragmites communis* under summer conditions in Death Valley. *Carnegie Inst. Washington Yearb.* **71,** 161–164.

Ridley, H. N. (1923). The distribution of plants. *Ann. Bot. London* **37,** 1–29.

Ródin, L. E., and Bazilevich, N. I. (1967). "Production and Mineral Cycling in Terrestrial Vegetation," (G. E. Fogg, ed.) Oliver & Boyd, Edinburgh. (Engl. transl.).

Smith, S. G. (1967). Experimental and natural hybrids in North America *Typha* (Typhaceae). *Amer. Midl. Natur.* **78,** 257–287.

Taylor, B. W. (1955). The flora, vegetation and soils of Macquarie Island. A.N.A.R.E. Depts. B2, 1, Melbourne, Antarctic Div. Dept. External Affairs.

Ugolini, F. (1970). Antarctic soils and their ecology. *In* "Antarctic Ecology," (N. W. Holdgate, ed.), Vol. 2, pp. 673–696. Academic Press, New York.

Some Genetic and Molecular Aspects of Enzyme Adaptations

Richard E. Tashian and William R. A. Osborne

Department of Human Genetics
University of Michigan Medical School
Ann Arbor, Michigan

Introduction

Enzymatic adaptations are usually considered as changes in the structure, function, or activity of an enzyme, induced by environmental stress, which are beneficial to the organisms in which they occur. Here, we would also like to discuss enzymatic adaptations from the standpoint of two general genetic mechanisms: (1) allelic variation; that is, adaptations resulting from single gene mutations, and (2) isozymic variation, or adaptations associated with the products of evolutionarily differentiated duplicated genes.

Since we will be discussing the genetic basis of enzyme preadaptation, preadaptation will be defined as those mutational changes in the structure of an enzyme for which no immediate adaptive value is apparent, but which could provide the organism in which it occurs with an adaptive advantage under certain conditions. Certainly, preadaptive variants which are polymorphic are of greater potential value to a species than those which are rare; nevertheless, rare variants obviously supply not only the raw material for polymorphisms, but, as we shall see, detailed studies of the structures and activities of some of these rare mutant enzymes may also provide valuable clues to the molecular mechanisms of enzyme adaptation.

37

A great many polymorphic enzyme systems and isozyme systems are now known for a wide variety of organisms; however, in only a few instances has any adaptive significance been associated either with a particular variant allele or with an individual isozyme. Thus, even though some examples of possible genuine enzyme adaptation will be discussed, many of the examples that we will use will be largely speculative.

Although hemoglobin is not an enzyme in the strictest sense, so much is known about its structure and function that it will be used occasionally in this review to demonstrate certain principles of enzyme adaptation.

Adaptive Single Gene Mutations

Some examples will now be given of single gene mutations (structural and regulatory) which have resulted in either a known adaptive function, or one for which an adaptive role might be postulated. Because of the limitations of this review, we will restrict the different kinds of environmental stress to low oxygen stress, chemical stresses such as toxic and carcinogenic agents, and temperature stress.

Perhaps the best known example of a structural gene mutation which gives an adaptive advantage (in heterozygous condition) to the organism in which it occurs is human hemoglobin S. Here, the ability of the hemoglobin S molecules to polymerize under low oxygen stress (i.e., the sickling process) is in some way deleterious to the falciparum malarial parasite (Livingstone, 1971). Apparently, the low oxygen tension brought about by the parasitic infestation actually induces the sickling process, which may cause the cell and its contained parasite to be destroyed. Thus, the amino acid substitution of valine for glutamic acid at position 6 in the β-chain of hemoglobin A has made, through the indirect mechanism of low oxygen stress, the organism resistant to malarial infection.

Oxygen Insufficiency Stress

Although no mutant enzymes are known which can be regarded as adaptive to low oxygen levels, the two enzyme variants which we will discuss next could in a sense be considered as preadaptive to hypoxemia.

It is known that under hypoxic stress (e.g., certain anemias, high altitude) that red blood cell 2,3-diphosphoglycerate (DPG) levels are increased (Brewer and Eaton, 1971). This appears to be an adaptive response which shifts the oxygen–hemoglobin dissociation curve to the right, thereby permitting the hemoglobin molecules to release their oxygen more readily. A possible example where an inherited increase in enzyme activity may be beneficial under conditions of low oxygen stress comes from the studies of Noble and Brewer (1972), who showed that high DPG levels were inherited in the hooded rat. These authors suggest that perhaps a mutant allele for a high activity form of the glycolytic enzyme phosphofructokinase might underlie the high DPG levels they observed. Some recent results (N. A. Noble, personal communication) indicate that the high DPG rats may be more tolerant to stress associated with increased oxygen need.

Another example of an inherited change in enzyme levels which might be preadaptive to hypoxic stress is the condition of carbonic anhydrase deficiency found in the pig-tailed macaque *(Macaca nemestrina)*. In all pig-tailed macaque populations examined, about one-third of the animals show an almost complete absence (5000-fold reduction) of one isozyme of carbonic anhydrase, CA I, and about a 60% reduction of the other isozyme, CA II (DeSimone *et al.*, 1973a). It appears that a mutation in a control gene for CA I has resulted in a marked suppression of the level of CA I, and a less marked reduction of CA II (DeSimone *et al.*, 1973b). If some adaptive value is found for this carbonic anhydrase deficiency, it would be a good example of how a reduced, rather than an increased, enzyme activity can be advantageous. It has been suggested that the inhibition of red blood cell carbonic anhydrase by acetazolamide confers a physiological advantage to humans at high altitudes (Forwand *et al.*, 1968). Whether or not active selection or random genetic drift is responsible for the high frequency (above 60%) of this CA I-deficiency gene (Tashian *et al.*, 1971), it is nevertheless tempting to speculate on its possible preadaptive potential for tolerance to low oxygen stress.

Abnormal human hemoglobins which show a reduced Bohr effect such as Hb Hiroshima, Hb Hirose, and Hb Yoshizuka have been reported (Morimoto *et al.*, 1971). Should a decreased Bohr effect be beneficial to the human organism under certain stress conditions, then these variant hemoglobins would represent yet another example of protein molecules with potential adaptive properties.

Chemical Stress

As an introduction to this section on adaptation to chemical stress, we will describe an interesting inherited variant of human carbonic anhydrase I, designated CA Ib Michigan, which seems to be an excellent example of a structural gene mutation that has given an entirely new property to an enzyme without altering its normal activity (Tashian, 1969). In fact, this latent property would have gone undetected if we had, for example, used a zinc-free azo dye-coupler rather than the zinc salt azo dye, Blue RR, in our staining reaction mixture. Or for that matter, it would have gone undetected if we had used *p*-nitrophenyl acetate or 2-hydroxy-nitro-α-toluene sulfonic acid sultone instead of α- or β-naphthyl acetate as our ester substrates. As it turned out, only the divalent cation zinc and not Mg^{++}, Co^{++}, Ni^{++}, or Cu^{++}, activated the hydrolysis of naphthyl acetate by the mutant enzyme. The hydrolysis of the phenyl acetate or sultone substrates by CA Ib was inhibited, rather than activated, by zinc. Increasing the concentration of zinc has the effect of decreasing the activity of the normal enzyme toward β-naphthyl acetate, thus, emphasizing the zinc activation of the mutant enzyme. In the reversible hydration of CO_2, supposedly the normal physiological function of carbonic anhydrase in the red blood cell, no differences were observed in the activities of the normal and variant enzyme at pH 7.3. Since the K_m values of the activated and inactivated enzyme are the same, the mechanism of activation appears to be an allosteric one. That is, the binding of zinc to the CA Ib variant enzyme somehow alters the orientation of the substrate in the active site cavity, effecting a more efficient hydrolysis of the naphthyl ester substrate.

The fact that this kind of mutational change in the activity of an enzyme was discovered more or less by chance suggests that "hidden" mutational changes of this type, which do not alter the normally accepted activity of an enzyme, may be far more common than previously thought, and may represent a rich source of preadaptive enzymes. One could speculate almost endlessly as to the potential adaptive value of this kind of mutant enzyme. One possibility is that it might represent a type of inherited drug resistance; on the other hand, it could just as well be a type of inherited drug sensitivity.

It is known that mutational alterations in the structure of certain enzymes can underlie the resistance of some bacterial strains to antibiotics (Benveniste and Davies, 1973). For example, two mutants of *Escherichia coli* are known—one which is resistant to rifampycin and the other to streptolydigin, and it appears that both mutations are located in the β subunit of its RNA polymerase. In higher organisms, examples of mutations either in structural or regulatory genes which confer resistance to chemical agents are not as well defined at the molecular level.

A number of examples of enzyme variants which produce resistance to pesticides in insects and mammals have been reported (Conney and Burns, 1972). A variant of microsomal oxidase in the housefly whose activity can be increased up to sixfold when exposed to sublethal doses of dieldrin, is a good example of an enzyme whose activity is inducible as the result of a mutation (Terriere *et al.*, 1971). It has not been determined, however, whether this mutation is in the structural gene for the oxidase or in its regulator gene.

Another enzyme variant whose activity is inducible is liver aldehyde dehydrogenase of the rat (Deitrich, 1971). The activity of this variant can be increased as much as 10-fold by phenobarbital. As with the inducible microsomal oxidase variant of the housefly, the mechanism of activation or the exact genetic control (or, for that matter, the mechanism of induction) has not been determined. However, by analogy with the metal ion activated mutant of human carbonic anhydrase just discussed, it is certainly possible that a structural gene mutation could underlie this type of inducible activation.

Most structural gene mutations result in either no change or a decrease in the level of the enzyme products. Once in a while, however, a structural gene mutation is found in which the level of an enzyme is increased. One such example is an inherited variant of human glucose-6-phosphate dehydrogenase (G6PD), G6PD Hektoen. It was at first thought that the increased activity of this mutant enzyme was due to a regulatory mechanism; however, it has now been shown that the single amino acid substitution of histidine to tyrosine is responsible for the increased production of the variant enzyme (Yoshida, 1970). So far as speculating about the possible adaptive significance of this increased activity mutation, one could say that because G6PD-deficient red blood cells are sensitive to the oxidant effects of certain drugs, such as primaquine, individuals who have increased levels of G6PD might be more resistant than normal to this type of drug induced hemolysis (Vesell, 1973).

The possibility that a decrease in the induction or activity of aryl hydrocarbon hydroxylase in man may provide protection from the carcinogenic effects of benzo[a]pyrene has been indicated in a recent report by Kellermann et al. (1973). These investigators present evidence that variation in the degree of inducibility of human aryl hydrocarbon hydroxylase may be under the control of a variant allele for the structural gene controlling this enzyme. Recent studies on the genetic specificity of the aromatic hydrocarbon-inducible hydroxylase activity in the mouse indicate that it is localized in one of the cytochrome P fractions associated with the hydroxylase enzyme complex (Nebert et al., 1973). The fact that the low-inducibility gene was found by Kellermann et al. (1973) to be present in high frequency (about 72%) in the normal United States white population they examined suggests that in certain human populations there may be a high percentage of individuals who possess a hereditary resistance to certain types of carcinogenic agents. If true, this would be another instance where reduced, rather than increased, enzyme activity is advantageous.

Temperature Stress

Although some structural gene mutations have the effect of making the variant enzyme less stable than the normal enzyme, sometimes a variant is discovered which is more stable than normal. An inherited

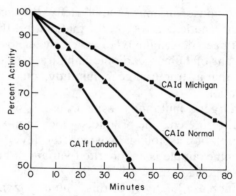

Figure 1 Heat inactivation plots of normal and two variants of human carbonic anhydrase I (CA I) at 55°C.

variant of human CA I, CA Id Michigan, appears to be just such a thermostable mutant (W. R. A. Osborne, unpublished results). At 55° C the first order rate constant for heat inactivation of CA Id Michigan is approximately half the value of another variant of CA I, CA If London, with the normal CA I giving an intermediate value. These heat inactivation plots are shown in Figure 1. An interesting comparative structural feature between the variant enzymes is that in both instances lysine has been substituted for the normal residue, and that these substitutions are only two residues apart (Tanis *et al.*, 1973; Carter *et al.*, 1973). In CA Id Michigan, threonine at position 100 has gone to lysine, and in CA If London, the glutamic acid at position 102 has also mutated to lysine. Now that the three-dimensional, high resolution structure of human CA I is almost completed (K. Kannan, personal communication), it may soon be possible to examine, and perhaps even understand, the molecular basis for this kind of alteration in conformational stability.

Although the adaptive value of the thermostable enzyme in a homeothermic animal is not obvious, it is possible that an increased stability of this type could be associated with an increased resistance either to proteolytic digestion or to conditions of high fever. In any event, it is a good molecular model of how an enzyme can become adaptive to increased temperature by a structural gene mutation.

The Mechanisms of Enzyme Adaptation to Temperature

This leads into a discussion of the temperature adaptation of enzymes. These have been classified by Somero and Hochachka (1971) on the time scale of the adaptive change, i.e., changes may occur on an evolutionary, seasonal, or more immediate time scale. These adaptive

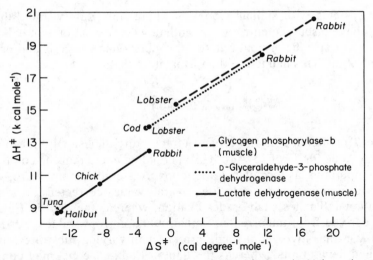

Figure 2 Compensation plots for the enthalpy ($\Delta H\dagger$) and entropy ($\Delta S\ddagger$) of activation of glycogen phosphorylase b (muscle), D-glyceraldehyde-3-phosphate dehydrogenase, and lactate dehydrogenase (muscle type or LDH-5), from various homeothermic and ectothermic animals. Data from Low *et al.* (1973).

changes have been investigated by studies of kinetic, physical, and thermodynamic properties, and as a general comment the experiments have displayed a wide range of sophistication. Nevertheless, the overall picture emerges that adaptive changes can be interpreted at the molecular level, involving changes in protein conformation and the structure–function consequences of amino acid substitutions.

A recent study by Low *et al.* (1973) of three enzyme systems, lactate dehydrogenase, glyceraldehyde dehydrogenase, and glycogen phosphorylase-b, from various homeothermic and ectothermic animals has indicated that the adaptation is derived from changes in the internal structures of the enzymes, as opposed to changes at the active site or in the reaction mechanisms. This statement is supported by the observation that homologous enzymes have similar active sites and reaction mechanisms, and similar values for the free energy of activation ($\Delta G\ddagger$). Therefore if, during the adaptive process, a constant free energy of activation ($\Delta G\ddagger$) has been maintained, this has been achieved by concomitant changes in enthalpy (heat of reaction), and entropy (conformation). This phenomenon of enthalpy ($\Delta H\ddagger$) and entropy ($\Delta S\ddagger$) compensation in enzymes from homeotherms and ectotherms is illustrated in Figure 2 where the data from Low *et al.* (1973) are plotted in the form of $\Delta H\ddagger$ versus $\Delta S\ddagger$. This plot shows a linear relationship within the three enzyme systems with similar slopes of about 43°. Lumry and Biltonen (1969) have discussed entropy and enthalpy compensation that exists for a variety of specific protein reactions, e.g., enzyme catalysis and protein denaturation. This had led to the formulation that:

$$\Delta H°_{\text{conformation}} = T_c \, \Delta S°_{\text{conformation}}$$

where T_c is defined as the critical temperature. These authors found a general value for T_c of 35°–40° C. It should be noted that the compensation temperature as formulated above involves enthalpy and entropy due to conformation changes only, i.e., overall values corrected for nonconformational changes such as desolvation, whereas the data in Figure 2 were derived from uncorrected enthalpy and entropy values. Also previous work has involved a single protein with varying substrates, inhibitors, and denaturants, whereas the data in Figure 1 concerned common substrates with enzymes from various species. This may well indicate the general applicability of a compensation principle. It is possible that the finding of similar critical temperatures is due to a fundamental property of aqueous solutions in general. Drost-Hansen (1965) has indicated the presence of phase transitions of water at temperatures of about 15°, 30°, 45°, and 60°C, and has postulated that this has been a selective force in the evolution of biological systems due to the variance in the behavior of aqueous systems in the regions of these temperatures.

The attainment of homeothermy by birds and mammals provides a system of relatively high heat and entropy content with respect to ectothermic systems. Therefore, it is probable that the homeotherms have evolved with different enthalpic versus entropic contributions in response to the energy characteristics of their cellular environment. The relatively low energy background of ectotherms has necessitated minimal enthalpy changes and the keeping of entropy changes to a minimum in the formation of the enzyme–substrate complex. The most likely method to achieve this is by the generation, in the interior of ectothermic enzymes, of a more rigid or ordered structure during catalysis. That relatively small differences in amino acid sequence can account for these required conformational changes has not only been demonstrated in a general way by the CA Id Michigan example just discussed, but also by the recent work of Kabat and Wu (1973), who compared nearest-neighbor frequencies of amino acids in relation to secondary protein structure.

A thermodynamic approach can also be applied to the phenomenon of discontinuities in Arrhenius plots of biological data, an example being the study by Kumamoto et al. (1971) of such discontinuities in mitochondrial oxidation. This has a bearing on the immediate response to temperature of an enzyme system. A good example is the temperature induced conformational change in rabbit muscle aldolase that has been investigated by Lehrer and Barker (1970). These workers found a discontinuity in the plots of log activity, K_m, and K_i, versus reciprocal temperature. In all plots a similar transition temperature was demonstrated. It was found that the values for the free energy of activation, inhibitor binding, and overall reaction, remained remarkably constant over the temperature range of the investigation. It is interesting that this complements the finding of a relatively constant free energy change for the overall reaction in the three enzyme systems from homeothermic and ectothermic organisms investigated by Low et al. (1973). A consideration of the thermodynamic data indicates that this temperature-dependent transition involved only the free enzyme. This conformational change is overcome by binding substrate, and the catalytic process involving the enzyme–substrate complex and the transition state are affected in a normal way by temperature.

It must be admitted that there is some debate as to the mode of these conformation transitions. Kumamoto et al. (1971) have supported a phase change theory, arguing that these intersecting discontinuities define isokinetic points, and consequently that the isothermal property of the phase change explains why the two independent processes function exclusively in their respective temperature regions. Alternatively, it is argued that the conformational states can exist in equilibrium over a range of temperature (Massey et al., 1966), or are a function of solvent and kinetic mechanisms (Dixon and Webb, 1964). However, it seems that a temperature-induced, protein conformational change is the basic rationale for both arguments.

It is appropriate to conclude this section by commenting on the large body of data concerning the temperature acclimation of ectothermic enzymes. For example, it has been suggested that warm and cold isozyme variants arise as a result of de novo protein synthesis that is temperature induced (Somero and Hochachka, 1971). It is unlikely that these are isozymes in the strict sense of different gene products, but are more likely to be temperature-induced conformational or secondary isozymes which are formed either by the types of structural changes just discussed, or by the binding of modifiers. It should also be stressed that thermodynamic parameters derived from the initial and final states of a system cannot be used to deduce reaction rates, i.e., kinetic properties. It can be argued that the method of investigation using crude tissue extracts is unable to provide information regarding enzymic mechanisms or structural changes that have occurred.

Isozymic Adaptation

Although studies of "true" isozyme systems such as the lactate dehy-drogenases (Vesell and Fritz, 1971) suggest that the different isozymic forms may have different adaptive roles, we feel at this time that the best examples of "isozymic" adaptation, which can be interpreted at the molecular level, come from the study of the different molecular forms of hemoglobin. The parameters usually investigated are the Bohr effect, i.e., the dependence of hemoglobin-oxygen affinity on pH, and the modifying effect of organic phosphates such as DPG on oxygen binding. Changes in these parameters have been elucidated at the molecular level permitting an interpretation of the hemoglobin isolated from different species from the viewpoint of their adaptive significance (Tomita and Riggs, 1971; Perutz, 1970). The investigation of hemoglobin adaptation in catostomid fish by Powers (1972) is an excellent example of the molecular approach. The subgenera *Pantosteus* and *Catostomus* can be distinguished from each other by the presence or absence, respectively, of cathodal components in the electrophoretic patterns of their hemoglobins. The hemoglobins of *Catostomus clarkii* have some components (20%) whose oxygen equilibria are independent of pH (i.e., they have no Bohr effect). The separation and partial sequence of the globin chains indicated that the chemical groups responsible for most of the Bohr effect were absent in the α- and β-chains of the cathodal components. Since the Bohr effect is normally a beneficial phenomenon, the maintenance of some hemoglobins which lack it probably confers a physiological advantage. The habitat of these fish is in swift moving streams where, as a consequence, the fish are hyperactive. Any violent excercise of these fish, e.g., in escaping a predator, can produce a high level of lactic acid that negates the normally beneficial consequences of the Bohr effect (i.e., releasing oxygen at the cellular level) by suppressing oxygen binding at the gills. This can produce the death of hyperactive fish. It would appear that the portion of hemoglobin lacking a Bohr effect provides a reserve system so that swimming may be maintained after emergency exertions. It is noteworthy that the catostomid fish without this adaptation predominantly inhabit slow-moving waters thus enabling these sympatric species to reduce competition by exploiting different ecological niches within the same stream.

There are several abnormal human hemoglobins such as Hb Hirose, Hb Malmö, Hb Yakima, Hb Kempsey, and Hb Zurich which show very high oxygen affinities (Morimoto *et al.*, 1971). As with the two examples of variant enzymes just described, we can again speculate as to the preadaptive significance to low oxygen stress for mutations of this type.

Summary

Several examples of single gene mutations, and an example of "iso-zymic" variation, have been discussed which appear to be either pres-ently adaptive, or which could be considered as preadaptive in the sense that the variant enzyme has the potential to respond in an adaptive way to certain hypothetical stress situations. It was shown that enzyme adap-tations could be achieved through a variety of mutational changes such as the increased or decreased levels of an enzyme, the capacity to be activated or induced, decreased inducibility, increased thermostability, and altered binding properties. It was pointed out that the frequency of preadaptive enzymes may be fairly high and could underlie the adaptive potential of an organism or a species.

The molecular mechanism of enzyme adaptation was discussed from the standpoint of the ability of enzymes to undergo conformational changes in response to temperature stress. The available evidence indi-cates that the process of this adaptation lies in the maintenance of a con-stant change in free energy of activation values which is achieved by concomitant changes in the heat of reaction (enthalpy) and conforma-tion (entropy).

Acknowledgment

Preparation of this paper supported by Grant GM-15419 of the U. S. Public Health Service.

References

Benveniste, R., and Davies, J. (1973). Mechanisms of antibiotic resistance in bacteria. *Annu. Rev. Biochem.* **42,** 471–506.

Brewer, G. J., and Eaton, J. W. (1971). Erythrocyte metabolism: Interaction with oxygen transport. *Science* **171,** 1205–1211.

Carter, N. D., Tanis, R. J., Tashian, R. E., and Ferrell, R. E. (1973). Characteri-zation of a new variant of human red cell carbonic anhydrase I, CA If Lon-don (102 Glu → Lys). *Biochem. Genet.* **10,** 399–408.

Conney, A. H., and Burns, J. J. (1972). Metabolic interactions among environ-mental chemical and drugs. *Science* **178,** 576–586.

Deitrich, R. A. (1971). Genetic aspects of increase in rat liver aldehyde dehy-drogenase induced by phenobarbital. *Science* **173,** 334–336.

DeSimone, J., Magid, E., and Tashian, R. E. (1973a). Genetic variation in the carbonic anhydrase isozymes of macaque monkeys. II. Inheritance of red cell carbonic anhydrase levels in different carbonic anhydrase I genotypes of the pig-tailed macaque, *Macaca nemestrina. Biochem. Genet.* **8,** 165–174.

DeSimone, J., Magid, E., Linde, M., and Tashian, R. E. (1973b). Genetic variation in the carbonic anhydrase isozymes of macaque monkeys. III. Biosynthesis of carbonic anhydrases in bone marrow erythroid cells and peripheral blood reticulocytes of *Macaca nemestrina. Arch. Biochem. Biophys.* **158**, 365–376.

Dixon, M., and Webb, E. C. (1964). "Enzymes," 2nd Ed. Academic Press, New York.

Drost-Hansen, W. (1965). The effects on biological systems of higher-order phase transitions in water. *Ann. N. Y. Acad. Sci.* **125**, 471–501.

Forwand, S., Landowne, M., Follansbee, J., and Hansen, J. (1968). Effect of acetazolamide on acute mountain sickness. *N. Engl. J. Med.* **279**, 838–845.

Kabat, E. A., and Wu, T. T. (1973). The influence of nearest-neighbor amino acids on the conformation of the middle amino acid in proteins: comparison of predicted and experimental determination of β-sheets in concanavalin A. *Proc. Nat. Acad. Sci.* **70**, 1473–1477.

Kellermann, G., Luyten-Kellermann, M., and Shaw, C. R. (1973). Genetic variation of aryl hydrocarbonchydroxylase in human lymphocytes. *Amer. J. Hum. Genet.* **25**, 327–331.

Kumamoto, J., Raison, J. K., and Lyons, J. M. (1971). Temperature "breaks" in Arrhenius plots: a thermodynamic consequence of a phase change. *J. Theor. Biol.* **31**, 47–51.

Lehrer, G. M., and Barker, R. (1970). Conformational changes in rabbit muscle aldolase. Kinetic studies. *Biochemistry* **9**, 1533–1539.

Livingstone, F. B. (1971). Malaria and human polymorphisms. *Annu. Rev. Genet.* **5**, 33–64.

Low, P. S., Bada, J. L., and Somero, G. N. (1973). Temperature adaptation of enzymes: roles of the free energy, the enthalpy, and the entropy of activation. *Proc. Nat. Acad. Sci.* **70**, 430–432.

Lumry, R., and Biltonen, R. (1969). Thermodynamic and kinetic aspects of protein conformations in relation to physiological function. *In* "Structure and Stability of Biological Macromolecules" (S. H. Timasheff and G. D. Fusman, eds.). Dekker, New York.

Massey, V., Curti, B., and Ganther, H. (1966). A temperature-dependent conformational change in d-amino acid oxidase and its effects on catalysis. *J. Biol. Chem.* **241**, 2347–2357.

Morimoto, H., Lehmann, H., and Perutz, M. F. (1971). Molecular pathology of human haemoglobin: stereochemical interpretation of abnormal oxygen affinities. *Nature London* **232**, 408–413.

Nebert, D., Heidema, J. K., Strobel, H. W., and Coon, M. J. (1973). Genetic expression of arylhydrocarbon hydroxylase induction. *J. Biol. Chem.* **248**, 7631–7636.

Noble, N. A., and Brewer, G. J. (1972). Studies of the metabolic basis of the ATP-DPG differences in genetically selected high and low ATP-DPG rat strains, *In* "Hemoglobin and Red Cell Structure and Function" (G. J. Brewer. ed.), pp. 155–164, Plenum, New York.

Perutz, M. F. (1970). Stereochemistry of cooperative effects in haemoglobin. *Nature London* **228,** 726–739.

Powers, D. (1972). Hemoglobin adaptation for fast and slow water habitats in sympatric catostomid fishes. *Science* **177,** 360–362.

Somero, G. N., and Hochackka, P. W. (1971). Biochemical adaptation to the environment. *Amer. Zool.* **11,** 159–167.

Tanis, R. J., Ferrell, R. E., and Tashian, R. E. (1973). Substitution of lysine for threonine at position 100 in human carbonic anhydrase Id Michigan. *Biochem. Biophys. Res. Commun.* **51,** 699–703.

Tashian, R. E. (1969). Specific zinc activation of naphthyl ester hydrolysis by a mutant erythrocyte carbonic anhydrase. *Fed. Eur. Biochem. Soc. Abstr. Madrid,* p. 161.

Tashian, R. E., Goodman, M., Headings, V. E., DeSimone, J., and Ward, R. H. (1971). Genetic variation and evolution in the red cell carbonic anhydrase isozymes of macaque monkeys. *Biochem. Genet.* **5,** 183–200.

Terriere, L. C., Yu, S. J., and Hoyer, R. F. (1971). Induction of microsomal oxidase in F_1 hybrids of a high and low oxidase housefly strain. *Science* **171,** 581–583.

Tomita, S., and Riggs, A. (1971). Studies of the interaction of 2,3-diphosphoglycerate and carbon dioxide with hemoglobins from mouse, man, and elephant. *J. Biol. Chem.* **246,** 547–554.

Vesell, E. S. (1973). Advances in pharmacogenetics. *Progr. Med. Genet.* **9,** 291–367.

Vesell, E. S., and Fritz, P. J. (1971). Factors effecting the activity, tissue distribution, synthesis and degradation of isozymes. *In* "Enzyme Synthesis and Degradation in Mamalian Systems" (M. Rechcigl, Jr., ed.), pp. 339–374. University Park Press, Baltimore, Maryland.

Yoshida, A. (1970). Amino acid substitution (histidine to tyrosine) in a glucose-6-phosphate dehydrogenase variant (G6PD Hektoen) associated with overproduction. *J. Mol. Biol.* **52,** 483–490.

Adaptation: The Ecosystem

G. M. Woodwell

Biology Department
Brookhaven National Laboratory
Upton, New York

Theory in ecology is evolutionary theory and the details of the science are the details of the evolutionary adaptations of organisms, or arrays of organisms, to their own special circumstances. These very circumstances are themselves, in large part, the product of evolution and, therefore, within the context of adaptations. But an approach, organism by organism, population by population, holds only a little more potential for significant simplification at the level of the ecosystem than the molecule-by-molecule approach has for predicting the pounce of the tiger. Two processes that are central to the theory of ecology seem to offer some vital insights. The processes are succession and retrogression, opposite sides of the same coin. They are important not only because they are at the core of ecology, the basis of most theory, but also because we are experiencing both processes now, worldwide, on a massive scale, often without recognizing them.

I shall use examples from terrestrial studies within my own program at Brookhaven, although I believe that the conclusions apply to aquatic and marine systems and I am well aware that there are other examples. The question we ask is the extent to which the theory of ecology is likely to require modification on the basis of current research. The answer appears to be that some modification seems appropriate, but that the broad theory is supported in ever greater detail.

Succession

Contemporary theory, developed largely on the basis of work by Clements (1928), Cowles (1899, 1901), Cooper (1926), Tansley (1935), and others, and articulated most concisely by Margalef (1963, 1968) and Odum (1971) suggests that the changes that occur with succession include an increase in diversity, net primary productivity and in the degree of differentiation of species, one with respect to another. The community, said Clements, is an organism; it has a phylogeny and an ontogeny. The ontogeny is, of course, succession. I shall use diversity, net primary productivity, and the distribution of nutrients to examine the current status of theory with respect to succession. The subject is the sere. I use these because they are the principal indices applicable at the ecosystem level.

In the field-to-forest sere of central Long Island, diversity follows the trend shown in Figure 1, taken from a study by Woodwell *et al.* (in press). Peak diversity occurred early in this sere. Diversity declined in midsere, and rose again in the forested stages without ever reaching the peak of the fifth year. One of the most important observations is the role of exotics. Plants were identified as exotics on the basis of Fernald's description (1950). Exotics formed an important segment of the total population initially, but did not occur in the later stages of succession. Elimination of exotics from the entire sere would not change the pattern of diversity appreciably; the peak would still occur in the fifth year after abandon-

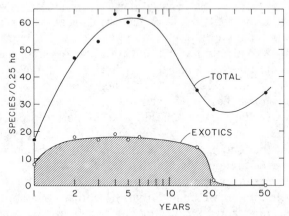

Figure 1 Diversity in the field-to-forest sere of Brookhaven, New York. Diversity was measured as the total number of higher plant species per quarter-hectare plot. Exotics were an appreciable fraction of the total diversity in early years of succession.

ment. Apparently there is in this sere no very pronounced tendency for diversity to increase consistently with age. The assumption seems reasonable that an increase in diversity would accompany further successional change toward oak – chestnut or oak – hickory. The theory in this instance, as in certain others, does not apply in a simple way. There is a substantial basis for belief that the earlier successional communities are more diverse.

The theory suggests that net primary productivity should increase along a sere as the number of species increases and resources in support of life accumulate. It appears to do so in the sere of central Long Island. The increase is correlated not simply with time, but with changes in the life form of the dominants. There is an abrupt rise in the herbaceous stage to 300 – 400 g of dry organic matter per $m^2 \cdot yr^{-1}$ and a subsequent rise with the transition to forest (Figure 2). The net primary production of the forest is about $1200 \ g \cdot m^{-2}$. Exotics contribute a major fraction of the total net production in the earliest stages of the sere, but their contribution drops rapidly in the third year, although the species persist for 20 years. It is not always true that net primary production is high in earlier stages of succession. Nor is it necessarily true that net production of successional forests approaches that of later successional or climax forests.

We might ask how net primary production itself is partitioned among species along this sere. Net primary production is the principal resource in support of life. We know that there are certain limits on its distribution, fixed in part by laws of thermodynamics. But it is reasonable to assume that the apportionment of the fixation of carbon among species

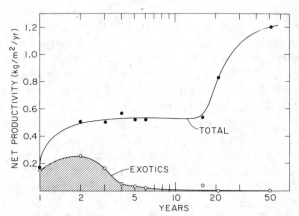

Figure 2 Net primary production in the field-to-forest sere of Brookhaven, New York. Net production of exotics declined abruptly after the second year, although exotics persisted through nearly two decades of succession.

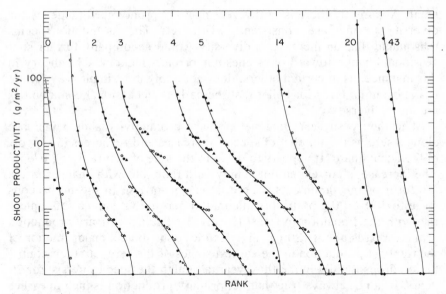

Figure 3 Dominance-diversity curves for the field-to-forest sere at Brookhaven, New York. The sigmoid forms of the intermediate stages of succession suggest a higher degree of evolutionary adaptation among the organisms of these stages. The adaptation has resulted in a wider, more nearly "equitable" distribution of net primary production. The linearity of the curves representing the later stages suggests that these stages may be impoverished in species (Woodwell *et al*, in press).

should show adaptive patterns as well. The dominance–diversity curves used most recently by R. H. Whittaker are one means of exploring these relationships (Figure 3). These are curves developed by plotting net primary production by species against the sequence of species from that with the largest net primary production to the smallest. The process was repeated for each stage in the sere studied.

The strongly linear, logarithmic series are characteristics of communities in which dominance is concentrated in a few species. Where diversity is higher, net production tends to be shared somewhat more equitably among several species and the curves acquire a hump. It is tempting to suggest that these communities are more mature in an evolutionary sense; that the species are more precisely integrated one with another. The graph lends limited support to that view. Certainly the most diverse communities show the greatest deviation from the logarithmic relationship and it is in these middle successional communities that the exotics, although present, diminish in importance as though excluded from a closed corporation. Perhaps in this sere the greatest degree of mutual adaptation among plants occurs in these more diverse intermediate stages of succession.

Additional support for the hypothesis that a tendency toward the sigmoid shape of dominance–diversity curves reflects a higher degree of mutual adaptation among plants comes from examination of synusia, small subcommunities that have considerable fidelity of structure and composition over large areas and are commonly thought to be especially durable, evolutionarily mature assemblages. The *Vaccinium–Gaylussacia* synusium of the oak–pine forest is one such example as is the com-

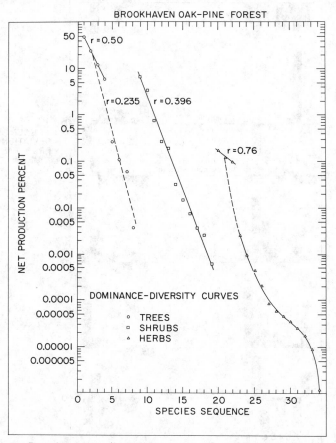

Figure 4 Dominance–diversity curves for the synusia of the oak–pine forest at Brookhaven. The shrub and herb synusia, which have considerable fidelity of composition over large areas in eastern North America and might be considered evolutionarily "mature" tend toward the sigmoid form (Whittaker and Woodwell, 1968).

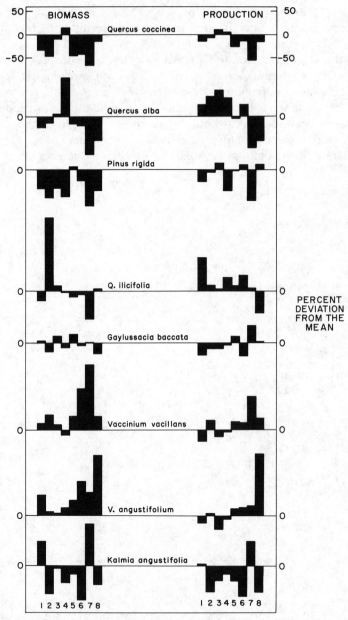

Figure 5 Relative distribution of nutrients among species of the Brookhaven Forest. Numbers refer to nutrients: 1, N; 2, P; 3, K; 4, Ca; 5, Mg; 6, Fe; 7, S; 8, Na.

munity of herbaceous species of the forest floor (Figure 4). Both these synusia tend to contribute toward a sigmoid flattening of the dominance – diversity curve for the forest.

If there is pattern in the distribution of net primary production, can there be pattern in the distribution of nutrients in an evolutionarily mature community? How are nutrients distributed among species in the oak – pine forest? If higher plant species are equal commensals at the nutrient feast, their mean nutrient concentrations, averaged over all tissues by species, should approximate the mean for the forest as a whole. Such does not appear to be the case according to Woodwell et al. (1974). The species of the oak – pine forest contain nutrients in strikingly different proportions. In Figure 5, taken from a detailed study by Woodwell et al. (1974), the nutrient content of species is expressed as deviations from the average for the forest as a whole. The differences apply to biomass and to net primary production; there is a consistency of pattern between the biomass and net production as might be expected, but the differences in the distribution of nutrients among species remain. If the species are commensals, their shares are disproportionate, not only among species, but also among nutrients. It is difficult to consider that such a relationship could be anything but "adaptive," reflecting the differential partitioning of nutrients.

The patterns in succession that I have examined here with greater detail than they have commonly been examined, but in much less detail than they deserve, simply reinforce the importance of the role that succession plays in ecology and the reason for examining succession as a touchstone of ecological theory. The story is incomplete without also examining retrogression: the patterns of change brought by chronic disturbance.

Retrogression

One of the very best examples of retrogression is the Irradiated Forest at Brookhaven National Laboratory, a decade-long experiment on the ecological effects of ionizing radiation. The forest appeared as shown in Figure 6(a) in September of 1961 when a large γ radiation source was being established in the center of it. In the spring of 1962, it appeared as shown in Figure 6(b) and eleven years later in May, 1973 it appeared as shown in Figure 6(c).

The most important observation in this experiment was that the changes in the structure of the vegetation followed patterns that are well

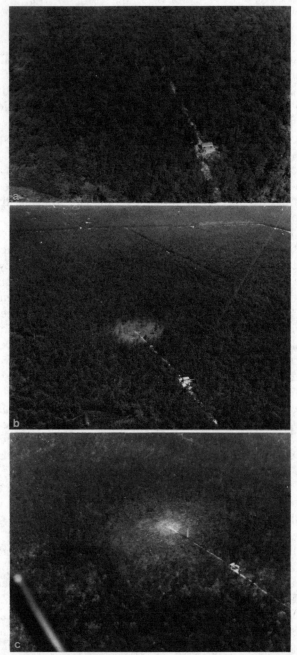

Figure 6 The Brookhaven Irradiated Forest during three stages of the experiment: in 1961 during establishment of the source prior to irradiation (a); in 1962 after 6 months' exposure to chronic irradiation (b); and in the spring of 1973 after 12 years' exposure (c).

known. They are not peculiar to the effect of ionizing radiation. The changes are representative of the changes that occur along virtually any gradient of increasing biotic stress, whether it be oxides of sulfur from a smelter, salt spray along a seashore, or the complex of factors called "exposure" on a mountain slope (Woodwell, 1970).

The pattern is developed through the progressive elimination of species, one or two at a time by higher and higher exposures. In the irradiated forest, the pine *(Pinus rigida)* was very much more sensitive to ionizing radiation than other plants and was eliminated first, leaving a forest that appears intact to a casual observer. Slightly higher exposures eliminated two more species, the two oaks *Quercus alba* and *Q. coccinea,* and left a community of shrubs and tree sprouts. At higher exposures the shrubs were eliminated, and then the herbs, leaving a devastated zone at highest exposures where no higher plants survive. Here certain populations of lichens, mosses, algae, and soil fungi persevered. These, too, are resistant forms that survive many insults, not simply ionizing radiation (Woodwell and Rebuck, 1967). This is the pattern of damage that was established in the first year of the experiment. Eleven years of chronic exposure has increased the circle of damage and given time for the invasion of successional species. But the changes over time have simply reinforced the broad pattern established initially.

The pattern is one of progressive simplification of structure: first, the trees are eliminated, then the shrubs; then the herbaceous plants. Within the lichen, moss, and soil fungus communities the same pattern holds. The more complex, taller statured forms are eliminated first, the simpler forms persist. An example provided by Dr. S. Gochenaur of Adelphi University, shows that among the soil microfungi those with simple fruiting structures persist at high radiation exposures. So do thick-walled, spore-forming, melanized forms (Figure 7).

Similarly, the successional species that have invaded the central devastated zone of the forest are species characteristic of disturbed sites: two species of *Rubus, Phytolacca americana, Comptonia peregrina, Erechtites hieracifolia* (fireweed), and very few others. These are hardy species of disturbed sites, characteristic of biotically and chemically impoverished communities.

I have suggested elsewhere that these changes are too familiar, too consistent among diverse types of disturbances, not to reflect a high degree of preadaptation (Woodwell, 1970). The mechanisms are several (Woodwell, 1967; Woodwell and Whittaker, 1968). What is important is that although in this instance the response has been elicited by ionizing radiation, the adaptations that ordained this pattern were probably not in response to ionizing radiation, but to a complex of environmental fac-

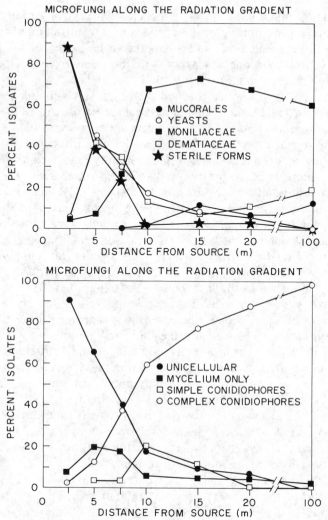

Figure 7 Distribution of soil microfungi along the gradient of ionizing radiation in the Brookhaven Irradiated Forest. The microfungi
surviving high exposures are the simpler forms that are common in
disturbed sites (Gochenaur and Woodwell, in press).

tors. The experiment tells us much about the effects of human activities
on the structure of the biota.

We ask what happens to diversity, net primary production, the the
pool of nutrients? The answer is clear in the broad context: all are reduced, approximately in proportion to the reduction in stature and complexity of the forest.

The availability of nutrients in soils follows the same pattern. After 7 years, exchangeable quantities of Na, K, and Mg were reduced appreciably along the gradient, and the evidence is that further reductions can be expected with continued reduction of the vegetation (Figure 8). Ca and P increased in soils, probably as a result of losses from the vegetation. A reestablishment of the forest will require succession, the rate of which will certainly be limited by the accumulation of nutrients.

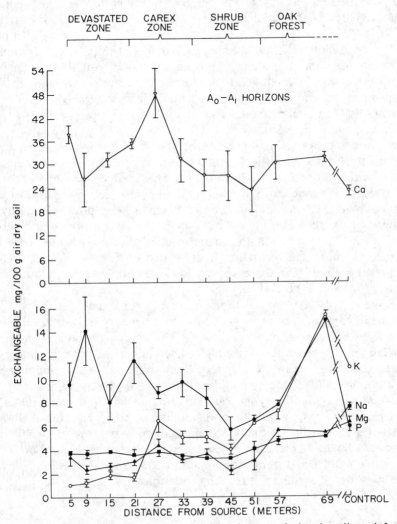

Figure 8 Nutrients in the A_0–A_1 horizons of the irradiated forest after 1 year's exposure to chronic γ irradiation (Horrill and Woodwell, 1973).

Succession and retrogression lie at the core of ecological theory and should lie at the core of theories of management of biotic resources. The broad basic theory that interprets succession toward maturity or climax as developmental and progressive leading toward an increased capacity for long-term support of life seems more rigorous today than ever before. The details of these adaptations include the partitioning of net production, the division of the nutrient pool, and, no less significantly, the chemical interactions lead to inhibition of nitrification and other changes suggested by E. Rice and his colleagues recently (Rice and Pancholy 1972).

Retrogression, articulated first by Clements (1928), is real. It implies a long-lasting impoverishment of the site including reductions in the biota, a shift in species, reductions in nutrient inventory, and reductions in net production, and reductions in potential for recovery. We see it more commonly than we recognize—in roadsides, hilltops, forests, rivers, lakes, and estuaries worldwide.

Nature appears resilient in that it springs back green after almost any treatment. But there is little question that the reduction of the biota associated with deforestation of large areas has reduced the potential of those sites for support of life. Plant communities occupy these sites, are well adapted to them, and sometimes channel large flows of energy to man's use. But the theory of ecology suggests that the more mature communities in the successional sequence would offer more support for life in general, more efficient and effective use of resources, and greater long-term stability for these resources. The rapidly accumulating evidence now supports this theory.

I like to hope that we are on the verge of a great new discovery. Biology made great advances around the cellular theory of life. Perhaps we are about to discover, now, very late in the history of the human being, that the environment, too, is cellular. The cells are ecosystems, forests, fields, estuaries, oceans; each basic biotic units, each in some stage of evolutionary and successional development, each containing species adapted in ways still beyond our ken to one another and interacting among themselves to provide for stability of their environment—and ours. And I like to hope that we shall recognize soon that the basic unit for management of the earth's resources is not energy, fish, food, oil— but whole units, ecosystems, that function according to a set of discoverable laws, not according to the whims of exploiters.

Acknowledgment

Research carried out at Brookhaven National Laboratory under the auspices of the U. S. Atomic Energy Commission.

References

Clements, F. E. (1928). "Plant Succession and Indicators." H. W. Wilson Co., New York.

Cooper, W. S. (1926). The fundamentals of vegetational change. *Ecology* **9**, 1–5.

Cowles, H. C. (1899). The ecological relations of the vegetation of the sand dunes of Lake Michigan. *Bot. Gaz. Chicago* **27**, 95.

Cowles, H. C. (1901). The physiographic ecology of Chicago and vicinity. *Bot. Gaz. Chicago* **31**, 73.

Fernald, M. L. (1950). "Gray's Manual of Botany," 8th Ed. American Book Co., New York.

Gochenaur, S. E., and Woodwell, G. M. (in press). The soil microfungi of an oak–pine forest receiving chronic ionizing radiation, *Ecology*.

Horrill, A. D., and Woodwell, G. M. (1973). Structure and cation content of a podzolic soil of Long Island, N. Y. seven years after destruction of the vegetation by chronic gamma irradiation. *Ecology* **54**, 439–444.

Margalef, R. (1963). On certain unifying principles in ecology. *Amer. Natur.* **97**, 357–374.

Margalef, R. (1968). "Perspectives in Ecological Theory." Univ. of Chicago Press, Chicago, Illinois.

Odum, E. P. (1971). "Principles of Ecology," 2nd Ed. Saunders, Philadelphia, Pennsylvania.

Rice, E. L., and Pancholy, S. K. (1972). Inhibition of nitrification by climax ecosystems. *Amer. J. Bot.* **59**, 1033–1040.

Tansley, A. G. (1935). The use and abuse of vegetational concepts and terms. *Ecology* **16**, 284.

Whittaker, R. H., and Woodwell, G. M. (1968). Dimension and production relations of trees and shrubs in the Brookhaven Forest, New York. *J. Ecol.* **56**, 1–25.

Woodwell, G. M. (1967). Radiation and the patterns of nature. *Science* **156**, 461.

Woodwell, G. M. (1970). Effects of pollution on the structure and physiology of ecosystems. *Science* **168**, 429.

Woodwell, G. M., and Rebuck, A. L. (1967). Effects of chronic gamma radiation on the structure and diversity of an oak–pine forest. *Ecol. Monogr.* **37**, 53–69.

Woodwell, G. M., and Whittaker, R. H. (1968). Effects of chronic gamma irradiation on plant communities. *Quart. Rev. Biol.* **43**, 42–55.

Woodwell, G. M., Holt, B. R., and Flaccus, E. (in press). Secondary succession: structure and production in the field-to-forest sere at Brookhaven, L. I., N. Y. *Ecology*.

Woodwell, G. M., Whittaker, R. H., and Houghton, R. A. (1974). Nutrient elements in terrestrial ecosystems: concentrations in plant tissues in the Brookhaven oak–pine forest. *Ecol. Monogr.* **44**, 255–277.

Part II
Adaptations of Desert Organisms

Water Vapor Absorption in *Prosopis*

F. W. Went

Laboratory of Desert Biology
Desert Research Institute
University of Nevada System
Reno, Nevada

The plant I want to discuss is *Prosopis tamarugo,* a mesquite from the Pampa del Tamarugal, a vast desert plain in the northern (tropical) part of Chile. This desert tree is truly exceptional, since it produces forests in a completely rainless and fogless area, where there is no underground liquid water source. I was guided to this area by Dr. Fusa Sudzuki, who had carried out much work on this remarkable tree. In my experience with desert plants I had become acquainted with phreatophytes, xerophytes, succulents, and drought avoiders, but not with a hydrophyte, which term we might apply to the tamarugo tree.

To set the scene, let me describe the Pampa del Tamarugal. It is located between 19° and 22° S latitude in the driest part of the Atacama Desert, behind a coastal mountain range, at 900–1000 m altitude, and bordered toward the east by the very slowly rising slopes of the Andes. This plain is utterly flat, with no depressions produced by washes or rises in the form of dunes. Most of the Pampa is covered with a few decimeters thick salt crust of $NaNO_3$ or Na_2SO_4, which, when cut into blocks, is used for building, such as house walls; they never disintegrate because of the complete lack of rain. The very limited amount of water run-off from the Andes is entirely underground, which in a few places (such as Matilla and Pica) is forced to the surface as springs. But, in the eastern part of the Pampa del Tamarugal, ground water is 40–100 m below the surface, and slightly lower in the western part where it is forced to near the surface as a brine. The forest of tamarugo trees (already greatly reduced due to cutting) occurs all over the plain, and is quite open, with trees as big as 15 m tall and 1 m diameter at the base. The lower branches spread over the ground, producing an umbrella-shaped canopy. The foliage is somewhat xeromorphic, much more so than that of *Prosopis chilensis* (closely related to our *P. juliflora*), which in some places with a sufficiently high water table, grows intermixed with tamarugo. There is no undergrowth of any sort, except where *Distichlis* grows in places with a salt seep.

The most outstanding difference between *Prosopis tamarugo* and all other *Prosopis* species is its root system. This does not penetrate deep into the soil: the longest roots penetrate only as far as 6 m, and even when all roots are cut off 2 m below the surface, the tamarugo tree does not suffer but continues to grow normally (Sudzuki, 1969). Therefore the tamarugo behaves entirely different from other mesquites, and does not obtain its water from the subsoil or ground water table.

The most remarkable characteristic of the tamarugo root system is the development of a dense mat of roots, 20–60 cm below the soil surface. The soil in this root-mat zone is sopping wet, and its water content is well above field capacity (Sudzuki, 1969). Since the soil above and below the root-mat is dry, this water cannot possibly have come from above or below through the soil. And the measurements of Dr. Sudzuki are not exceptional. In the half-dozen root systems I have dug up, both in natural tamarugo forests and in plantations, I always found the root-mat zone soaking wet. It was easy to squeeze water droplets from the cortex of these roots by applying only mild pressure.

The roots of tamarugo in the root-mat zone are quite exceptional in that they occupy about 10% of the soil volume and are all of about the same diameter (1–2 mm), and retain their dead cortex of which the cells have thickened brown cell walls which act as blotting paper. In this way any water excreted by the stele of the root remains in or around the root, and is available for immediate reabsorption. Thus the root-mat zone provides a most effective water storage system; no living water storage tissue of the plant is required, and none of this water can escape into the air through a 20- to 40-cm thick layer of soil or a solid salt layer.

The source of this root-mat water is the main problem confronting the scientist trying to understand the occurrence of these tamarugo trees in an area where no liquid water is available from rain or underground reservoirs. Yet, the fact of their occurrence has to be accepted. Not only do these trees occur here naturally, but about 8000 hectares of tamarugo have been planted there, requiring not more than 4–6 months of artificial watering after the 3-month-old seedlings have been placed in plant holes. After this period, they no longer need liquid water, and they grow at a rate of 40 cm or more per year, becoming 10–15 m tall trees in 20–30 years, with a stem diameter of up to 30 cm. They are economically important since four to six sheep can be raised per hectare of such tamarugo forests. Several villages in the Pampa del Tamarugal, such as Tirana and La Huayca, exist exclusively on sheep and goat raising in tamarugo forests.

Sudzuki (1969) has provided the necessary experimental evidence to establish the source of this water in the root-mat of tamarugo. She found that during the summer, when the relative humidity of the air rises almost every night to over 80%, tritiated water, when applied to the foliage, is taken up during night, and is translocated to the root system. On such humid nights the direction of the normal transpiration stream is reversed, and water flows in the stem from the foliage downward into the root system. Since such massive water vapor uptake has never before been found to occur in plants, this case deserves special attention.

We will first analyze the water vapor uptake energetically. Table 1 summarizes a thermo-hygrograph record for summer nights in the Pampa del Tamarugal. Immediately after sunset the air temperature starts to decrease rapidly due to the then negative radiation balance. By assuming an outgoing radiation rate at ground level of 0.2 cal $\cdot$ cm^2 $\cdot$ min^{-1} at 10°C, this surface cooling can reduce the temperature of a 100-m column of air plus the soil to the observed 6.7°C during the first 2 night hr. This rate of cooling continues until about midnight, when the dew point is reached. Then the rate of cooling drops sharply, because the radiative cooling not only must lower the air temperature, but also must condense water vapor. This is evidenced by the lowering of the dew point of the air. From Table 1 we see that on the 6 nights which are averaged, a total of 0.12 g of water was condensed per night per cm^2 ground surface, or the equivalent of 1.2 mm of rain. Table 2 summarizes a thermo-hygrograph record for a week during winter. During 5 of the 6 nights the dew point was not reached by the dry-bulb thermometer and the lowering of the dew point was due to dry upper air mixing with air near the surface. Only during the last night of this winter week did water condensation near the ground occur as the dry bulb thermometer reached the dew point.

These two tables show that the critical condition, which allows the reaching of the dew point during the night and the condensing of water vapor to liquid water, is the absence of wind which would bring in dry upper air. The dew point of the air layer covering the Pampa del Tamarugal equals about the temperature of the seawater off the coast. Since there are no surface winds in that area, the only air movements are rising

Table 1[a] Summary of a Thermo-hygrograph Record for Summer Nights

	Parameter	Results								
Line										
1	Time of night	1800	2000	2200	2400	0200	0400	0600	0800	1000
2	Air temperature (°C)	32.2	25.5	19.8	15.8	13.2	11.2	9.2	7.7	15.8
3	Relative humidity (%)	26.3	34.7	54.2	69.0	78.9	84.0	82.0	89.5	72.5
4	Dew point (°C)	10.2	9.7	10.2	10.0	9.6	8.6	6.2	6.0	10.9
5	Decrease in temperature per 2 hr (°C)	–	6.7	5.7	4.0	2.6	2.0	2.0	1.5	–8.1
6	Outgoing radiation in (cal · cm⁻² · 2 hr⁻¹)	–	30	28	26	25	24	23	22	–
7	Height of air column cooled (m)	–	100	100	80	60	60	60	60	–
8	Radiation needed for air cooling (cal · cm⁻² · 2 hr⁻¹)	–	17	14	12	3	3	3	3	–
9	Radiation needed for soil cooling	–	13	14	14	5	3	2	2	–
10	Radiation available for water condensation (cal · cm⁻² · 2 hr⁻¹)	–	0	0	0	17	18	18	17	–
11	Amount of water condensed	–	0	0	0	0.029	0.031	0.031	0.029	–

[a]Meteorological data (lines 2 and 3) from 12–18 March 1970 as measured in Canchones (Pampa del Tamarugal). All other data calculated from this weather record and from estimates of outgoing radiation. (0.2 cal · cm⁻² · min⁻¹ at 10°C).

thermal columns during the day and subsidence of that same air during the night. Therefore there is no overall water vapor loss from the air mass over the Pampa del Tamarugal, and the same water which is lost by transpiration during the day is available again during the night for condensation. In the other desert areas I am acquainted with, surface winds bring in dry air preventing the recovery of the moisture lost during the day. Only in the Negev desert in Israel does a regular amount of water condensation occur as dew during the summer (Duvdevani, 1953) and it is in Israel that water vapor absorption by trees and subsequent excretion by their roots has been shown to occur (Gindel, 1973).

The same value for water vapor condensation, which was calculated from dew point depression and from radiative cooling at night, is obtained when the nightly increase in soil moisture is measured. This was also done by Dr. Sudzuki, and she found that the upper layer of the soil in the desert surrounding the tamarugo forest absorbed 0.12 g of water per cm² per night (equivalent to 1.2 mm rain).

During September 1971 the transpiration of a 30-year-old tamarugo tree was measured, by multiplying the water loss per branch (measured over a 40-hr period for five branches) with the number of branches on the tree. This transpiration loss amounted to 0.12 g · cm² of ground surface, the same value as calculated for water vapor condensation per night. This establishes that energetically and quantitatively condensation of water vapor at night can account for enough water to satisfy the transpirational needs of the tamarugo tree.

Meteorologically the situation on the Pampa del Tamarugal is quite interesting. Over this area a high pressure condition preserves the same air mass, originating over the nearby Pacific Ocean (with a water content in equilibrium with a water temperature of 11°C), for at least the whole summer season. The amount of water vapor condensing each night due to radiative cooling is returned to the air by evaporation and transpiration the next day. But at any time that winds bring in air with a lower water vapor content (typically during winter) this equilibrium is broken, and a new supply of moist air (from the ocean) has to reestablish the equilibrium. This apparently happened on 25 July 1970 (see Table 2), making the following night a dew night.

The complete flatness of the Pampa del Tamarugal apparently discourages surface winds, which makes it possible for a high dew point to be maintained without importation of new moisture (of which there is no local source). Dr. Carlos Lopez (1973) failed to establish tamarugo trees in our southwestern deserts, apparently because frequent night winds lower the dew point so far that no water vapor condensation can occur.

Table 2[a] Summary of a Thermo-hygrograph Record for Winter Nights

Parameter	Results							
20–25 July 1970								
1 Time of night	1800	2000	2200	2400	0200	0400	0600	0800
2 Air temperature (°C)	27.6	19.8	14.8	9.8	7.2	4.8	3.2	1.8
3 Relative humidity (%)	19.0	24.2	32.0	37.0	43.0	47.0	50.6	52.2
4 Dew point (°C)	2.6	−1.7	−2.2	−4.7	−4.8	−6.2	−6.7	−7.6
25–26 July 1970								
12 Air temperature in (°C)	27	19.5	13	9	6	4	2	0
13 Relative humidity (%)	30	45	75	84	87	90	90	95
14 Dew point (°C)	9	9	9	6.6	4.0	2.6	0.6	−0.5

[a]Meteorological data from 20–26 July 1970 as measured in Canchones (same recorder as Table I). Data from the first 5 windy nights (lines 2–4) contrasted with the last quiet night (lines 12–14).

This would restrict the area where tamarugo or other water vapor absorbing plants can grow to windless deserts.

Although we have evidence that energetically and factually water vapor uptake can occur in *Prosopis tamarugo*, its uptake mechanism is still a mystery. Since dew has never been seen on tamarugo leaves, we only can assume that internal dew formation occurs. Dr. Sudzuki has pointed out that in the epidermis and subepidermis of tamarugo slime cells occur. Perhaps water condensation occurs inside these cells, producing a gel with a very low matrix pressure, which would easily give up its water of inbibition upon hydrostatic suction. This water would then be drawn by gravity to the root system, where it then would ooze out into the dead cells of the root cortex and into the surrounding soil. Lopez (1973) has actually observed liquid water excretion from tamarugo roots, supplied with liquid water 1 m above the region of excretion.

Why has the tamarugo mechanism of water vapor uptake from the air not been reported in other plants? In the first place, experiments on water vapor uptake in the laboratory have always been carried out under isothermal conditions. They either failed, or accounted for such a slow rate that its role in water uptake in nature could be discounted. Let me give a few examples.

In experiments carried out in 1957 and 1958 (together with Dr. L. Overland Sheps) I found that when Southern California leafy *Peucephyllum schottii* branches were placed in a container with air drier than 60%, they lost water through normal transpiration, but when placed in an atmosphere above 70% (relative humidity), they continued (for at least $1/2 - 1$ hr) to absorb water from this relatively moist air. More recently Dr. N. Stark, using a different technique, failed to observe such water vapor uptake by *Peucephyllum* in Death Valley.

In addition I observed an epiphyte, *Schoenorchis juncifolia*, in the tropical rain forest of Tjibodas in Java, which I grew for 4 years (1929–1932) under a glass roof in the forest atmosphere of 92–99% R H. Their rootless stems, carrying about 10 leaves, were suspended with brass wire under the glass, with no access at any time to liquid water. When they were attached to recording balances, they were found to lose about 1% of their weight during the day, which they largely recovered each following night, apparently through water vapor uptake. At an average relative humidity of 96%, this would require a water tension of 60 atm in their tissues. Even though the osmotic concentration of the cell sap of the leaf cells was found to be only 19 atm by the plasmolytic method, their water tension was much higher because of a negative turgor, which in leaf sections submerged in paraffin oil caused abnormal plasmolysis (with the cell sap released from cut cells). Occasionally (apparently when the cell wall was just barely cut) paraffin oil was observed to be avidly absorbed as tiny droplets between the cytoplasm and cell wall, proving the existence of a negative turgor. This also would allow water vapor uptake at relative humidities above 96%. However, this process was extremely slow, enabling the *Schoenorchis* plants to produce only three to four new leaves each year. Therefore isothermal water vapor uptake is possible under natural conditions, but it is very slow, and probably plays no significant part in nature. With the exception of Renner (1942), who demonstrated water vapor uptake by epiphytic mosses in the same rain forest in Java, no other investigators found that isothermal water vapor uptake played a significant role in plant growth.

In experiments carried out in 1926–1927, I found that seeds of *Avena sativa* failed to germinate in a saturated atmosphere (suspended in a constant temperature darkroom in a container over pure water), but dead seeds soon became overgrown by mycelium, which could take up water vapor from the air and use it for growth.

Another reason that water vapor uptake was not reported for desert plants could be because it seems to be only effective under the special meteorological conditions existing in windless deserts, such as the Pampa del Tamarugal.

The possibility exists that plants have basically the ability to absorb water vapor from a moist atmosphere when a negative radiation balance lowers their temperature below the dewpoint of the surrounding air. This is most likely insufficient to maintain a positive water balance.

The final reason for the success of the tamarugo plant in keeping a positive waterbalance, while depending exclusively on water vapor uptake, may lie in its special adaptations, such as the slime cells in its leaves, its root-mat, and possible other properties allowing water excretion into a dead root cortex.

Whatever the ultimate solution of the water balance of the tamarugo tree is, a detailed study of all aspects of its life in a waterless desert is highly interesting and very much worthwhile. But let nobody dismiss this botanical paradox with a shrug of the shoulder, or the mental excuse that someone must have made wrong observations: this absolute desert forest exists and may produce many new and unexpected phenomena and mechanisms concerning growth and water economy of plants in general, and may provide us with new insights in adaptation.

References

Duvdevani, S. (1953). Dew gradients in relation to climate, soil, and topography. *Desert Res. Proc. Int. Symp.*, May 7–14, Jerusalem.

Gindel, I. (1973). A new ecophysiological approach to forest – water relationships in arid climates. Dr. W. Junk B. V.-The Hague, The Netherlands.

Lopez, C. E. O. (1973). Effect of thermoperiod on *Prosopis tamarugo* Phil.
Doctoral Dissertation, University of Nevada, Reno, Nevada.

Renner, O. (1942). Hydrostatischer Druck und Gasgehalt. *Ber. Deut. Bot. Ges.*
60, 292 – 294.

Sudzuki, F. H. (1969). Absorcion foliar de humedad atomsferica en tamarugo,
Prosopis tamarugo Phil. Universidad de Chile, Facultad de Agronomia, Bol.
Tech. NO. 30, Maipu-Chile.

Absorption of Water Vapor from Unsaturated Air

E. B. Edney

*University of California
Los Angeles, California*

Introduction

Maintenance of water balance is an important problem for most land arthropods, and the mechanisms involved have received much attention from arthropod physiologists and ecologists. Of these mechanisms one of the most intriguing is that whereby water vapor is absorbed from unsaturated air, sometimes against very impressive water activity gradients. Although the title of the section of this volume refers to desert organisms, I hope to be forgiven for considering water vapor uptake in general, not only as a process of significance for arthropods that live in places marked as deserts on maps, but for all arthropods living in environments where water may be in short supply. Some recent reviews are those of Beament (1961, 1964, 1965), Locke (1964), Berridge (1970), and Maddrell (1971).

Historical Overview

In 1930 P. A. Buxton described how the larvae of the meal worm *Tenebrio molitor* increased in weight, even though starved, at high humidities, and ascribed this to the overproduction of metabolic water.

Mellanby (1932) found that production of metabolic water was insufficient to account for the increases in weight and water content observed,
and suggested that water vapor is condensed and absorbed through the
tracheae. Soon thereafter Ludwig (1937) observed uptake in nymphs of
the grasshopper *Chortophaga* (above 92% RH); Lees (1946) observed it
in various ticks with lower limits from 84% to 94% RH; and Edney
(1947) found uptake in flea prepupae *(Xenopsylla brasiliensis)* down to
50% RH.

Since then several species of arthropods have been found to take up
water vapor in a variety of cricumstances, and it is worth considering
these species to see whether any regularities or trends appear. Table 1,
which is based on a list prepared by Berridge (1970) with some later
additions, shows that all the arthropods reported to take up water vapor
are either acarines (ticks or mites) or insects. Furthermore, none of the
insects included is winged. This sometimes means that the faculty is restricted to the immature forms, as it is in beetles and orthopterans. However it does occur in some imagines, but, if so, they are wingless, as are
psocids, mallophagans, thysanurans, and the neotenic adult females of
the desert cockroach *Arenivaga*. However, by no means all wingless
insects possess this faculty; caterpillars, for example, so far as they have
been studied, do not. The restriction to wingless forms is probably more
than a mere coincidence—it may be an indirect reflection of the adaptive
significance of the process whereby insects are able to live in environments where free water either is not available or is in short supply. This
is true for the following groups: the stored-products arthropods (whose
original habitat was often birds' nests), such as *Tenebrio* larvae, the
mites, such as *Acarus* and *Laelaps*, flea larvae and prepupae, firebrats,
desert thysanurans, and sand cockroaches. We note that adult fleas are
wingless, but they do not have much difficulty in obtaining water in the
blood of their hosts, while flea pupae may have to wait a long time in
dry places before the adults which emerge find a host. Most adult fleas
do not take up water vapor: the hen flea, *Ceratophyllus gallinae*, which
apparently does during the first day of adult life (Humphries, 1967) is
an exception. Ticks obtain water from the blood of their hosts, and if
the tick spends most of its life on the host, the need for water vapor
uptake is less immediate. However, many ticks drop off and have to
find a new host after each molt.

The adaptive significance of uptake may be seen in the fact that the
lowest humidity that permits survival in culture is the same as that which
permits uptake both in the mallophagan *Goniodas colchici* (Williams
1970, 1971) and in the psocid *Liposcellis rufus* (Knulle and Spadafora,
1969). The limits for these species is about 60% RH.

Table 1 Arthropods That Are Known to Take Up Water Vapor from Unsaturated Air and Their Critical Equilibrium Humidities[a]

Arthropod	RH%	Authority
Arachnida		
Acarini		
Ixodes ricinus	92.0	Lees (1946)
Ixodes canisuga	94.0	Lees (1946)
Ixodes hexagonus	94.0	Lees (1946)
Ornithodorus moubata	85.5	Lees (1946)
Rhipicephalus sanguineus	84.0–90.0	Lees (1946)
Dermacentor andersoni		
Larvae	80.0–85.0	Knulle (1965)
Adults	85.0	Lees (1946)
Dermacentor variabilis	80.0–85.0	Knulle (1965)
Dermacentor reticulatus	86.0–88.0	Knulle (1965)
Amblyomma cajennense		
Larvae	80.0–85.0	Knulle (1965)
Adults	91.0	Lees (1946)
Amblyomma maculatum	88.0–90.0	Lees (1946)
Acarus siro	75.0	Knulle (1962)
Laelaps echidnina	90.0	Wharton and Kanungo (1962)
Insecta		
Thysanura		
Thermobia domestica	45.0	Beament *et al.* (1964)
Ctenolepisma longicaudata	≈70.0	Lindsay (1940)
Ctenolepisma terebrans	47.5	Edney (1971)
Mallophaga		
Goniodes colchici	60.0	Williams (1971)
Psocoptera		
Liposcellis rufus	58.0	Knulle and Spadafora (1969)
Liposcellis bostrychophilus	60.0	Knulle and Spadafora (1969)
Liposcellis knulleri	≈70.0	Knulle and Spadafora (1969)
Siphonaptera		
Xenopsylla brasilinensis	50.0	Edney (1947)
Xenopsylla cheopis	65.0	Knulle (1967)
Ceratophyllus gallinae	82.0	Humphries (1967)
Coleoptera		
Tenebrio molitor larvae	88.0	Mellanby (1932)
Orthoptera		
Chortophaga viridifasciata	92.0	Ludwig (1937)
Arenivaga investigata	82.5	Edney (1966)

[a]Water activity in the vapor phase (a_v) is equal to relative humidity percent divided by 100, and the approximate osmotic pressure is osmoles corresponding to each a_v can be obtained from the relationship: Osmoles $= (55.5/a_v) - 55.5$. (After Berridge, 1970, with additions).

In *Arenivaga*, the nymphs and adult females (which are larviform) live in sand dunes. The adult males become winged and can presumably find water more easily; in any event, they lose the capacity to absorb. The nymphs and females feed on dead leaves of desert shrubs. They become active at night just below the surface, presumably searching for food. Even at night the surface is hot — we have measured 35°C where the nymphs were feeding — and in the summer, very dry — below 10% RH. But the insects have only to move downward, usually 10 cm, at the most 45 cm, to find an area where the RH is above 80%, and where they can reabsorb lost water as vapor.

In *Ixodes* too, the faculty is closely linked with behavior (Lees, 1948a). These sheep ticks crawl to the top of tall grasses and "quest" for hosts. In so doing they may be exposed to dehydration. But after losing a certain amount of water their behavior changes and they move downward, returning to an area of high humidity at the base of the grass, where they can absorb water vapor to make up for that lost.

There are, of course, many wingless insects, termites for example (Edney, unpublished) and adult tenebrionid beetles with fused elytra, that live in dry areas and do not possess the faculty. So the reason for the limitation of the faculty to certain species within the phylum Arthropoda, and particularly within the Insecta, is by no means clear. In general, however, where it does occur, the adaptive significance of uptake is abundantly clear, and we need not labor the point further.

Limiting Conditions

It became clear early on that for any one species, uptake would occur only if (a) the individual was to some degree dehydrated (there is an important qualification to this to be considered later) and (b) if the relative humidity is above a critical equilibrium humidity (c.e.h. — a term coined by Knulle and Wharton, 1964).

Satisfaction of the second criterion can be seen clearly in some work on flea prepupae (Edney, 1947). Figure 1 shows that these insects gained about 14% of their wet weight during the first 3 – 4 days after ceasing to feed and evacuating the gut. The amount of water gained was not determined by RH provided the latter was at 50% or above. After the pupal molt (which usually occurs inside the cocoon), the insects began to lose weight, and they did so faster in lower humidities, so that the adults which finally emerged started life with water contents determined by the RH during the pupal period. That the changes in weight were indeed due to changes in water content was demonstrated by measuring

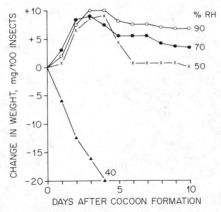

Figure 1 Change in weight caused by uptake (or loss) of water by prepupae of the flea *Xenopsylla brasiliensis*. The prepupal period lasts for 3 days after cocoon formation. (Redrawn from Edney, 1947.)

the water contents of aliquot batches of fleas before, during, and after exposure.

When this experiment was done at different temperatures and over a narrower range of humidities, about half the fleas avoided desiccation at 45% RH; nearly all fleas died of desiccation at 40% and nearly all survived and gained water at 50%, irrespective of temperature (12°, 24°, or 35°C) in each case (Table 2).

To clinch the matter of the lower humidity limit, 50 prepupae were enclosed in about 90 ml of air at 70% RH in an airtight container with a paper hygrometer. The humidity was quickly reduced to 50% by the prepupae, and held there until after the third day, when the insects pupated and lost the power to absorb water. This result is shown in Figure 2.

Table 2 Percentage of Batches of About 30 *Xenopsylla brasiliensis* Prepupae Each, Which Avoided Desiccation during the First 3 Days of the Prepupal Period at Temperatures and Humidities Shown[a]

Temperature (°C)	Percent prepupae avoiding desiccation at different RH%				
	35	40	45	50	55
12	0	0	45	90	95
24	0	0	50	95	100
35	0	0	20	95	95

[a]Percentage given at nearest 5%. (From Edney, 1947.)

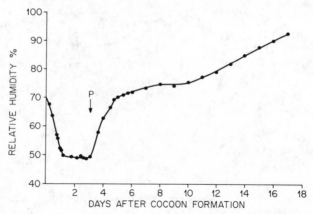

Figure 2 The variation in relative humidity in a closed vessel containing about 90 ml air and 50 *Xenopsylla* prepupae. The fleas took up water vapor and reduced the humidity to 50%. At P the prepupae molted to become pupae and began to lose water. (Redrawn from Edney, 1947.)

In a somewhat similar experiment, Kalmus (1936) put *Tenebrio* larvae in a small enclosed space and found that they generated a RH of 90% until they died; and, in a rather different but relevant experiment, Solomon (1966) found that *Acarus siro* maintained RH's of 90%, 87%, or 76% when kept in a small closed vials. These values correspond with the humidities at which they had been previously cultured.

In flea prepupae, as we have seen, and in several other arthropods, e.g., the psocid *Liposcellis* (Knulle and Spadafora, 1969), and *Thermobia domestica* (Noble-Nesbitt, 1969), the final water content is uninfluenced by humidity during rehydration. This is not always so however, as Solomon (1966) found for the flour mite *Acarus siro*, which had body water contents of 70% at 95% RH and 66% at 75% RH, and as Knulle (1967) found for *Xenopsylla cheopis* larvae, where the equilibrium body water content increased or decreased as the larvae were transferred to higher or lower humidities, provided these were above the c.e.h. (These are important exceptions to the general statement made above that all arthropods which exhibit water vapor uptake gain water at all humidities above the c.e.h.) Knulle also found that as soon as the prepupae were formed they took up more water, irrespective of the humidity to which they had previously equilibrated. This would account for the fact that Edney (1947) found that prepupae absorbed much water even though the larvae from which they developed had not been dehydrated.

An example of the combined effects of temperature and RH on vapor

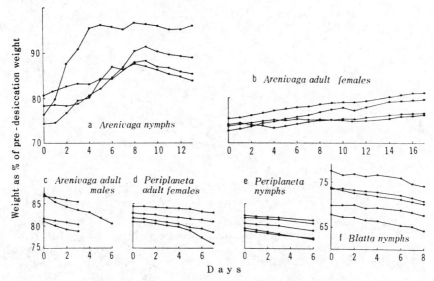

Figure 3 Change in weight of *Arenivaga investigata* and other cock-roaches in 95% RH after previous dehydration to between 75% and 85% of their original wet weight. *Arenivaga* nymphs and adult females gained weight by water uptake, the remainder lost weight. (From Edney, 1966.)

uptake is shown by the desert cockroach *Arenivaga investigata* (Edney, 1966). Figure 3 shows that after dehydration to about 80% of their origi-nal weight, both sexes of nymphs and adult females (but not males) re-gained water at 95% RH. *Periplaneta* or *Blatta* nymphs, however, did not. Figure 4 shows further that nymphs took up water at 82.5% or above regardless of temperature, although the rate was faster at higher temperatures. Molting inhibited uptake, and so did mild abrasion of the cuticle, although the damage was repaired in a day or so.

In *Arenivaga* the gain in weight at high humidities was indeed due to water uptake because the volume of the body water increased by about 15.7% of original weight, while metabolically produced water during the same time would have been only about 3%. The effects of vapor uptake on the osmotic concentration of the hemolymph was to reduce this from 452 to 373 mOsm-liter^{-1}, which is less than the expected reduction in the absence of regulation (Figure 5). Further work (Edney, 1968) showed that regulation during dehydration and rehydration occurred as the result of removal from or addition to the hemolymph of osmotically active substances. Okasha (1973) has recently found a similar effect in *Thermobia*.

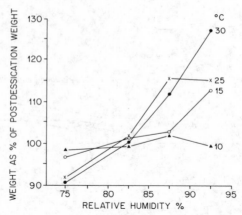

Figure 4 The effect of temperature and humidity on direction and rate of water exchange in *Arenivaga investigata* nymphs. The critical equilibrium humidity is about 82.5% RH irrespective of temperature and, therefore, of vapor pressure deficit. (From Edney, 1966.)

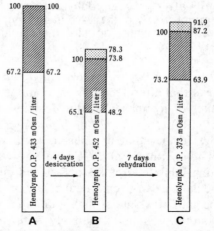

Figure 5 Absolute and relative proportions by weight of dry material, water and fecal material. (A) insects before dehydration; (B) other insects after dehydration for 4 days; (C) other insects after dehydration and subsequent rehydration for 7 days. Open areas, water; hatched areas, dry material; stippled areas, fecal material. Numbers to the right of each column represent mean amounts of the various materials concerned in arbitrary units of weight. Numbers to the left of each column express the amounts present as percentages of the net weight (excluding fecal material) of insects in each group. (From Edney, 1966.)

Before closing this section we may note that the critical equilibrium humidities present a very wide range — from 94% RH in some *Ixodes* species, to 47.5% in *Ctenolepisma terebrans* (Edney, 1971) and even 45% RH in *Thermobia domestica*. The thysanurans seem to be particularly good at absorbing from low humidities, but there is no obvious correlation in this respect with phyletic position.

The Energetics of Water Vapor Uptake

So far we have considered the distribution, extent, limits, and some of the effects of vapor uptake. In some cases the process takes place against very steep gradients, and this raises the question of the amount of energy involved. The process is certainly an active one, since it ceases at death (Kalmus, 1936; Edney, 1947), is inhibited by anesthesia (Lees, 1946; Browning, 1954) or by poisoning (Lees, 1946; Belazerov and Sevarin, 1960).

One of the earliest estimates was that of Lees (1948b) who found that the actual amount of energy required was small compared with the energy resources of the ticks concerned (about 1 part in 3800 of stored fat per day), and Ramsay (1964) reached a similar conclusion for the larval meal worm, *Tenebrio molitor*. Kanungo (1965) compared O_2 uptake by mites which were or were not absorbing water and found no significant difference. Calculations also showed that such a difference would be very small, for the observed O_2 uptake was $0.17 \ \mu l \ O_2 \cdot hr^{-1}$ by a standard female mite *(Laelaps echidnina)*, while the O_2 necessary to supply the energy needed to concentrate water from an activity of 0.90 to one of 0.99 ($a_v = 0.90$ to a_w 0.99) is only $0.0006 \ \mu l \cdot mite^{-1} \cdot hr^{-1}$.

For *Arenivaga*, calculations based on the well-known relationship $G = RT \ln P_2/P_1$ showed that a 100-mg insect, absorbing 6 mg water $\cdot$ day^{-1} expends about $0.036 \ cal \cdot day^{-1}$ in doing so, while its basal metabolic rate is $2.6 \ cal \cdot day^{-1}$. The extra energy necessary for uptake is, therefore, relatively very small.

Maddrell (1971) considered the energetics of uptake of water vapor by *Thermobia*, and calculated that to move $5 \ \mu g \cdot min^{-1}$ of water from $a_v = 0.5$ (in the air) to $a_w = 0.99$ (in the hemolymph) takes $0.006 \ cal \cdot hr^{-1}$. Even at 10% efficiency this represents only $18 \ \mu g \cdot hr^{-1}$ of glucose — less than 0.07% of the body weight. For comparison, a flying insect uses up to 20% of its body weight $\cdot hr^{-1}$ (Weis-Fogh, 1967).

Thus, although the gradient is often very steep, the energy required to concentrate the quantities involved is comparatively small. However, this is not to say that the problem is solved, for although the energy is demonstrably available, the mechanism is still an open question.

The Site of Absorption

In order to discover the mechanisms involved we must first be clear about the site or sites where uptake occurs. Mellanby (1932) was inclined to implicate the tracheae, but most subsequent workers have favored the whole cuticle as the site of uptake. The reasons for this are compelling in the case of those mites and ticks where a tracheal system is absent, but such reasoning need not be extrapolated to arthropods which possess a tracheal system. Lees (1946) observed absorption in *Ixodes* (a tick which does have tracheae) even when the spiracles were blocked, and he also observed that damage by abrasion to one part of the cuticle put the whole cuticle out of action so far as uptake was concerned. In *Arenivaga,* successful blocking of the spiracles led to death, so that experiment was inconclusive; but abrasion, which of course leads to a great increase in water loss and might therefore mask absorption, did not damage the cuticle as a whole because covering the abrasion with nail polish immediately restored net absorption (Edney, 1966).

In fact, it is difficult to see how tracheoles, which usually contain some fluid which is probably nearly in equilibrium with the hemolymph ($a_w = 0.99$) could absorb water vapor from air down to $a_v = 0.5$.

Recently Noble-Nesbitt (1970) found that blocking the anus of *Thermobia* prevented uptake, and proposed that the rectum is the usual site of uptake at least in that species. The suggestion is very attractive, particularly when seen in conjunction with the work of Ramsay (1964, 1971) and of Grimstone *et al.* (1968) on the rectal complex of *Tenebrio molitor* larvae. This is an insect known to absorb water vapor down to about 88% RH ($a_v = 0.88$), and fecal material in its rectum can be dehydrated (by a complex system involving cryptonephridial tubules and rectal cells) by the net transport of water from the lumen to the hemocoele, until it is in equilibrium with $a_v = 0.9$ (air at 90% RH).

Recent observations suggest that in ticks the site for water vapor uptake is not the rectum (McEnroe, 1972), but the mouth (Rudolph and Knulle, 1974).

In *Thermobia,* of course, unlike *Tenebrio* larvae, absorption occurs from $a_v = 0.5$; so while the rectal complex of *Tenebrio* may explain that insect's ability to dehydrate fecal material, some other process must occur in *Thermobia,* which does not even have a crytonephridial system, and has rectal cells with a structure quite different from those of *Tenebrio*.

In any case, the further work of Okasha (1971, 1972) has shown that uptake by *Thermobia* continues until the insect's original volume has been reached. Thus after several cycles of dehydration followed by rehydration while starving, a final volume equal to the original is reached, but the water content percent is much higher. Okasha supposes that the sensory input concerning volume necessary to activate or suppress the uptake process may be inhibited by anal blockage, and that it is therefore unnecessary to implicate the rectal walls as the site of uptake.

In *Arenivaga*, rectal blocking with beeswax also inhibited uptake but so did oral blockage, so that experiment was also inconclusive (Edney, unpublished observation).

The Rate of Uptake

Another area of information needed before we can understand the mechanism concerns the rate at which uptake occurs, and the relationship of this to water loss by transpiration. It seems to be generally true that uptake is faster than loss. For example, Knulle and Spadafora (1969) found that in *Liposcellis* the ratio (rate in to rate out) was 38. In *Arenivaga* the ratio was up to 20. Noble-Nesbitt (1969) and Locke (1964) found similar ratios for *Thermobia* and *Tenebrio* larvae, respectively.

But these figures are not very helpful because they are the net result of several contemporaneous processes, and if we are to understand the mechanisms involved, all the components of gain and loss must be separated and measured. The recent work of Wharton and his associates Knulle, Kanungo, and Devine, has been useful in this respect.

By using tritiated water, Wharton and Devine (1968) showed that in the spiny rat mite *Laelaps echidnina*, under conditions above the c.e.h., where no change in weight occurs, (i) the time taken to turn over half the total water contents was 18.6 hr, (ii) transpiration and sorption both occurred at the same rate, according to first-order kinetics, with a coefficient $k_T = k_S = 0.0373 \cdot hr^{-1}$ (i.e., transpiration and sorption both proceed at a rate of 3.73% of the total water mass per hour). For mites weighing 100 μg, this works out at a turnover rate of 7.46 μg $\cdot$ hr^{-1} under equilibrium conditions. When this is compared with the net rate reported earlier (Wharton and Kanungo, 1962), of up to 1.2 μg water $\cdot$ hr^{-1}, the conclusion is clear that measurements of net water movement leads to serious underestimation of cuticle permeability.

It has for long been a debatable question as to whether the mechanism involved in uptake at higher humidities ceases to function below the c.e.h. (which of course varies from one species to another), or whether it continues to function, and, although overshadowed by the much greater rate of transpiration at lower humidities, nevertheless restricts net water loss to a lower rate than would otherwise be the case. Lees (1947), Edney (1957), Winston and Nelson (1965), and Knulle (1967) have taken the view that restriction of water loss by living insects (as compared with loss from dead ones) below the c.e.h. may indeed reflect the continued action of the uptake mechanism.

Using tritiated water, Knulle and Devine (1972) measured the net water movement and its components in the tick *Dermacentor variabilis* over a wide range of humidities, and reached the conclusion that transpiration occurred according to first-order kinetics, with a rate constant k_T of about $1\% \cdot hr^{-1}$ throughout the humidity range from 0% to 92.5%, while uptake occurred according to zero order kinetics, at rates which were nearly proportional to ambient a_V. Thus they argue that the reason why net loss increases with decreased humidity is not that the rate of movement of water molecules outward increases, but rather that the rate of diffusion of water molecules inward decreases.

By comparing rates of uptake in CO_2-anesthetized and control ticks, they obtained data suggesting that inward movement occurs by passive diffusion over the whole humidity range, but is reinforced by an active uptake mechanism (inactivated by CO_2) at or above 85% RH ($a_V = 0.85$).

Assuming zero-order kinetics for poth passive and active uptake, the rates above $a_V = 0.85$ are (in terms of $\mu g \cdot larva^{-1} \cdot hr^{-1}$), 0.200 for total sorption, 0.156 for passive sorption, and, therefore, 0.044 for active sorption. The answer to the initial question then, is that in these animals the uptake mechanism is inactive below the c.e.h.

Meanwhile Noble-Nesbitt (1969) obtained confirmatory evidence, by different methods, with *Thermobia*. He found that net water loss from this insect at humidities below its c.e.h. was proportional to $1 - a_V$, which is a function of vapor pressure deficit, and not to $0.5 - a_V$ as it should be if the active uptake mechanism was reducing the a_w at the insects' surface to equilibrium with 50% RH, i.e., to $a_w = 0.5$. Noble-Nesbitt's data are compatible with the ideas of water movement proposed by Knulle and Devine, but because we do not know the rates of each component of net water movement further comparison is not possible.

Recently Devine and Wharton (1973) have obtained further data about water exchange in *Laelaps*, this time in conditions other than those ensuring zero net weight change. Their results suggest that, as in

Dermacentor (Knulle and Devine, 1972), transpiration in *Laelaps* obeys first-order kinetics, and occurs through the tracheal system, while uptake follows zero-order kinetics and takes place through the cuticle. No distinction was looked for between passive inward diffusion and active uptake.

The physiological significance of the observed first order rate process for water loss is not clear. Devine and Wharton (1973) propose that it is related to a progressive decrease in water mass in the arthropod. Decreases in rates of water with time during anything but short periods of desiccation have often been observed (Edney, 1951; Bursell, 1955; Loveridge, 1968; among others). Such decreases have been ascribed to changes in the permeability of one or another layer of the cuticle, or of the apical membrane of the epidermal cells, or to exhaustion of hygroscopic water in the cuticle and failure to replace it owing to a constant high impermeability of the apical membrane (Berridge, 1970). Any of these mechanisms could play a part in determining the effects observed, and further work is necessary to identify and measure the factors involved.

Cuticular Structure

Another area of knowledge necessary for understanding vapor uptake is the structure of arthropod cuticles. Much is now known about this, and good reviews of one or another aspect are available (Beament, 1964; Locke, 1964; Neville, 1970; Weis-Fogh, 1970; Hackman, 1971). Here we shall be concerned only with those aspects that affect water exchange — and only briefly. Acquaintance with the general structure of arthropod cuticles will be assumed in what follows.

Until recently it has been thought that differences in permeability to water are associated with differences in form and structure of the epicuticle, particularly with the outermost lipid layers, molecules of which are believed to form a monolayer over the hydrophilic cuticle surface and thus to confer relative impermeability (Beament, 1964). However, as Berridge (1970) and others have pointed out, it is possible that we have been neglecting a most important part of the integument and that control of permeability may be exercised by the apical membrane of the epidermal cells. One consequence of this would be that the cuticle itself may have a low a_w not because a pump moves water from it to the cells inside but because a relatively impermeable apical membrane permits cuticle a_w to come into equilibrium with air a_v. These relationships are well shown in a diagram by Berridge (1970), which is reproduced as Figure 6.

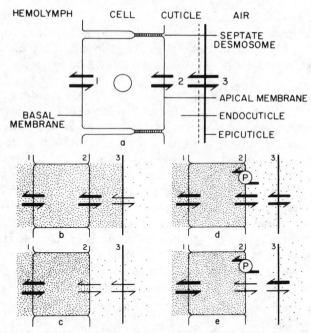

Figure 6 Berridge's formulation of mechanisms which may be responsible for regulating water movement through the integument of arthropods. (a) The major barriers are (1) the basal membrane of the epidermal cell, (2) the apical membrane, (3) the cuticle. (b) to (e) show how the activity of water in the cuticular compartment can be reduced by decreasing the permeability of the apical membrane as in (c) or by imposing a water pump (P) as in (d) and (e). Water would move passively from an area of higher activity (heavy stippling) to one of lower activity (lighter stippling). (From Berridge, 1970.)

However, if active uptake is to occur, then cuticle a_w must be maintained below air a_v, and this can be achieved only by an energy consuming process (a pump) which moves water against an activity gradient from the cuticle to the epidermal cells, and to the hemolymph. Any satisfactory model must include some device which ensures that the pump withdraws water from the outside air, not from the cell or hemolymph, and conversely, it must release water in the opposite direction.

Models, based on morphological observations, to explain the movement of water against osmotic gradients from the insect rectal lumen to the hemolymph have been proposed (e.g., Berridge and Gupta, 1967). These models depend on the secretion and recycling of solutes in numerous very fine intercellular channels, and would work well against fairly low osmotic gradients, but is is difficult to see how gradients of over 55 Osm could be overcome in this way.

Possible Mechanisms for Active Uptake of Water Vapor

Several mechanisms to explain uptake have been proposed. We shall consider two of the most reasonable — one due to Locke (1964) the other to Beament (1964, 1965). Locke notes that the secretion of lytic enzymes by the epidermal cells into the endocuticle occurs during preparation for molting, and when insects are starved. These enzymes depolymerize glycoproteins of the endocuticle, converting them to smaller molecules such as amino acids and glucosamine units. Such smaller molecules, Locke proposes, generate locally osmotic concentrations high enough to cause the absorption of water molecules from outside the insect. These concentrated solutions could then be taken into the cells by pinocytosis (a process which normally forms part of the preparation for a molt), and subsequent repolymerization of the solutes would release water. A highly impermeable apical membrane would prevent water from moving out of the cell in the wrong direction.

One difficulty is that release and solution of molecules the size of even small amino acids would probably generate no more than 1 or 2 Osm and yet insects are known to take up water from air at $a_v = 0.5$, against a gradient of 55.5 Osm.

Beament's hypothesis uses the fact that protein molecules, if moved away from their isoelectric point, expose hydratable polar groups which have a high attraction for water molecules. If cyclic changes in the pH of the cuticle could be effected, water would be absorbed onto the protein chains during one phase of the cycle and released at another. This, combined with a valve permitting the movement of water inward but not out, would ensure that water was released to cells and not to the outside (Figure 7).

Such valves may exist in the fine capillaries observed by Locke in electron micrographs of the epicuticle of the caterpillar *Calpodes*. These so called wax canals are much narrower than pore canals, down to about 30 Å in *Calpodes,* and about 80 Å in *Thermobia* (Noble-Nesbitt, 1967). During one phase of the cycle, water would be withdrawn by suction from such a capillary, a meniscus would form, at the surface of which there would be a low a_w. Calculations by Beament (1964) and Noble-Nesbitt (1969) based on extrapolations from the properties of larger capillaries, and therefore not necessarily applicable, suggest that water at the meniscus of a 30 Å capillary may have $a_w = 0.5$, and could thus cause condensation of water molecules from air with $a_v > 0.5$. During the other phase of the cycle, when suction is released, water in the capillary would rise, flatten at the surface, and become covered by a monolayer of lipid molecules, thus preventing rapid evaporation. As the suction increased again, water would be drawn down the capillary and the

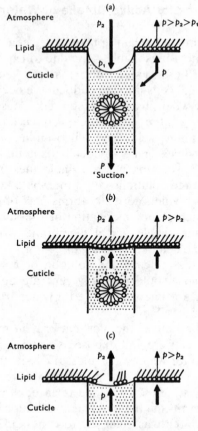

Figure 7 Beament's microcapillary valve model, modified by Noble-Nesbitt. In (a) suction from below produced a meniscus, breaking the superficial impermeable lipid monolayer, and causing lowered water activity at its surface, so that water molecules from the air (higher water activity) condense on the meniscus. In (b), suction from below decreases, and the water rises to the surface, where it is covered by a lipid monolayer which prevents rapid evaporation. In (c), the arthropod is dead and supposedly incapable of producing new lipid material to cover the exposed water surface, so that evaporation is rapid. (From Noble-Nesbitt, 1969.)

lipid monolayer would be broken, so that water molecules could move rapidly into the capillary and condense on the meniscus surface.

This model has certain advantages. It accounts for a lower impedance to flow inward than outward, and explains why transpiration is greater after death by assuming that a supply of lipid molecules necessary for the formation of the barrier over the capillary pores is no longer available. It also could explain why the limiting a_v for uptake is species specific, if indeed the size of the microcapillaries differs between species in an appropriate manner.

The weaknesses of the model are (i) that we do not know how a cyclic change in pH of the cuticle could be brought about, and (ii) we do not know whether the surface lipids behave in the manner required. It is also rather inconvenient for the hypothesis (though by no means fatal) that the fine capillaries necessary for uptake from $a_v = 0.5$ (30 Å) exist in *Calpodes* (which has never been shown to absorb water vapor), while in *Thermobia* (which does absorb from $a_v = 0.5$) the capillaries are 80 Å in diameter.

Summary

It would be gratifying to be able to synthesize the available information into an acceptable explanation of water vapor uptake, but such cannot as yet be done, at least by the present writer. The process has been known for 40 years, but the mechanism is still virtually a mystery. The crux of the problem is how to generate a water activity as low as 0.5 somewhere in the cuticle to bring about the movement of water inwards from $a_v > 0.5$ outside, and then to release it for general use at $a_w = 0.99$. The existence of fine capillaries by themselves does not solve the problem — there must be suction forces to remove water from them to generate appropriately low water activities within them.

We need to know much more about the fine structure and function of cuticles, and about the properties of the epidermal cell membranes. A comparative study of the fine structure of cuticles of arthropods that do and those that do not show vapor uptake, or of different stages in the same insect (e.g., *Xenopsylla* larvae and prepupae), where the conditions of uptake are different might be productive. We also need much more information about the components of net water exchange in a variety of arthropods, and of the laws that govern them.

Finally we need the corporation of biophysicists. I am very clearly not one, yet it is my belief that the problem will finally yield only to biophysical analysis. I commend it as an intriguing interdisciplinary puzzle.

References

Beament, J. W. L. (1961). The water relations of the insect cuticle. *Biol. Rev.* **36,** 281–320.

Beament, J. W. L. (1964). Active transport and passive movement of water in insects. *Advan. Insect Physiol.* **2,** 67–129.

Beament, J. W. L. (1965). The active transport of water: evidence, models and mechanisms. *In* "Water in Living Organisms" (G. E. Fogg, ed.), *Symp. Soc. Exp. Biol.* **19**, 273–298.

Beament, J. W. L., Noble-Nesbitt, J., and Watson, J. A. L. (1964). The water-proofing mechanism of arthropods. III. Cuticular permeability in the firebrat, *Thermobia domestica* (Packard). *J. Exp. Biol.* **41**, 323–330.

Belazerov, V. N., and Sevarin, L. N. (1960). Water balance in *Alectrobius tholozani* at different atmospheric humidities. *Medskaya Parazit.* **3**, 308–313.

Berridge, M. J. (1970). Osmoregulation in terrestrial anthropods. *In* "Chemical Zoology," Vol. 5 (M. Florkin and B. T. Scheer, eds.), pp. 287–320. Academic Press, New York.

Berridge, M. J., and Gupta, B. L. (1967). Fine structural changes in relation to ion and water transport in the rectal papillae of the blowfly, *Calliphora*. *J. Cell Sci.* **2**, 89–112.

Browning, T. O. (1954). Water balance in the tick *Ornithodoros moubata* Murray, with particular reference to the influence of carbon dioxide on the uptake and loss of water. *J. Exp. Biol.* **31**, 331–340.

Bursell, E. (1955). The transpiration of terrestrial isopods. *J. Exp. Biol.* **32**, 238–255.

Buxton, P. A. (1930). Evaporation from the mealworm (*Tenebrio*, Coleoptera) and atmospheric humidity. *Proc. Roy. Soc. London* **B 106**, 560–577.

Devine, T. L., and Wharton, G. W. (1973). Kinetics of water exchange between a mite, *Laelaps echidnina,* and the surrounding air. *J. Insect Physiol.* **19**, 243–254.

Edney, E. B. (1947). Laboratory studies on the bionomics of the rat fleas *Xenopsylla brasiliensis* Baker and *X. cheopsis* Roths. II. Water relations during the cocoon period. *Bull. Entomol. Res.* **38**, 263–280.

Edney, E. B. (1951). The evaporation of water from woodlice and the millipede *Glomeris*. *J. Exp. Biol.* **28**, 91–115.

Edney, E. B. (1957). The water relations of terrestrial arthropods. *Monogr. Exp. Biol. Cambridge* **5**.

Edney, E. B. (1966). Absorption of water vapor from unsaturated air by *Arenivaga* sp. (Polyphagidae, Dictyoptera). *Comp. Biochem. Physiol.* **19**, 387–408.

Edney, E. B. (1968). The effect of water loss of the haemolymph of *Arenivaga* sp. and *Periplaneta americana*. *Comp. Biochem. Physiol.* **25**, 149–158.

Edney, E. B. (1971). Some aspects of water balance in tenebrionid beetles and a thysanuran from the Namib Desert of Southern Africa. *Physiol. Zool.* **44**, 61–76.

Grimstone, A. V., Mullinger, A. M., and Ramsay, J. A. (1968). Further studies on the rectal complex of the mealworm *Tenebrio molitor,* L. (Coleoptera Tenebrionidae). *Phil. Trans. Roy. Soc. London* **253**, 343–382.

Hackman, R. H. (1971). The integument of Arthropoda. *In* "Chemical Zoology," (M. Florkin and B. T. Scheer, eds.), Vol. 6, pp. 1–62. Academic Press, New York.

Humphries, D. A. (1967). Uptake of atmospheric water by the hen flea *Ceratophyllus gallinae* (Schrank). *Nature London* **214**, 426.

Kalmus, H. (1936). Die Verwendung der Tracheeblasen der Corethra-larve als Mikrohygrometer. *Z. Wiss. Mikrosk.* **53**, 215–219.

Kanungo, K. (1965). Oxygen uptake in relation to water balance of a mite *(Echinolaelaps echidninus)* in unsaturated air. *J. Insect Physiol.* **11**, 557–568.

Knulle, W. (1962). Die Abhängigkeit der Luftfeuchtereaktionen der Mehlmilbe *(Acarus siro* L.) vom Wassergehalt des kröpers, *Z. Vergl. Physiol.* **45**, 233–246.

Knulle, W. (1965). Equilibrium humidities and survival of some tick larvae. *J. Med. Entomol.* **2**(4), 335–338.

Knulle, W. (1967). Physiological properties and biological implications of the water vapour sorption mechanism in larvae of the oriental rat flea, *Xenopsylla cheopis* (Roths). *J. Insect Physiol.* **13**, 333–357.

Knulle, W., and Devine, T. L. (1972). Evidence for active and passive components of sorption of atmospheric water vapour by larvae of the tick *Dermacentor variabilis. J. Insect Physiol.* **18**, 1653–1664.

Knulle, W., and Spadafora, R. R. (1969). Water vapor sorption and humidity relationships in *Liposcelis* (Insecta: Psocoptera). *J. Stored Prod. Res.* **5**, 49–55.

Knulle, W., and Wharton, G. W. (1964). Equilibrium humidities in arthropods and their ecological significance. *Acarologia* **6**, 299–306.

Lees, A. D. (1946). The water balance in *Ixodes ricinus* L. and certain other species of ticks. *Parasitology* **37**, 1–20.

Lees, A. D. (1947). Transpiration and the structure of the epicuticle in ticks. *J. Exp., Biol.* **23**, 379–410.

Lees, A. D. (1948a). The sensory physiology of the sheep tick, *Ixodes ricinus* L. *J. Exp. Biol.* **25**, 145–207.

Lees, A. D. (1948b). Passive and active water exchange through the cuticle of ticks. *Disc. Faraday Soc.* **3**, 187–192.

Lindsay, E. (1940). The biology of the silverfish *Ctenolepisma longicaudata* Esch. with particular reference to its feeding habits. *Proc. Roy. Soc. Victoria* **52**, 35–83.

Locke, M. (1964). The structure and formation of the integument in insects. *In* "The Physiology of Insecta," (M. Rockstein, ed.), Vol. 3, pp. 379–470. Academic Press, New York.

Loveridge, J. P. (1968). The control of water loss in *Locusta migratoria migratorioides* R. and F. *J. Exp. Biol.* **49**, 1–29.

Ludwig, D. (1937). The effect of different relative humidities on respiratory metabolism and survival of the grasshopper *Chortophaga viridifasciata* de Geer. *Physiol. Zool.* **10**, 342–351.

Maddrell, S. H. P. (1971). The mechanisms of insect excretory systems. *Advan. Insect Physiol.* **8**, 199–331.

McEnroe, D. (1972). The rectum is not the site of water vapor uptake by *Dermacentor variabilis* Say (Acarina: Ixodidae). *Acarologia* **14**, 562–563.

Mellanby, K. (1932). The effect of atmospheric humidity on the metabolism of the fasting mealworm (*Tenebrio molitor* L., Coleoptera). *Proc. Roy. Soc. London B* **111**, 376–390.

Neville, A. C. (1970). Cuticle ultrastructure in relation to the whole insect. *In*

"Insect Ultrastructure," (A. C. Neville, ed.), *Symp. Roy. Entomol. Soc. London* **5**, 17–39.

Noble-Nesbitt, J. (1967). Aspects of the structure, formation and function of some insect cuticles. *In* "Insects and Physiology," (J. W. L. Beament and J. E. Treherne, eds.), pp. 3–16. Oliver & Boyd, Edinburgh.

Noble-Nesbitt, J. (1969). Water balance in the firebrat, *Thermobia domestica* (Packard). Exchanges of water with the atmosphere. *J. Exp. Biol.* **50**, 745–769.

Noble-Nesbitt, J. (1970). Water balance in the firebrat, *Thermobia domestica* (Packard). The site of uptake of water from the atmosphere. *J. Exp. Biol.* **52**, 193–200.

Okasha, A. Y. K. (1971). Water relations of an insect, *Thermobia domestica*. I. Water uptake from sub-saturated atmosphere as a means of volume regulation. *J. Exp. Biol.* **55**, 435–448.

Okasha, A. Y. K. (1972). Water relations in an insect. *Thermobia domestica*. II. Relationships between water content, water uptake from sub-saturated atmosphere and water loss. *J. Exp. Biol.* **57**, 285–296.

Okasha, A. Y. K. (1973). Water relations in the insect *Thermobia domestica*. III. Effects of desiccation and rehydration on the haemolymph. *J. Exp. Biol.* **58**, 385–400.

Ramsay, J. A. (1964). The rectal complex of the mealworm, *Tenebrio molitor* L. (Coleoptera, Tenebrionidae). *Trans. Roy. Soc. London B* **248**, 279–314.

Ramsay, J. A. (1971). Insect rectum. *Phil. Trans. Roy. Soc. London B* **262**, 251–260.

Rudolph, D. and Knulle, W. (1974). Site and mechanism of water vapour uptake from the atmosphere in ixodid ticks. *Nature* **249**, 84–85.

Solomon, M. E. (1966). Moisture gains, losses and equilibria of flour mites, *Acarus siro* L., in comparison with larger arthropods. *Entomol. Exp. Appl.* **9**, 25–41.

Weis-Fogh, T. (1967). Metabolism and weight economy in migrating animals, particularly birds and insects. *In* "Insects and Physiology," (J. W. L. Beament and J. E. Treherne, eds.). Oliver & Boyd, Edinburgh.

Weis-Fogh, T. (1970). Structure and formation of insect cuticle. *In* "Infrastructure," (A. C. Neville, ed.), pp. 165–185. Blackwell, Oxford.

Wharton, G. W., and Kanungo, K. (1962). Some effects of temperature and relative humidity on water-balance in females of the spiny rat mite, *Echinolaelaps echidninus* (Acarina: Laelaptidae). *Ann. Entomol. Soc. Amer.* **55**, 483–492.

Wharton, G. W., and Devine, T. L. (1968). Exchange of water between a mite, *Laelaps echidnina,* and the surrounding air under equilibrium conditions. *J. Insect Physiol.* **14**, 1303–1318.

Williams, R. T. (1970). *In vitro* studies on the environmental biology of *Goniodes colchici* (Denny) (Mallophaga: Ischnocera). II. The effect of temperature and humidity on water loss. *Aust. J. Zool.* **18**, 391–398.

Williams, R. T. (1971). *In vitro* studies on the environmental biology of *Goniodes colchici* (Denny) (Mallophaga: Ischnocera). III. The effect of temperature and humidity on the uptake of water vapor. *J. Exp. Biol.* **55,** 553 – 568.

Winston, P. W., and Nelson, V. E. (1965). Regulation of transpiration in the clover mite *Bryobia praetiosa* Koch (Acarina: Tetranychidae). *J. Exp. Biol.* **43,** 257 – 269.

Physiological Adaptation to Water Stress in Desert Plants

Irwin P. Ting

Department of Biology
University of California
Riverside, California

Introduction

A major problem encountered by land plants growing under arid conditions is unfavorable water balance because of excessive temperatures and frequently hot, dry winds. These factors create water potential differences between leaf evaporating surfaces and the air far in excess of that encountered in most environments. By and large, desert plants are covered by a thick cuticle which impedes the loss of water. The problem, however, arises because the major portals of carbon dioxide entry are the stomates, the same pathways through which most water is lost. Because of the absolute necessity for uptake of atmospheric carbon dioxide, transpiration has been referred to in the past as a "necessary evil." Desert plants have evolved a variety of mechanisms by which they can exist under arid conditions and yet maintain favorable internal water status (Fahn, 1964). In some instances, arid conditions are largely avoided by growth during wet, cool periods or by growth along water courses and washes which have deep, but available water. In some, there is a marked capability of drying without cellular tissue collapse. Others may reduce surface area by shedding leaves and photosynthesize largely with green stem tissue (Adams *et al.*, 1967). An interesting adaptation which will be discussed in detail is a modification of the mechanism for carbon

99

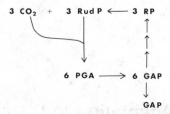

Figure 1 Abbreviated C_3 photosynthetic CO_2 assimilation pathway as outlined by Calvin and co-workers (Hatch and Slack, 1970). For each three CO_2 molecules assimilated, one net glyceraldehyde phosphate (GAP) can result. RudP= ribulose diphosphate, PGA= phosphoglycerate, RP= ribose phosphate.

dioxide assimilation such that the ratio of water loss to carbon dioxide assimilated (transpiration ratio) is much reduced.

This modification of carbon assimilation appears to have evolved by coupling of two sequential carboxylation reactions. By way of introduction, we can say that plants which photosynthesize largely via the Calvin photosynthetic cycle are referred to as C_3 plants (Hatch and Slack, 1970). A schematic of the metabolic pathway elucidated by Calvin and his co-workers is shown in Figure 1. Here the initial carbon assimilatory step is the carboxylation of ribulose diphosphate (RudP) by the enzyme ribulose diphosphate carboxylase:

$$RudP + CO_2 \rightarrow 2\,PGA \tag{1}$$

It is believed that two molecules of phosphoglyceric acid (PGA), a three-carbon phosphorylated acid, are formed. Hence, these plants have recently been referred to as C_3 plants. Subsequent to PGA formation, through a series of sugar transformations known as the Calvin cycle, the RudP acceptor is regenerated and for each three CO_2 molecules assimilated, there will result one reduced sugar, glyceraldehyde phosphate (GAP).

The carbon dioxide assimilatory modification under discussion here involves a precarboxylation by the ubiquitous plant enzyme, phosphoenolpyruvate carboxylase (Ting and Osmond, 1973a, b). In C_4 plants (differentiated from C_3 plants in that the first stable intermediate is a four-carbon acid, malate or aspartate), and during crassulacean acid metabolism (CAM) by succulent plants, the initial assimilation reaction is a carboxylation of phosphoenolpyruvate (PEP) to form oxaloacetate OAA):

$$PEP + CO_2 \rightarrow OAA + P_i \tag{2}$$

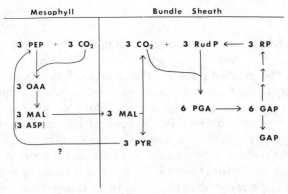

Figure 2 The C$_4$ photosynthetic CO$_2$ assimilation pathway as outlined by Hatch and Slack (1970). A carboxylation of three phosphoenol-pyruvate (PEP) molecules in the undifferentiated mesophyll cells results in three oxaloacetates (OAA) and ultimately in three malates (MAL) or aspartates (ASP). The C$_4$ acids, malate or aspartate, are transported to the photosynthetic bundle sheath cells where malate is decarboxylated to form CO$_2$ and pyruvate (PYR). The pyruvate or other C$_3$ compound is transported back to the mesophyll and converted to PEP whereas the CO$_2$ enters into a Calvin-type photosynthetic cycle (see Figure 1).

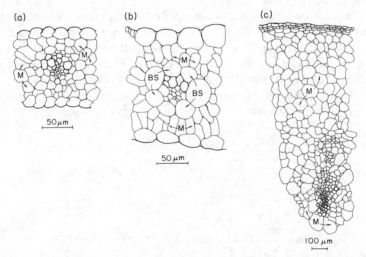

Figure 3 Diagrams of C$_3$ [wheat, (a)], C$_4$ [maize, (b)], and CAM [*Sedum* (c)] leaf anatomy. In wheat, photosynthesis of the Calvin cycle type (see Figure 1) occurs primarily in the undifferentiated mesophyll (M) or in the case of dicots in the entire mesophyll. In C$_4$ grasses such as maize and comparable dicots, the PEP to malate step occurs in the mesophyll (M) whereas the remaining portion of the cycle including malate decarboxylation and the Calvin cycle occur largely in the photosynthetic bundle sheath cells (BS). In CAM plants, the entire sequence from PEP carboxylation to GAP synthesis is assumed to occur in the undifferentiated mesophyll cells (M).

101

The C_4 photosynthetic cycle as outlined by Hatch and Slack (1970) is summarized in Figure 2. C_4 plants are characterized by Kranz anatomy in which the internal photosynthetic parenchyma cells are differentiated into an outer undifferentiated mesophyll and an inner enlarged bundle sheath arrangement (Figure 3). Both mesophyll and bundle sheath cells have chloroplasts. In the light during photosynthesis, in the mesophyll cells PEP is carboxylated to form oxaloacetate. The oxaloacetate is rapidly reduced to malate or aminated to form aspartate. The malate or aspartate is therefore the first stable intermediate of C_4 photosynthesis. It is believed that the C_4 acid is transported to the bundle sheath cells where it is decarboxylated to form free CO_2. This CO_2 which is effectively transported and concentrated in the bundle sheath cells reacts in a standard Calvin cycle-type photosynthesis to result in phosphoglyceric acid and ultimately in glyceraldehyde phosphate. The three-carbon fragment arising from the decarboxylation of malate is believed to be transported back to the mesophyll and reduced to PEP by a specific enzyme, pyruvate P_i, dikinase (Hatch and Slack, 1967). The entire sequence is light-driven and believed to be the mandatory photosynthetic sequence in C_4 plants.

In crassulacean acid metabolism plants, the general sequence of pre-carboxylation via PEP carboxylase and primary carboxylation with RudP carboxylase appears to be virtually the same as in C_4 plants (Figure 4; Ting, 1971). Here, however, the PEP carboxylase reaction takes place largely in the dark and malate is stored in succulent, vacuolated cells (Figure 3). The source of PEP for carboxylation appears to be via glycolysis from stored starch. In the dark, malate steadily builds

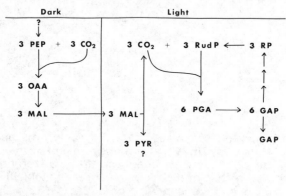

Figure 4 The CAM photosynthetic pathway similar to the C_4 pathway except that the PEP carboxylase to malate step occurs at night and the decarboxylation of malate to form CO_2 for photosynthetic assimilation occurs in the light (refer to Figures 1 and 2). Presumably, all reactions occur in the same succulent cells.

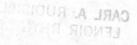

up approaching 200 μEq $\cdot$ g^{-1} fresh weight. At the onset of the light period, malate rapidly decreases as the result of some unknown light-driven
reaction. It is believed that malate is decarboxylated, perhaps by the
malate enzyme, to form free CO_2 and pyruvate, not unlike that in C_4
plants. Carbon dioxide released through the decarboxylation of malate
enters into a carbon assimilation reaction with RudP carboxylase in a
standard Calvin cycle-type sequence. Theoretically, one GAP results
for every three carbon dioxide molecules assimilated or for every three
malate molecules decarboxylated. The fate of the three-carbon fragment,
pyruvate, is not known.

In both C_4 plants and CAM plants, the basic photosynthetic sequences appear to be virtually the same; a precarboxylation with PEP
carboxylase to form a C_4 acid, usually malate, with a subsequent decarboxylation of malate to form CO_2 which enters into the Calvin cycle.
The major apparent difference between C_4 and CAM plants is that in C_4
plants the two sequential carboxylation reactions are separated spatially,
that is, in mesophyll cells and bundle sheath cells; whereas in CAM
plants the two sequential carboxylation reactions are separated in time,
that is, in dark and light. The physiological adaptation to arid environments which will be detailed below appears to be centered around a
more efficient carboxylation by these two mechanisms than in the case
of C_3 plants. C_4 plants have a greater efficiency of carboxylation and a
higher leaf resistance to gas transfer than C_3 plants. Hence, relatively
more carbon dioxide is assimilated per unit of water loss. In CAM
plants the adaptation is more straightforward. Here, under arid conditions stomates are largely open in the dark and closed in the light. Hence,
carbon dioxide is assimilated during that period of the day when evaporative demand is lowest. For these reasons, water loss to carbon assimilation ratios in CAM plants are also quite low, albeit quite variable.

Comparative Carbon Assimilation

C_4 Plants

The capacity for carbon dioxide assimilation by C_4 plants exceeds
that for C_3 plants by two- to three-fold ($\sim$ 60 mg $\cdot$ dm^{-2} $\cdot$ hr^{-1} for C_4 plants
compared to 20 mg $\cdot$ dm^{-2} $\cdot$ hr^{-1} for C_3 plants (Kanai and Black, 1972;
Osmond *et al.*, 1969; Slack and Hatch, 1967; Ting *et al.*, 1972)). Car-
bon dioxide compensation points of C_4 photosynthetic plants are less
than 5 ppm and approach zero with the result that apparent photorespiration is nil, whereas carbon dioxide compensation points for C_3 plants
are in the range 50–100 ppm (Moss, 1971; see Table 1). At ambient
oxygen concentrations, CO_2 assimilation by intact leaves of C_4 plants is

Table 1 Some Physiological Parameters of C_3, C_4, and CAM Plants[a]

Parameter[b]	C_3	C_4	CAM
Ps	15–35	40–60	1–20
TR	600	300	<300
£	>30[c]	≥5[c]	1–100[d]
R_1 minimum	<1.0[e]	>1.0[e]	2–10[f]
R_m minimum	3.0[e]	0.5–1.5[e]	VAR[g]

[a]Data presented are of a summary nature.

[b]Abbreviations: Ps = photosynthesis rate, mg $CO_2 \cdot dm^{+2} \cdot hr.^{-1}$. Estimates are from our own data and a variety of published sources see text). TR = transpiration ratio = ratio of water lost to carbon assimilated based on Kanai and Black, 1972; Neales et al., 1968; Shantz and Piemeisel, 1927; and Ting et al., 1972). £ = CO_2 compensation point in ppm CO_2.

[c]Data of various authors.

[d]Data from Jones and Mansfield, 1972.

[e]Data from Osmond et al., 1969, and Slatyer, 1971.

[f]Data from Ting et al., 1967.

[g]Assumed from variable £ estimates.

not light saturated up to full sunlight, whereas C_3 plant photosynthesis frequently saturates at about 20% of full sunlight (Björkman, 1971). The optimum temperature for photosynthesis in C_4 plants may be about 10°– 20° higher than for photosynthesis in C_3 plants (Björkman, 1971). These observations, well documented in the literature, clearly indicate that when grown under the proper environmental conditions, C_4 plants have a greater photosynthetic efficiency than C_3 plants. The exact reason for this greater capacity of CO_2 assimilation is not entirely clear; however, it may be related to low photorespiration (Tolbert, 1971) or high PEP carboxylase activity (Ting and Osmond, 1973a) or a combination of the two. It is worth noting that despite the fact that C_4 plants have high PEP carboxylase activity, dark fixation is not greater than in C_3 plants (Ting and Osmond, 1973a).

Crassulacean Acid Metabolism Plants

Because of the difficulty of working with crassulacean acid metabolism plants and the complication of both dark and light net CO_2 fixation, comparable data on carbon dioxide assimilation are less generally available. With intact plants, we estimated that dark CO_2 fixation rates could average 0.5–5.0 mg $CO_2 \cdot dm^{-2} \cdot hr^{-1}$ (Ting et al., 1972). Neales et al. (1968) have estimated a maximum rate of 11.8 mg $CO_2 \cdot dm^{-2} \cdot hr^{-1}$ for *Agave*. In the light under conditions of acid metabolism, exogenous CO_2 fixation is usually nil. However, with stomates open and photosynthetic activity proceeding, estimations from the literature suggest that photosynthetic CO_2 fixation of CAM plants can approach that of C_3 plants and perhaps be on the order of 20 mg $\cdot$ dm^{-2} $\cdot$ hr^{-1}. On a chlorophyll basis, Slack and Hatch (1967) estimated maximum rates for C_4 plants of 180–300 μmoles CO_2 $\cdot$ hr^{-1} $\cdot$ mg^{-1} chlorophyll and for C_3 plants of 90–120 μmoles $\cdot$ hr^{-1} $\cdot$ mg^{-1} chlorophyll. Rouhani et al. (1973) estimated a rate of 70–85 μmoles $\cdot$ hr^{-1} $\cdot$ mg^{-1} chlorophyll for isolated Sedum cells. Little is known concerning photorespiration in CAM plants; however, it has been reported that CO_2 compensation points vary from zero to 100 ppm (Jones and Mansfield, 1972). These data suggest that photorespiration is variable depending upon the available substrates or perhaps they simply reflect changing capacities of CO_2 fixation by PEP carboxylase (Queiroz, 1969). Optimum temperature for dark CO_2 fixation by crassulacean plants is low, on the order of 5° – 10°. The effect of light saturation and temperature on succulent plant photosynthesis is poorly understood.

Resistances to Gas Transfer

Overall gas transfer (H_2O and CO_2) can conveniently be evaluated with the standard gas transfer equation,

$$Q = \frac{D\Delta e}{R_a + R_1 + R_m}$$

where Q is the rate of gas transfer (e.g., CO_2 uptake or water loss); e is the gas concentration differential; R_a, the boundary layer resistance to gas transfer; R_1, the leaf or stomatal resistance to gas transfer, either CO_2 or H_2O; R_m, the remaining resistances to gas transfer; here, $R_m = O$ for water and $R_m = CO_2$ diffusion within photosynthetic cells and biochemical events for photosynthesis; and D is the diffusion coefficient for H_2O or CO_2 depending on the gas in question. An evaluation of the parameters R_a, R_1, and R_m for C_3, C_4, and CAM plants suggests significant differences which markedly effect water and carbon balance. R_a is largely a function of the leaf or plant surface and will not be discussed further. In the case of C_3 plants, published measurements indicate that R_1 may be less than 1.0 sec $\cdot$ cm^{-1}, whereas in C_4 plants minima are above 1.0 sec $\cdot$ cm^{-1} (Slatyer, 1971). Minimum R_1 values for CAM plants usually exceed those of C_3 plants and are in the range of 2–10 sec $\cdot$ cm^{-1} (Ting et al., 1967). Hence, other factors being equal, the data predict that the order of transpiration rates would be: $C_3 > C_4 >$ CAM.

Stomatal opening in CAM plants is, of course, special, since under most ambient conditions R_1 estimates are high in the light and low in the dark. In a variety of CAM species tested, under greenhouse conditions, Nishida (1963) found that stomates may be open during the day or night. In our own work with *Kalanchoe blossfeldiana,* we found that if day temperatures were low with little diurnal fluctuation, R_1 values were low in the light and high in the dark (Ting *et al.,* 1967). However, if day temperatures were high with large diurnal fluctuations, leaf resistances were lower in the dark than in the light. With *Opuntia* species under natural field conditions, R_1 estimates, except after precipitation, were always very high in the light (greater than 200 sec · cm⁻¹) and frequently high in the dark. After precipitation, night R_1 estimates were low and exogenous CO_2 was taken up. The increased CO_2 uptake was accompanied by a marked diurnal fluctuation of organic acids indicating a renewed photosynthetic activity after an idling period.

The reverse diurnal fluctuation of stomatal opening and capability to hermatically seal for extended periods allows CAM plants to continually recycle respired CO_2. If stomates are closed, CO_2 evolved into the intercellular spaces at night is refixed through the PEP carboxylase system. During the subsequent light period, this same CO_2 of respiration is refixed photosynthetically. Therefore, a low level of photosynthetic metabolism is possible without uptake of exogenous CO_2. Small diurnal fluctuations of acidity in the range of 25 μEq · g⁻¹ fresh weight are a direct measure of this sustaining metabolism. After precipitation, exogenous CO_2 is taken up at night, and an enhanced diurnal acidity occurs up to 200 μEq · g⁻¹ fresh weight (unpublished data of our own research with cactus).

Minimum R_m estimates for C_3 plants are apparently higher than for C_4 plants (Osmond *et al.,* 1969; Slatyer, 1971) accounting for the generally higher CO_2 assimilation rates of C_4 plants. Further evidence of the low R_m values of C_4 plants are the low estimates of CO_2 compensation points mentioned previously. Few R_m values for CAM plants have been published (Ting *et al.,* 1967), but data indicate that the estimates are variable and highly dependent on the metabolic state of the plant. We estimated R_m for *Opuntia* under a variety of conditions from 13 to over 200 sec · cm⁻¹ (unpublished).

The apparent result of the different resistance values in C_3, C_4, and CAM plants is a greater water use efficiency of C_4 and CAM plants in comparison with C_3 plants. Average transpiration ratios (unit of water loss to carbon assimilation) are in the range of 600 for C_3 plants, 300 for C_4, and less than 300 for CAM (Table 1). Of course, for CAM plants transpiration ratio estimates can be quite high if based on CO_2 assimilation since at any one time during portions of the diurnal CO_2 cycle, CO_2 may be lost quite rapidly.

Summary

C_4 and CAM plants, assumed to be of tropical origin (see Evans, 1971, for a phylogenetic analysis), have a photosynthetic metabolism adaptive to arid environments. C_4 plants, because of a high capacity for CO_2 assimilation through the PEP carboxylase system, and an apparent high leaf resistance to water loss, lose considerably less water per unit of carbon gained than C_3 plants. These plants are therefore adapted to tropical regions with variable or extended dry periods and to arid, desert-type environments. The C_4 plants are largely tropical grasses and sedges occurring in environments with seasonal dry periods or are summer growing herbaceous dicots of the Amaranthaceae, Aizoaceae, Chenopodiaceae, Compositae, Euphorbiaceae, Nyctaginaceae, Portulaceae, and Zygophyllaceae. Black (1971) discussed the high productivity of many C_4 plant groups in relation to their high yielding potentials in agriculture and aggressive weedy nature.

In CAM plants, the metabolic adaptation to aridity is much the same as in C_4 plants except that the PEP carboxylase sequence occurs during the dark period while evaporative demands are low (Kunitake and Saltman, 1958; Shreve, 1916; Ting and Dugger, 1968). Therefore, these plants assimilate CO_2 maximally when water loss potentials are lowest. Photosynthetic assimilation of carbon dioxide occurs during the subsequent light period from stored CO_2. Since stomates are closed, water loss is low. The CAM plants are largely succulent in the families Cactaceae, Crassulaceae, Euphorbiaceae, Liliaceae, Agavaceae, and Aizoaceae, but include epiphytic members of the Orchidaceae and Bromiliaceae. These families, among some others, flourish in warm environments with extended dry periods. The CAM plants can withstand extreme aridity for lengthy periods by recycling CO_2 if occasional water is available.

It is concluded, therefore, that at least in part, the C_4 and CAM photosynthetic metabolism is adaptive to arid, water-stressed environments.

Acknowledgment

Research supported in part by USNSF Grants GB 6735, 2547, and 25878, and GB-15886 administered through the US/IBP Desert Biome.

References

Adams, M. S., Strain, B. R. and Ting, I. P. (1967). Photosynthesis in chlorophyllous stem tissue and leaves of *Cercidium floridum:* accumulation and distribution of ^{14}C from $^{14}CO_2$. *Plant Physiol.* **42**, 1797–1799.

Björkman, O. (1971). Comparative photosynthetic CO_2 exchange in higher plants. *In* "Photosynthesis and Photorespiration," (M. D. Hatch, C. B. Osmond, and R. O. Slatyer, eds.), pp. 18–32. Wiley-Interscience, New York.

Black, C. C. (1971). Ecological implications of dividing plants into groups with distinct photosynthetic production capacities. *Advan. Ecol. Res.* **7**, 87–114.

Evans, L. T. (1971). Evolutionary, adaptive, and environmental aspects of the photosynthetic pathway: assessment. *In* "Photosynthesis and Photorespiration," (M. D. Hatch, C. B. Osmond, and R. O. Slatyer, eds.), pp. 130–136. Wiley-Interscience, New York.

Fahn, A. (1964). Some anatomical adaptations of desert plants. *Phytomorphology* **14**, 93–102.

Hatch, M. D., and Slack, C. R. (1967). Studies on the mechanism of activation and interaction of pyruvate, phosphate dikinase. *Biochem. J.* **112**, 549–558.

Hatch, M. D., and Slack, C. R. (1970). Photosynthetic CO_2 fixation pathways. *Annu. Rev. Plant Physiol.* **21**, 141–162.

Jones, M. B., and Mansfield, T. A. (1972). A circadian rhythm in the level of carbon dioxide compensation in *Bryophyllum fedtschenkoi* with zero values during the transit. *Planta* **103**, 134–146.

Kanai, R. H., and Black, C. C. (1972). Biochemical basis for net CO_2 assimilation in C_4-plants. *In* "Net carbon dioxide assimilation in higher plants," (C. C. Black, ed.). *Proc. Symp. South. Sect. Amer. Soc. Plant Physiol./Cotton Incorp.*, pp. 75–93.

Kunitake, G., and Saltman, P. (1958). Dark fixation of CO_2 by succulent leaves; conservation of the dark fixed CO_2 under diurnal conditions. *Plant Physiol.* **33**, 400–403.

Moss, D. N. (1971). Carbon dioxide compensation in plants with C_4 characteristics. *In* "Photosynthesis and Photorespiration," (M. D. Hatch, C. B. Osmond, and R. O. Slatyer, eds.), pp. 120–123. Wiley-Interscience, New York.

Neales, T. F., Patterson, A. A., and Hartney, V. J. (1968). Physiological adaptation to drought in the carbon assimilation and water loss of xerophytes. *Nature London* **219**, 469–472.

Nishida, K. (1963). Studies on stomatal movement of Crassulacean plants in relation to the acid metabolism. *Physiol. Plantarum* **16**, 281–298.

Osmond, C. B., Troughton, J. H., and Goodchild, D. J. (1969). Physiological, biochemical, and structural studies of photosynthesis and photorespiration in two species of Atriplex. *Z. Pflanzenphysiology* **61**, 218–237.

Queiroz, O. (1969). Photoperiodisime et activitie enzymatique (PEP carboxylase et enzyme malique) dans les feuilles de *Kalanchoë blossfeldiana*. *Phytochemistry* **8**, 1655–1663.

Rouhani, I., Vines, H. M., and Black, C. C. (1973). Isolation of mesophyll cells from *Sedum telephinum* leaves. *Plant Physiol.* **51**, 97–103.

Shantz, H. L., and Piemeisel, L. N. (1927). The water requirement of plants at Akron, Ohio. *J. Agr. Res.* **34**, 1093–1190.

Shreve, E. B. (1916). An analysis of the causes of variations in the transpiring power of cacti. *Physiol. Res.* **2,** 73–127.

Slack, C. R., and Hatch, M. D. (1967). Comparative studies on the activity of carboxylases and other enzymes in relation to the new pathway of photosynthetic carbon dioxide fixation in tropical grasses. *Biochem. J.* **103,** 660–665.

Slatyer, R. O. (1971). Relationship between plant growth and leaf photosynthesis in C_3 and C_4 species of Atriplex. *In* "Photosynthesis and Photorespiration," (M. D. Hatch, C. B. Osmond, and R. O. Slatyer, eds.), pp. 76–81. Wiley-Interscience, New York.

Ting, I. P. (1971). Nonautotrophic CO_2 fixation and crassulacean acid metabolism. *In* "Photosynthesis and Photorespiration," (M. D. Hatch, C. B. Osmond, and R. O. Slatyer, eds.), pp. 169–185. Wiley-Interscience, New York.

Ting, I. P., and Dugger, W. M. (1968). Nonautotrophic carbon dioxide metabolism in cacti. *Bot. Gaz. Chicago* **129,** 9–15.

Ting, I. P. and Osmond, C. B. (1973a). Multiple forms of plant phosphoenolpyruvate carboxylase associated with different metabolic pathways. *Plant Physiol.* **51,** 448–453.

Ting, I. P. and Osmond, C. B. (1973b). Photosynthetic phosphoenolpyruvate carboxylases. *Plant Physiol.* **51,** 439–447.

Ting, I. P., Thompson, M. L. D., and Dugger, W. M. (1967). Leaf resistance to water vapor transfer in succulent plants: effect of thermoperiod. *Amer. J. Bot.* **54,** 245–251.

Ting, I. P., Johnson, H. B., and Szarek, S. R. (1972). Net CO_2 fixation in crassulacean acid metabolism plants. *In* "Net Carbon Dioxide Assimilation in Higher Plants," (C. C. Black, ed.). *Proc. Symp. South. Sect. Amer. Soc. Plant Physiol./Cotton Incorp.,* pp. 26–53.

Tolbert, N. E. (1971). Leaf peroxisomes and photorespiration. *In* "Photosynthesis and Photorespiration," (M. D. Hatch, C. B. Osmond, and R. O. Slatyer, eds.), pp. 458–471. Wiley-Interscience, New York.

Adaptive Mechanisms in Desert Plants

M. Evenari

Department of Botany
The Hebrew University of Jerusalem

E. D. Schulze, L. Kappen, U. Buschbom, and O. L. Lange

Botanisches Institut II
Botanische Anstalten der Universität
Würzburg

Plants have adapted in many different ways to desert conditions. It would take much more than a short chapter to describe the many different strategies evolved during evolution which permit plants to survive in deserts. Therefore, this discussion has been restricted to deal mainly with adaptations of desert plants to water stress; these adaptations will be summarized and examples will be given to illustrate only the most important points. The desert we are concerned with in this chapter is the Negev, an area with an average annual rainfall of about 20–100 mm of winter rain (for detailed description of its climatic conditions, see Evenari *et al.,* 1971, and Zohary, 1962, 1973).

In relation to water stress, terrestrial plants have developed two basically different ways of life, a poikilohydrous and a homeohydrous one. Drought-resistant poikilohydrous plants can tolerate repeated, extreme, and prolonged dehydration without any damage. Homeohydrous plants must always maintain a certain minimum hydration level in order to survive (Walter, 1962, 1972). There is only one phase in their life cycle where they dehydrate one of their organs, the seeds, which enables them to endure adverse external conditions. But in contrast to drought-resistant poikilohydrous plants, once the seeds are for some time fully hydrated they cannot withstand a second dehydration.

Table 1 Main types of Poikilo- and Homoiohydrous Plants of the Negev Desert

| Poikilohydrous plants | Homoiohydrous plants | |
	Aridopassive plants	Aridoactive plants
Algae	All geophytes	Most phanerophytes
Lichens	Most hemicryptophytes	Most chamaephytes
Mosses	All pluviotherophytes	All biseasonal therophytes

Poikilohydry is with few exceptions restricted to lower plants (Table 1). It is probably the oldest surviving evolutionary strategy to deal with environmental water stress.

The homeohydrous desert plants, according to their reaction to the changes of dry and wet seasons of their environment, can be divided into two main groups: aridopassive and aridoactive plants (Table 1). The aridopassive plants are metabolically active only during the wet season. The geophytes, being aridopassive, and the hemicryptophytes survive the dry period individually since their bulbs, corms, rhizomes, or similar organs become dormant when water stress develops. The pluviotherophytes fulfill their complete individual life cycle during the rainy season. But, before they die at the start of the dry season, they form dormant propagules which can survive several dry periods bridging in this way the generation gap.

The aridoactive plants are metabolically active throughout the year, including the whole dry season. In the Negev this group is composed almost entirely of phanerophytes, chamaephytes, and biseasonal therophytes. The chamaephytic dwarf shrubs are the most important compo-

Table 2 Main Adaptive Features of Aerial Poikilohydrous Plants of the Negev Desert

a. Capacity to equilibrate with hydration level of environment and to tolerate extreme and prolonged desiccation.
b. Capacity to enter anabiotic state when desiccated.
c. Extreme cold and heat resistance in anabiotic state.
d. Capacity of the thallus to take up water directly and instantaneously from water vapor of the air, dew, and rain.
e. Instantaneous switching on of metabolic activity when water is available and vice versa.
f. Capacity to go through repeated periods of hydration and dehydration without injury.
g. Relatively high rates of photosynthesis at low temperatures (lichens) and low light intensities (algae).

nent of this group since they are the dominant element in the Negev ecosystems. There are only a few biseasonal therophytes in the Negev. Their seeds germinate immediately after the first rain; the plants grow and develop during the wet and dry period and die at the end of the dry season after having formed seeds. The borderline between aridoactive and passive plants is not always sharply drawn. In extremely bad years, plants normally aridoactive may become aridopassive toward the end of the dry season.

The main adaptive features of poikilohydrous Negev plants (Berner,

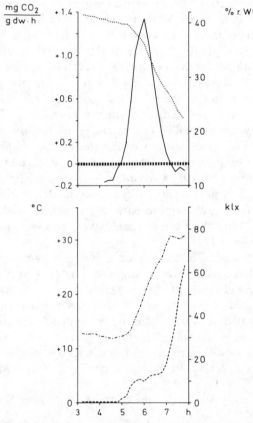

Figure 1 CO_2 gas exchange of *Ramalina maciformis* (solid line) related to day weight (dw); relative water content of its thallus (% rWC, dotted line) in percent of thallus dry weight; light intensity (dashed line, kilolux); thallus temperature (dot-dash line, °C) during the morning hours after uptake of dew during the night.

1973; Lange, 1969; Lange *et al.,* 1970a,b) are listed in Table 2. Figure 1 illustrates some of the points made in Table 2, showing the activity of the Negev lichen *Ramalina maciformis* during one day as measured in the field under natural conditions.

During a dewy night the thallus imbibed water up to 40% of its dry weight and started to respire. In the early morning hours with the start of illumination, photosynthesis began and its light compensation point was passed at a relatively low temperature. Photosynthesis reached a short, steep peak around 6:00 A.M. followed by a sharp decline due to increasing desiccation of the thallus. When the relative water content was down to about 20%, the moisture compensation point was reached and photosynthesis stopped. With further increased desiccation, the thallus became metabolically inactive around 8 A.M. This example shows that poikilohydrous plants can live under severe external conditions provided that the temperature during a certain minimum number of nights drops to the dew point causing dew formation (the average annual number of dewy nights in the Negev is 198). In addition to dew as a water source, the Negev lichens can also take up water from air with a relative humidity above 80%. The capacity to remain in an anabiotic state for a very long time, during which the thallus is most resistant to extreme low and high temperatures, is most advantageous in deserts for all of which extreme climatic variability is characteristic. But since with the exception of a very few rainy days poikilohydrous plants can photosynthesize only for a few hours in early morning after nights with dew or high relative humidity their growth rate is very low (Kappen *et al.,* 1974; Lange and Evenari, 1971).

The main adaptation of the aridopassive geophytes and hemicryptophytes (Table 3) consists in restricting the time of their physiological activity to the optimal ambient thermoperiodic, photoperiodic, and water conditions. But water stress according to its severity may modify or even suppress those photo- and thermoperiodically controlled reactions which would occur when water stress would be absent.

In years with insufficient rainfall, some geophytes and hemicryptophytes remain completely dormant, as shown in Figure 2 for *Ornithoga-*

Table 3 Main Adaptive Features of the Aridopassive Negev Geophytes and Hemicryptophytes

a. Capacity to tolerate prolonged dormancy
b. Modification of the photo- and thermoperiodically controlled length of the active period by the water stress of the habitat.
c. Suppression of flowering in years with high water stress.
d. Fast growth of rootlets and shoots after rain.

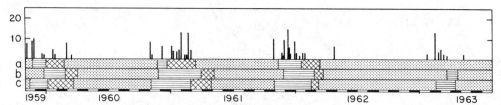

Figure 2 Phenology of (a) *Ornithogalum trichophyllum,* (b) *Poa sinai-ca,* (c) *Carex pachystilis.* Hatching, plants with leaves; crosshatching, plants flowering and fruiting; stippling, plants dormant. Vertical black bars above a rainfall in millimeters.

lum trichophyllum. In consecutive bad years this dormancy may last for 2 or even 3 years as observed for the Negev tulip *(Tulipa polychroma)* and the desert rhubarb *(Rheum palaestinum).* Under the same circumstances other geophytes will suppress flowering and grow vegetatively only for a few weeks *(Carex pachystilis* and *Poa sinaica* in Figure 2). In "normal" years inside the limits imposed by the ambient thermo- and photoperiod the length of the active period is determined by the availability of water (Evenari *et al.,* 1971).

The pluviotherophytes (Table 4) evince their most pronounced adaptations to the desert environment in their germination behavior since this is the most critical phase for survival of the individual and of the species. They have a great variety of mechanisms permitting them to correlate seed dispersal and germination in time and space to the water status of their environment and at the same time to retain always a great number of viable seeds of each species in the soil as a seed reserve (Koller, 1968). One mechanism involved is heteroblasty. Because each seed of

Table 4 Main Adaptive Features of Negev Pluviotherophytes

a. Mechanisms for formation of heterogeneous dispersal units on one mother plant
 1. Heteromorphous dispersal units (e.g., telechoric and antitelechoric, as in *Gymnarrhena micrantha*)
 2. Heteroblastic dispersal units
  (e.g., *Pteranthus dichotomus*)
b. Special mechanisms for seed dispersal
 (e.g., restricting seed dispersal to periods of rain or high relative humidity as in *Anastatica*)
c. Prolonged viability of seeds
d. Special germination mechanisms
 1. Internal water clock of seeds
 2. Extreme heteroblasty of seed populations
e. Large-scale modification of the photo- and thermoperiodically determined length of life cycle by water state of habitat
f. Proportional regulation of body size as a function of available soil water

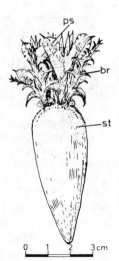

Figure 3 Dispersal unit of *Pteranthus dichotomus* carrying on its stalk (st) spiny branches (br), bearing pseudocarps (ps). (After Zohary, 1962.)

the seed population produced by one plant during 1 year has its own specific germination requirements different from those of any other seed, the seeds of one year's population will never germinate in total in one single year. This is to a certain degree true for all plants with the exception of cultivated species, but in desert plants heteroblasty is much more pronounced. Therefore, the probability that during one year a combination of ambient conditions could occur which would trigger off the germination of all seeds of one year's seed population is very small. *Pteranthus dichotomus* is a good example (Evenari, 1963). Its dispersal unit is a whole fruiting head (Figure 3) carrying seven pseudocarps each containing one seed. The pseudocarps are arranged in three orders (Figure 4). We never found a single case in the field where more than one or two pseudocarps had germinated in the same year out of one dispersal unit. The reason can be seen in Table 5 which shows that the pseudocarps of each order have different germination requirements concerning light and temperature. In addition to heteroblasty, desert pluviotherophytes have developed dispersal units which are at the same time heteroblastic and heteromorphous. For example, *Gymnarrhena micrantha* forms two kinds of dispersal units: small achenes with a pappus which develops in aboveground inflorescences (aerial, telechoric achenes) and large achenes with a rudimentary pappus which develop in below-ground inflorescenes (subterranean, antitelechoric achenes). The subterranean achenes are antitelechoric since they never disperse, but germinate out of the dead mother plant, the telechoric achenes disperse and germinate away

Figure 4 Schematic drawing of a dispersal unit of *Pteranthus di-chotomus* showing the arrangement of the one first-order pseudo-carp, the two second-order pseudocarps, and the four third-order pseudocarps.

from the mother plant. The biological function of the antitelechoric achenes is to guarantee survival of the species. Under desert conditions the probability to be able to complete a full life cycle at a habitat where a previous generation had already succeeded is relatively high. The tele-choric achenes are responsible for the spatial propagation of the species. In good years they will succeed in establishing themselves in new habitats, in bad years they will fail (Evenari, 1963; Evenari *et al.*, 1971; Koller and Roth, 1964).

Another adaptation of desert pluviotherophytes is their ability to regulate their total body size according to the water conditions of their

Table 5 Germination of Fruits of *Pteranthus dichotomus* Derived from Different Orders of Pseudocarps at Different Temperatures in Light and in Darkness

Temperature (°C)	% Germination of different orders of pseudocarp					
	I		II		III	
	Light	Dark	Light	Dark	Light	Dark
8	18	12	72	58	90	99
15	50	23	89	83	98	97
26	65	8	97	90	100	95
30	72	16	97	84	100	96
35	12	4	66	20	100	89
37	0	0	65	24	91	82

habitat. In very dry localities they are tiny with very few small leaves and fruits, in habitats with a good water supply they are big with many proportionally large leaves and fruits (see, e.g., Evenari *et al.*, 1971; Fig. 176 of *Anastatica hierochuntica*). The variable body size is also an indication of the great variability of the length of their life cycle since the small individuals complete theirs in much shorter time than the large ones. This is clearly advantageous for their survival because in a habitat with little available water, the time during which conditions are optimal for development is shorter than in well-watered ones. The question arises how the signal on the water status of the soil (soil water potential) which must be received by the roots is transmitted to the growing points of the shoots and what is the nature of this information which leads to the regulation of growth and of the length of their life cycles. Went as early as 1938 proposed the hypothesis that roots produce a hormone (caulocaline) which regulates shoot growth. This idea can today be reformulated based on a growing body of evidence. Cytokinins are formed in the root tips (Kende and Sitton, 1967; Weiss and Vaadia, 1965). Under water stress the amount of cytokinins produced by the roots decreases (Itai and Vaadia, 1965). The cytokinins move with the transpiration stream to the shoots (Carr and Burrows, 1966; Kende, 1965) where they act in various ways. They affect protein metabolism of the leaves (Richmond and Lang, 1957; Shah and Loomis, 1965), they affect the water balance through their influence on stomatal movements (Tal and

Table 6 Schematic Representation of the Main Adaptive Features of Negev Aridoactive Plants

---

a. Tendency to develop xeromorphic structures
b. High root:shoot ratio
c. Reduction of metabolically active surface.
   1. Constitutionally small surface in relation to dry weight
      (e.g., *Retama raetam, Anabasis articulate*)
   2. Seasonal surface reduction mainly as a function of water stress
      (e.g., *Artemisia herba-alba, Zygophyllum dumosum*)
   3. "Partial death" (e.g., *Zygophyllum dumosum*)
d. Capacity to tolerate high soil water stress
   1. Tolerance of high internal water saturation deficits
   2. Capacity to create and tolerate low plant water potentials
   3. Photosynthetic activity even at low osmotic potentials
e. Reduction of transpiration rate through morphological and anatomic changes
f. Sensitive stomatal regulation as a function of ambient conditions
   1. Regulation by water stress
   2. Regulation by temperature
   3. Regulation by air humidity
g. Adaptation of gas exchange mechanisms to high temperatures

---

Imber, 1970; Tal *et al.*, 1970), and they affect the auxin-mediated growth (Hartung and Witt, 1968; Hemberg, 1972). Any one or a combination of these processes could regulate growth.

The main adaptive features of the aridoactive plants are summarized in Table 6. With very few exceptions the aridoactive plants have a constitutionally small surface in relation to their dry weight. They are either leafless or their leaves are very small, belonging to the size class of nanophytes and leptophytes (Taylor, 1971). In addition they have also the ability of seasonal reduction of their metabolically active surface which in limits set by photo- and thermoperiods is mainly a function of increasing water stress. This reduction is done in various ways. As examples, *Zygophyllum dumosum* throws off its leaf blades and only the green photosynthesizing petioles remain; *Hammada scoparia* sheds parts of its green cortex; *Artemisia herba-alba* loses its large winter leaves, and at the end of the dry season only very small summer leaves and flower bracts remain as metabolically active organs; *Reaumuria negevensis* sheds whole branches (Evenari and Richter, 1937; Orshan, 1954; Orshan and Zand, 1962; Evenari *et al.*, 1971). The degree which surface reduction may attain can be seen in Figure 5 which also shows that it is more pronounced in "bad" years with scanty rainfall than in "good" ones. One of the results of the seasonal reduction of the metabolically

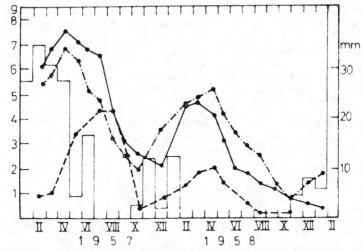

Figure 5 Annual march of dry weight (g) of the transpiring body of three aridoactive dwarf shrubs: *Artemisia herba-alba* (solid line), *Noea mucronata* (dashed line), *Hammada scoparia* (dash-dot line). Average monthly rainfall (mm, light solid line). (After Orshan and Zand, 1962.)

active surface is a considerable reduction of the amount of water lost by a whole plant (Evenari, 1953; Table 7).

Surface reduction has also another interesting aspect which was termed "survival by partial death" (Evenari *et al.,* 1971). In drought years when stress is very high, whole branches of the aridoactive dwarf shrubs die and only a restricted number of branches remain alive, retaining just as much photosynthesizing tissue as can be supplied with the little available water. In very bad years in the driest habitat only a single branch out of many may survive. In following "good" years the plants may slowly regenerate themselves from dormant renewal buds.

Survival through partial death is only possible because the individual branches of those aridoactive dwarf shrubs in which this phenomenon has been observed are largely physiologically independent. Stem splitting, which is typical for some dwarf shrubs, corroborates this fact. At a certain age their primary undivided stems split into a number of daughter stems which are only loosely attached to each other or are completely separated. The mechanism by which stem splitting is accomplished has been described for *Zygophyllum dumosum* (Evenari *et al.,* 1971; Fahn, 1964; Ginzburg, 1963). In this way an older dwarf shrub represents more of a colony than one individual plant.

Of the various physiological adaptations of aridoactive Negev plants which have been investigated (Evenari and Richter, 1937; Evenari *et al.,* 1972; Koch *et al.,* 1971; Lange and Schulze, 1972; Schulze *et al.,* 1971, 1972a,b,c; Stocker, 1970–1972, in press) and are listed in Table 6 we

Table 7 Monthly Output of Water per Plant

Plant:	*Retama raetam*		*Heliotropium rotundifolium*		*Haplophyllum tuberculatum*	
Month	Average output (kg/plant)	Percentage of max. output	Average output (kg/plant)	Percentage of max. output	Average output (kg/plant)	Percentage of max. output
I	180	47	1.2	16	6.2	26.6
II	350	92	5.6	75	10.5	48.5
III	380	100	6.1	81	21.6	100
IV	360	95	7.5	100	16.3	80
V	108	28	1.8	24	2.2	10.2
VI	23	6.1	0.55	7.5	1.2	5.5
VII	9	2.4	0.6	8	0.8	4.2
VIII	10	2.6	0.4	5.3	0.6	2.8
IX	11	2.9	0.34	4.5	0.6	2.8
X	7	1.8	0.23	3.5	0.45	2.2
XI	21	5.5	0.7	9.3	1.8	8.3
XII	130	34	0.9	12	5.1	26.5

can illustrate only a few.* These concern the movement of stomata and photosynthesis. During the dry season aridoactive Negev plants find themselves in a permanent dilemma. When during the day the stomata are open for CO_2 supply, the plant may lose too much water by transpiration and cannot keep up a hydration level necessary for metabolic activity. When they close their stomata to save water, they cannot take up CO_2 and produce sufficient organic material needed as raw material for growth and as a source of energy. Their stomatal movements must therefore be very carefully balanced. This is achieved by highly sensitive regulatory mechanisms controlled directly or indirectly by plant water stress, temperature, and ambient air humidity (Schulze *et al.*, 1972 b,c, 1973). The example given in Figure 6 illustrates this concerning water

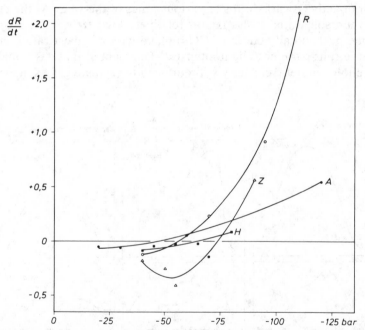

Figure 6 The change in total diffusion resistance per 1°C increase in leaf temperature ($\Delta R/\Delta T$) as related to the minimal water potential (bar) in the experimental plants during the day. A positive value of $\Delta R/\Delta T$ designates stomatal closure, and negative values indicate stomatal opening with increasing temperature.
A, Artemisia herba-alba; H, Hammada scoparia; R, Reaumuria negevensis; Z, Zygophyllum dumosum.

*See Walter (1973) for the relationship between water stress, osmotic potential, and xeromorphy as a feedback system, a topic with which we do not deal in this chapter.

stress and temperature. When in the experiment at low water stress leaf temperature was raised, the stomata opened. When the same was done at high water stress, the stomata closed. The water stress at which the opening response was reversed to a closing one was different for each species. The ecological advantages of this behavior are obvious. At low water stress water is available and can be lost by transpiration through the open stomata which at the same time take up CO_2. Through increased transpiration the leaf is cooled and leaf temperature becomes more favorable. At high water stress water is most scarce and must be saved. Water loss is restricted by closing the stomata. The ecological disadvantage of the closing reaction (overheating, no uptake of CO_2) must be tolerated since under these conditions the overriding danger is loss of too much water. Figure 7 shows the photosynthetic activity of three aridoactive dwarf shrubs at various times of the year. At the end of April when soil water stress is still relatively low, *Hammada scoparia* has a one-peaked daily curve of CO_2 uptake with a highest rate at noon. The curve runs parallel to light intensity. The plant at that day could use its full photosynthetic capacity without need to regulate gas exchange by

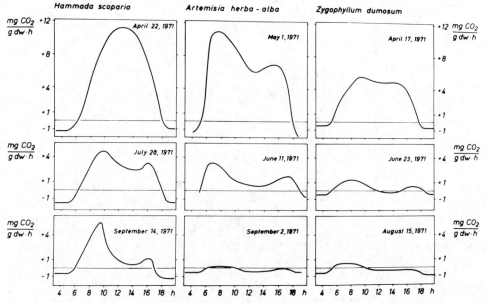

Figure 7 The diurnal course of net photosynthesis of three aridoactive dwarf shrubs in the different seasons. Ordinate: CO_2 exchange per gram dry weight; Abscissa: time of day.

stomatal closure. The curve of *Artemisia herba-alba* however at about the same time of the year shows a midday depression, obviously indicating that gas exchange was regulated by stomatal movement. The curve of *Zygophyllum dumosum* has only a slight noon depression but runs all day long on a lower level than those of the two other dwarf shrubs. The curves for all three plants in midsummer show clearly how much the ambient conditions had worsened and to what degree the plants had to use their regulating mechanisms. The curves of all three plants are sharply two-peaked. At noon the curve of *Z. dumosum* is depressed below the compensation point. At the same time the curves of all three plants are on a much lower level than the corresponding curves in April–May. At the end of the dry season only *H. scoparia* was able to keep up a positive net photosynthesis during the whole day. The two other plants have only a very low rate of net photosynthesis in the morning hours. During the rest of the day their curves lie below the compensation point indicating respiratory loss and a negative dry matter balance for that day.

Figure 8 shows the daily photosynthetic gain of two aridoactive dwarf shrubs over a period of 8 months together with their minimal daily xylem pressure potential. *Hammada scoparia* shows gains over the whole period. But from July onward the gains become smaller although the internal water stress remains the same as shown by the fact that the minimum water potential stays more or less on the same level. The overall decrease in gain is mainly due to the increasing dry weight of the photosynthesizing organs which become more xeromorphic as the dry season progresses. This must appear in Figure 8 as a decrease in photosynthetic gains since the CO_2 uptake is related to dry weight. The behavior of *Z. dumosum* is quite different. From July onward there are mainly respiratory losses clearly related to the sharply decreasing xylem water potentials. These losses are not very important for the overall annual dry matter production since they occur when the plant has already reduced its metabolically active surface by 85–95% through leaf blade shedding, and the gains occur when *Z. dumosum* still possesses all its active surface. Figure 8 demonstrates another interesting fact which is valid for both plants. There are pronounced day-to-day differences in daily gains. These are not caused by water stress but are due to temperature and air humidity controlled stomatal reactions (Schulze *et al.*, 1972b,c, 1973). Figure 8 shows also that these plants can tolerate low xylem water potentials (−90 and −110 bars). *Artemisia herba-alba* is still photosynthetically active at −125 bar (Kappen *et al.*, 1972).

The few aridoactive biseasonal therophytes of the Negev represent an interesting problem. *Salsola inermis* will serve as an example. After

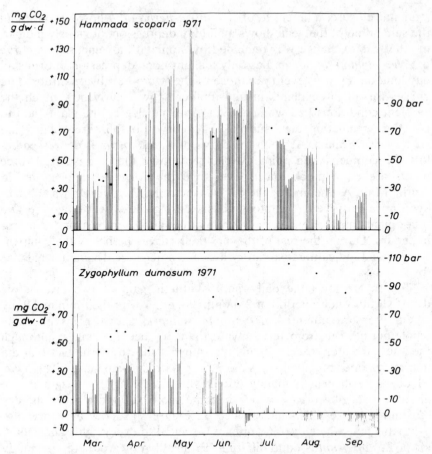

Figure 8 The annual course of the daily gain of net photosynthesis (vertical lines) together with the minimal daily water potentials (dots) for two aridoactive dwarf shrubs. Abscissa: time of year.

germination, the seedlings remain for most of the rainy season in a rosette stage. With the onset of the dry season the stems start to elongate and the main development of the plant including flowering and fruit set takes place during the dry season. As with all desert annuals their root system is shallow and not very extensive. How can these plants procure enough water throughout the dry summer enabling them to be aridoactive? The bulk of the soil depth in which they root does not contain available water from June–July onward. Is dew, which is taken up by the plant, the water source? The amounts seem to be insufficient (Evenari *et al.*, 1971). If the water pockets which are found below the stones even during the late summer months are the main water source (Evenari *et al.,* 1971), how can they persist and how are they recharged? Through subterranean dew formation? Through condensation of water vapors caused by nightly soil temperature conversion? Through uptake of dew from the air by the plant during night and transport of this water to the roots (negative transpiration) and its excretion into the water pockets from where the roots take it up in daytime to cover transpirational losses? These questions cannot be answered yet and the problem remains.

All the controls used by the aridoactive Negev plants in order to balance their water economy restrict their dry matter production and hence their phytomass. It can be seen from Table 8 that the peak standing phytomass of three most important aridoactive dwarf shrubs of the Negev as measured in the Avdat desert station in 1971 is very small. The same is true for the total standing phytomass of three vegetation types of which *Z. dumosum, A. herba-alba,* and *H. scoparia* are the dominant plants (Table 9, details in Evenari *et al.,* 1974). These figures are between the very lowest reported for any desert plant community. Table 9 relates only to the higher plants of the three vegetation types and the phytomass of the poikilohydrous lichens and algae must be added. It is estimated (Kappen *et al.,* 1974) that the standing biomass of *Ramalina maciformis* in habitats where it grows abundantly amounts to 73 g dry matter · m^{-2} and that of the crustaceous lichen *Diploschistes calcareus* on northerly exposed rocks to 141 g dry matter · m^{-2}. Other species of crustaceous lichens in the same type of habitats are estimated to have a biomass about two to three times as high as that of *D. calcareus.* Since these figures relate only to special habitats most favorable to the growth of lichens, we do not know how much standing lichen biomass has to be added to the figures given in Table 9 for the various vegetation types. In the Hammadetum, lichens are very rare because of the action of floods in the wadis and floodplains and relatively few rocks and stones serving as substrates. An estimate of an overall standing lichen phytomass of at

Table 8 Standing Peak Shoot, Root Biomass, and Total Plant Phytomass in g · m^{-2}

Plants	Shoot[a]			Root	Total plant
	ap	pp	Total		
Zygophyllum dumosum	10	54	64	54	118
Artemisia herba alba	17	18	35	32	67
Hammada scoparia	12	23	35	37	72

[a]ap, annual parts; pp, perennial parts.

Table 9 Standing Peak Phytomass in g · m⁻²
of Three Vegetation Types of the Negev
Desert

Vegetation type	Total phytomass
Zygophylletum dumosi	146
Artemisietum herbae albae	161
Hammadetum scopariae	323

least $5-10$ g of dry matter · m⁻² for the other two plants communities is possibly not far off the mark. The standing phytomass of the hypolithic desert algae is estimated to be 1.88 g dry matter · m⁻² (Berner, 1973). The figures for lichens and algae do not include soil lichens and algae since there are no measurements of their phytomass.

The figures of the standing biomass do not indicate the annual production, i.e., how much *permanent* phytomass is added each year. It is estimated that this figure for the above-ground parts of the *Zygophyllum* is 3.5% (Evenari *et al.*, 1974) and it may be assumed that the corresponding figure for the *Artemisietum* is of the same order of magnitude. We do not know how much permanent phytomass is produced each year by the below-ground parts of the plants concerned but most probably it is of the same order of magnitude as the figure given for the above ground parts. Such a low annual increase of the biomass shows that the primary production of at least these two desert vegetation types is extremely low. Under the stress conditions prevailing in the Negev for the greatest part of the year, the low primary production is the end result of all the climate- and water stress-controlled morphological and physiological reactions of the plants which keep the water economy balanced but only at the price of a very low primary production. The desert by its very nature could not sustain plants or ecosystems with high production rates. The lichens of the desert apparently have a productivity of the same order of magnitude as the higher plants. The annual primary production of the lichens is estimated to amount to $5-10\%$ of their standing biomass (Kappen *et al.*, 1974). Thus the two completely different strategies of desert plants, namely the poikilohydrous way of life of the lichens and the homoiohydrous one of the aridoactive phanerogams, are equally successful concerning the production of permanent biomass.

References

Berner, T. (1973). Ecological and physiological problems of the hypolithic algae on flint stone in Avdat and Sde Boker. Ph.D. thesis, Hebrew University (Hebrew with English summary).

Carr, D. J., and Burrows, W. J. (1966). Evidence of the presence in xylem sap of substances with kinetin-like activity. *Life Sci.* **5**, 2061–2077.

Evenari, M. (1953). The water balance of plants in desert conditions. *Desert Res. Proc. Symp. Jerusalem*, pp. 266–274.

Evenari, M. (1963). Zur Keimungsoekologie zweier Wüstenpflanzen. *Mitteil. Floris. Soziol. Arbeitsgemeinschaft N.F.*, **10**, 70–81.

Evenari, M., and Richter, R. (1937). Physiological-ecological investigation in the wilderness of Judaea. *J. Linn. Soc. London* **51**, 333–351.

Evenari, M., Schulze, E. D., and Lange, O. L. (1972). Ecophysiological investigation in the Negev desert. III. The diurnal course of carbon dioxide exchange and transpiration and its balance in regard to primary production. *Symp. U.S.S.R. Acad. Sci. Leningrad Ecophys. Found. of Ecosyst. Product. in Arid Zone*, pp. 66–70.

Evenari, M., Shanan, L., and Tadmor, N. (1971). "The Negev: The Challenge of a Desert," Harvard Univ. Press, Cambridge, Massachusetts.

Evenari, M., Bamberg, S., Schulze, E. D., Kappen, L., Lange, O. L., and Buschbom, U. (1974). Primary production of deserts. II. The biomass production of some higher plants in Near Eastern and American deserts. "Symp. Photosynthesis and Productivity in Different Environments," (J. P. Cooper, ed.). Cambridge Univ. Press.

Fahn, A. (1964). Some anatomical adaptations of desert plants. *Phytomorphology* **14**, 93–102.

Ginzburg, C. (1963). Some anatomical features of splitting of desert shrubs. *Phytomorphology* **13**, 92–97.

Hartung, W., and J. Witt. (1968). Über den Einfluss der Bodenfeuchtigkeit auf den Wuchsstoffgehalt von Anastatica hierochuntica und Helianthus annuus. *Flora Jena Abt. B* **157**, 603–614.

Hemberg, T. (1972). The effect of kinetin on the occurrence of acid auxin in *Coleus blumei*. *Physiol. Plant* **26**, 98–103.

Itai, Ch.; and Vaadia, Y. (1965). Kinetin-like activity in root exudate of water-stressed sunflower plants. *Physiol. Plant.* **18**, 941–944.

Kappen, L., Lange, O. L., Schulze, E. D., Evenari, M., and Buschbom, U. (1972). Extreme water stress and photosynthetic activity of the desert plant *Artemisia herba-alba*. *Oecologia Berl.* **10**, 177–182.

Kappen, L., Lange, O. L., Schulze, E. D., Evenari, M., and Buschbom, U. (1974). Primary production of deserts. IV. Primary production of lower plants (lichens) in the desert and its physiological basis. "Symp. Photosynthesis and Productivity in Different Environments, (J. P. Cooper, ed.). Cambridge Univ. Press.

Kende, H. (1965). Kinetin-like factors in the root exudate of sunflowers. *Proc. Nat. Acad. Sci. Wash.* **53**, 1302–1307.

Kende, H., and Sitton, D. (1967). The physiological significance of kinetin- and gibberellin-like root hormones. *Ann. N. Y. Acad. Sci.* **144**, 235–243.

Koch, W., Lange, O. L., and Schulze, E. D. (1971). Ecophysiological investigations on wild and cultivated plants in the Negev desert. I. Methods: A mobile laboratory for measuring carbon dioxide and water vapour exchange. *Oecologia Berl.* **8**, 296–309.

Koller, D. (1968). The physiology of dormancy and survival of plants in desert environments. *Soc. Exp. Biol. Symp. 23* Dormancy and survival, pp. 449–469.

Koller, D., and Roth, N. (1964). Studies on the ecological and physiological significance of amphicarpy in *Gymnarrhena micrantha* (Compositae). *Amer. J. Bot.* **51**, 26–35.

Lange, O. L. (1969). Experimentell ökologische Untersuchungen an Flechten der Negev-Wüste. I. CO_2-Gaswechsel von *Ramalina maciformis* (Del.) Bory unter kontrollierten Bedingungen im Laboratorium. *Flora Jena Abt. B* **158**, 324–359.

Lange, O. L., and Evenari, M. (1971). Experimentell-ökologische Untersuchungen an Flechten der Negev-Wüste, IV. Wachstumsmessungen an *Caloplaca aurantia Flora Jena Abt. B* **160**, 100–104.

Lange, O. L., and Schulze, E. D. (1972). Ecophysiological investigations in the Negev desert. I. The relationship between transpiration and net photosynthesis measured with a mobile field laboratory. *Symp. U.S.S.R. Acad. Sci. Leningrad Ecophys. Found. of Ecosyst. Product. in Arid Zone*, pp. 57–62.

Lange, O. L., Schulze, E. D., and Koch, W. (1970a). Experimentell ökologische Untersuchungen an Flechten der Negev-Wüste. II. CO_2 Gaswechsel und Wasserhaushalt von *Ramalina maciformis* (Del.) Bory am natürlichen Standort während der sommerlichen Trockenperiode. *Fora Jena Abt. B* **159**, 38–62.

Lange, O. L., Schulze, E. D., and Koch, W. (1970b). Experimentell ökologische Untersuchungen an Flechten der Negev-Wüste. III. CO_2 Gaswechsel und Wasserhaushalt von Krusten- und Blattflechten am natürlichen Standort während der sommerlichen Trockenperiode. *Flora Jena Abt. B* **159**, 525–528.

Orshan, G. (1954). Surface reduction and its significance as a hydro-ecological factor. *J. Ecol.* **42**, 442–444.

Orshan, G., and Zand, G. (1962). Seasonal body reduction of certain desert halfshrubs. *Bull. Res. Counc. Israel* **11D**, 35–42.

Richmond, A. E., and Lang. A. (1957). Effect of kinetin on protein content and survival of detached Xanthium leaves. *Science* **125**, 650–651.

Schulze, E. D., Lange, O. L. and Koch, W. (1971). Oekophysiologische Untersuchungen an Wild- und Kulturpflanzen der Negev Wüste. II. Die Wirkung der Ausserfaktoren auf CO_2-Gaswechsel und Transpiration am Ende der Trockenzeit. *Oecologia Berl.* **8**, 334–355.

Schulze, E. D., Lange, O. L., and Koch, W. (1972a). Oekophysiologische Untersuchungen an Wild- und Kulturpflanzen der Negev Wüste. III. Tagesläufe von Nettophotosynthese und Transpiration am Ende der Trockenzeit. *Oecologia Berl.* **9**, 317–340.

Schulze, E. D., Lange, O. L., Buschbom, U., Kappen, L., and Evenari, M. (1972b). Eco-physiological investigations in the Negev desert. II. The stomatal response to air humidity as a factor influencing plant productivity. *Symp. U.S.S.R. Acad. Sci. Leningrad Ecophys. Found. of Ecosyst. Product. in Arid Zone*, pp. 62–66.

Schulze, E. D., Lange, O. L., Buschbom, U., Kappen, L., and Evenari, M. (1972c). Stomatal responses to changes in humidity in plants growing in the desert. *Planta* **108**, 259–270.

Schulze, E. D., Lange, O. L., Kappen, L., Buschbom, U., and Evenari, M. (1973). Stomatal responses to changes in temperature at increasing water stress. *Planta* **110**, 29–42.

Shah, C. B., and Loomis, R. S. (1965). Ribonucleic acid and protein metabolism in sugar beet during drought. *Physiol. Plant.* **18**, 240–254.

Stocker, O. (1970–1972). Der Wasser- und Photosynthese-Haushalt von Wüstenpflanzen der mauretanischen Sahara I-III. *Flora Jena Abt. B* **159**, 539–572; **160**, 445–494; **161**, 46–110.

Stocker, O. (in press). Der Wasser- und Photosynthesehaushalt von Wüstenpflanzen der südalgerischen Sahara. I. Standorte und Versuchspflanzen. *Flora Jena.*

Tal, M., and Imber, D. (1970). Abnormal stomatal behavior and hormonal imbalance in flacca, a wilt mutant of tomato. II. Auxin and abscissic-like activity. *Plant Physiol.* **46**, 373–376.

Tal, M., Imber, D., and Itai, C. (1970). Abnormal stomatal behavior and hormonal imbalance in flacca, a wilt mutant of tomato. I. Root effect and kinetin-like activity. *Plant Physiol.* **46**, 367–372.

Taylor, E. S. (1971). Ecological implications of leaf morphology considered from the standpoint of energy relations and productivity. Ph.D. Thesis, Washington University.

Walter, H. (1962). Die Vegetation der Erde in ökologischer Betrachtung. Vol. 1. Die tropischen und subtropischen Zonen. Fischer, *Jena.*

Walter, H. (1972). Die Hydratur der Pflanze als Indikator ihres Wasserhaushaltes. *Handb. Pfl. Ernährung* und *Düngung Bd.* 1, Wien.

Walter, H. (1973). Der Wasserhaushalt der Pflanzen in kausaler und kybernetischer Betrachtung. *100 Jahre Hochsch. Bodenkultur Wien* **2**, 315–331.

Weiss, C., and Vaadia, Y. (1965). Kinetin like activity in root apices of sunflower plants. *Life Sci.* **4**, 1323–1326.

Went, F. W. (1938). Specific factors other than auxin affecting growth and root formation. *Plant Physiol.* **13**, 55–80.

Zohary, M. (1962). "Plant Life of Palestine." Ronald Press, New York.

Zohary, M. (1973). "Geobotanical foundations of the Middle East," (2 Vols.). Fischer and Swets and Zeitlinger, Stuttgart-Amsterdam.

Temperature Regulation and Water Requirements of Desert Mammals: Physiological Strategies and Constraints of Domestication

C. Richard Taylor

Museum of Comparative Zoology
and
Biological Laboratories
Harvard University
Cambridge, Massachusetts

Introduction

Two serious physiological problems are posed for mammals that live in hot deserts: heat and lack of water. These problems are related, for to avoid overheating, animals must either escape from the desert heat or use evaporation to keep cool. Some of the most familiar and obvious inhabitants of the hot deserts of Africa and Asia are domesticated mammals: camels, goats, sheep, donkeys, and cattle. In this chapter I should like to develop the thesis that domestication has (1) limited the potential physiological solutions for dealing with heat and lack of water; (2) created a serious new problem, lack of food; and (3) resulted in basic differences in the physiological mechanisms which wild and domestic ungulates have adopted to cope with these problems.

The domestic ungulates which inhabit hot deserts are (1) watered regularly, even during droughts; (2) corralled at night to protect them from thieves and predators; and (3) maintained at high population densities. As a result of these husbandry procedures, availability of food becomes at least as important a problem for domestic animals as availability of water. In marked contrast, wild ungulates that live in these regions are (1) able to survive droughts without drinking; (2) appear to graze at night when the free water content of their food plants is high; and (3)

131

have a low population density. Since they are neither tied to the availability of surface water, nor are herded in high densities, they should seldom, if ever, encounter food shortages.

I should like to rely heavily on data from the humped African zebu cattle *(Bos indicus)* to develop my thesis about constraints of domestication. In general terms, however, it also applies to other domestic animals which inhabit deserts. Zebu cattle are herded by pastoral nomads in arid, semiarid, and marginal lands throughout Africa and are one of the most abundant ungulates in these regions. They were first introduced into Africa about 2000 years ago (Payne, 1963). Since their introduction they have been subjected to a heavy selection pressure for survival by droughts which have regularly decimated their populations. Toward the end of one of these droughts the landscape is dominated by zebu carcasses, and watering points can be found by following a gradient of increasing density of carcasses. The magnitude of this decimation can be appreciated from records of the drought of 1961, where in the Kajiado District of Kenya, an area of about 5 million acres, 300,000 cattle out of a total population of 450,000 died (Fallon, 1962). During droughts large areas around watering points are reduced to barren ground and the sources of water can be located easily from the air by barren circles of earth. As droughts progress the circles expand. This is simply a reflection of the fact that domestic animals are watered regularly even during droughts. Many watering points dry up during droughts and the number of animals relying on those that remain increases dramatically. As the drought progresses all of the food close to the watering points is eaten and the distance between water and food becomes greater and greater. After a prolonged drought an animal may walk 2 days over almost completely barren ground from a watering point to an area with pasture, graze for a day, and walk 2 days back to the watering point, a period of 5 days having elapsed between watering.

I should like to compare data from zebu cattle with data from five other ungulates:

1. The eland *(Taurotragus oryx)*, a tractable animal that occupies a variety of habitats including very arid regions. It is easily tamed and has often been proposed as a candidate for efficient ranching of hot arid regions (Skinner, 1971; Talbot *et al.*, 1965). Adults weigh about the same as zebu cattle, 150–1000 kg.
2. The oryx *(Oryx beisa)*, a true desert-dwelling antelope. It is intermediate in size and adults weigh 70–300 kg. It inhabits most of the deserts of Africa. It can be found standing in the open sun at midday.
3. The Grant's gazelle *(Gazella granti)*, a small antelope which inhabits

the arid regions of East Africa. Similar gazelles inhabit the other deserts of Africa. Adults weigh 10–50 kg. Like the oryx, they can be found in the open sun at midday.

4. The haired sheep *(Ovis aires)*, an animal herded in African deserts which is characterized by its hair and fat tail. Adults weigh 15–40 kg.
5. The Hereford steer *(Bos taurus)*, a familiar meat-producing animal. Adults weigh 170–1100 kg.

First I should like to consider the physiological mechanisms which desert dwelling ungulates utilize to reduce water loss; then I would like to examine how the wild desert ungulates manage to survive droughts without drinking; and finally I should like to argue that the physiological mechanisms adopted by domestic ungulates for survival in deserts suggest that shortage of food has been at least as great a problem for them as shortage of water.

Physiological Mechanisms Desert Ungulates Use to Reduce Water Loss

Variable Body Temperature

At the beginning of this chapter I mentioned that desert mammals must evaporate large amounts of water in order to maintain a constant body temperature. A variable rather than a constant body temperature can result in large savings of water. This was first pointed out by Schmidt-Nielsen and his colleagues in their classic study of the camel (Schmidt-Nielsen *et al.,* 1957). They found that the hydrated camel increased evaporation by sweating and maintained a relatively constant body temperature even during the hottest days in the Sahara. When the camel's water intake was restricted and it became dehydrated, then its body temperature fell to very low levels early in the morning. It warmed slowly during the day as a result of its relatively small surface area and low metabolic rate per unit mass, and seldom reached a body temperature where sweating was necessary to avoid overheating.

The eland has adopted a strategy almost identical to that of the camel. Its body temperature falls each morning and rises slowly during the day (Taylor and Lyman, 1967). In a simulated desert its temperature increases as much as 7°C during the course of a day (from 33.9° to 41.2°C). An eland weighing a 1000 kg would store about 6000 kcal as its temperature rose 7°C and this heat could be lost nonevaporatively during the cool night. To dissipate this amount of heat evaporatively would require more than 10 liters of water. There is one important difference between the variable body temperature of the eland and that of the camel. The eland exhibits large excursions of body temperature regardless of whether it is hydrated or dehydrated, while the camel maintains a nearly constant body temperature when it is hydrated. The eland's variable body temperature, coupled with its moist diet of *Acacia* leaves, probably enables it to avoid dehydration even during severe droughts.

Hyperthermia is another possibility for reducing evaporation in the heat. When dehydrated, both the oryx and the Grant's gazelle make use of an extreme hyperthermia to reduce evaporation in the heat (Taylor, 1970a,b). Hydrated animals maintain a nearly constant body tempera-

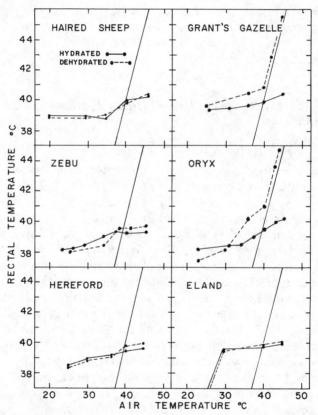

Figure 1 Steady state rectal temperatures of hydrated (solid lines) and dehydrated (dashed lines) ungulates at air temperatures between 20° and 45°C. Thin diagonal lines indicate equal air and rectal temperatures. Data on haired sheep is from Maloiy and Taylor (1971); on Grant's gazelle, oryx, and zebu is from Taylor (1970b); and on Hereford and eland is from Taylor and Lyman (1967).

Table 1 Oxygen Consumption of Hydrated and Dehydrated Ungulates[a]

Animal	% Hydrated	Dehydrated (80–85%)	% Reduction
Hereford	113	96	15
Zebu	77	58	26
Haired sheep	105	88	16
Eland	137	125	99
Oryx	128	83	35
Grant's gazelle	115	83	23

[a]Expressed as percentage of standard metabolic rate of the hydrated animal. The standard metabolic rate is predicted from Kleiber's equation: $M = 14.6\ W^{0.75}$, where M is liters $O_2 \cdot day^{-1}$ and W is weight in kg. Measurements were made at 22°–27°C. Data are unpublished observations from my laboratory.

ture of about 39°C even when air temperature exceeds 45°C (Figure 1). However, when dehydrated their body temperature may reach 47°C and exceed air temperature by 1°–2°C even when air temperature is 45°C (Figure 1). It is interesting to note that while all three of the wild desert dwelling ungulates utilize a variable body temperature to minimize water loss, none of the three domestic animals do.

Low Metabolic Rate

A low metabolic rate would be another way for an animal to reduce water loss. This would reduce all three avenues of water loss: fecal, urinary, and evaporative. Table 1 gives the resting metabolic rates for the six ungulates. Two things are immediately obvious on examining the oxygen consumption values of hydrated animals: (1) wild ungulates, particularly the eland and oryx, have a metabolic rate of about a third greater than would be predicted from Kleiber's equation; and (2) the zebu steer has a metabolic rate of about a third less than would be predicted from Kleiber's equation. The high metabolic rate of the wild ungulates has also been observed by Rogerson (1968) in long-term metabolic studies. It should result in a higher rate of water loss from hydrated animals while the lower metabolic rate in the zebu should result in a lower rate of water loss.

A variable metabolism, analogous to a variable body temperature, would be one way of reducing water loss during a drought. Metabolic rate fell when ungulates were dehydrated (Table 1). The effect of dehydration on metabolism of Hereford cattle, haired sheep, and eland was the same as had been previously observed in the camel (Schmidt-Nielsen *et al.*, 1967): metabolic rate decreased in direct proportion to the amount of water lost during dehydration. Thus an animal which had lost

15% of its weight during dehydration had a metabolic rate which was approximately 15% less than the rate observed when the animal was fully hydrated. Three animals, the zebu, the oryx, and the Grant's gazelle showed a reduction in metabolic rate with dehydration about twice that found in the other animals. The zebu started with a low metabolic rate when hydrated and the dehydrated zebu had a metabolic rate of only 58% of the level predicted for a mammal of its weight. This extremely low metabolism appears to be the key physiological mechanism which enables the zebu to survive in these desert regions.

Survival in Hot Deserts without Drinking

The eland, the oryx, and the gazelle can apparently survive in hot deserts without having to drink (Taylor, 1969, 1972). To understand how they accomplish this feat and to evaluate whether domestic animals might also be able to survive without drinking, we need to know how much water these animals require under desert conditions and then to find out how they obtain the water.

How Much Water Do Desert Ungulates Require?

An animal takes in water by drinking and as free water in its food; and it creates water by oxidation of its food to carbon dioxide and water. It loses water in its urine, with its feces, and through respiratory and cutaneous evaporation. Quantifying these avenues of water intake and loss in the desert would be very difficult. In the laboratory they can be easily measured. Laboratory studies also have the advantage that animals can be compared with one another under identical conditions. The problem then is to simulate desert conditions in the laboratory. Heat and aridity are the two environmental parameters which are necessary to include in any simulated desert. It is very hot during the middle of the day in the desert, but it cools off in the night, thus animals are subjected to a periodic rather than a constant heat load. A number of the physiological mechanisms take advantage of this day – night change in temperature. For these reasons, I selected a periodic heat load to simulate desert conditions in the laboratory: 12 hours at 40°C alternating with 12 hours at 22°C.

To determine the minimum amount of water that animals required in this simulated desert, I gradually reduced the amount of water that I gave to an animal until it weighed 85% of its initial weight. I then gave

Table 2 Minimum Water Requirements
of Ungulates in Simulated Desert[a]

Ungulate	Liters H_2O (100 kg · day^{-1})
Hereford	6.4
Zebu	3.2
Haired sheep	3.6
Eland	5.5
Oryx	3.0
Grant's gazelle	3.9

[a]Data from Taylor (1968b) and Maloiy and Taylor (1971)

just enough water to maintain this weight. If I gave any more water the animal gained weight and if I gave any less it lost weight. Then all of the avenues of water intake and loss were determined for 2 weeks while maintaining this 85% weight (Taylor, 1968b). It seems reasonable to assume that any water-conserving mechanisms would be maximally stimulated under these conditions and the water requirements determined in this manner would be close to minimal.

Table 2 compares the minimal water requirements of the six ungulates in the simulated desert environment. The Hereford steer and the eland required about twice as much water as the other ungulates whose requirements were similar.

How the Ungulates Meet their Requirements for Water in Hot Deserts

The eland requires water amounting to over 5% of its body weight each day, yet this animal is able to survive in hot arid regions without drinking. How is this possible? Three things are important: (1) the eland inhabits the edges of the deserts where there are *Acacia* trees and it eats their moist leaves; (2) during the middle of the day it seeks shade; and (3) it would seldom need to use evaporation to keep cool as a result of its size and variable body temperature when fully hydrated. I collected *Acacia* leaves during a severe drought and found that they contained 59% water. By calculating the weight of the leaves the eland would eat to meet its normal metabolic requirements, I found that the leaves would provide 5.3 liters of water per 100 kg of body weight per day, or almost exactly the amount of water needed by an eland for it to survive without drinking. An eland that obtains this much water by browsing can probably live indefinitely without having to drink, and reports to this effect are apparently true (Taylor, 1969). Other browsing ungulates that eat moist leaves and seek shade at midday, such as the gerenuk and lesser kudu, are probably also independent of surface water.

The oryx and the gazelle, however, neither seek shade at midday nor eat the moist leaves of the *Acacia*. I followed herds of both animals during droughts and collected the plants which they ate. Both ate dry grasses and shrubs which at midday contained as little as 1% water. The leaves were so dry that they often disintegrated into a powder when I tried to collect them. At first I was extremely puzzled. The only source of water which appeared to be available to these animals was oxidation water. I calculated that this would provide the oryx and the gazelle with only about 10–20% of their minimum water requirement. In thinking over this enigma, I realized that I made all of my collections of grass for determining moisture content during the middle of the day. As long ago as 1924, Buxton had observed that dried grass collects moisture from desert air at night, even when there is no dew. I made some measurements on the plants which the oryx and gazelle were eating during a severe drought in the arid Northern Frontier of Kenya. Their water content could increase from 1% to 42% in 10 hours under temperature and humidity conditions similar to those observed in nature (Taylor, 1968a). It seems very likely that by eating mainly by night, the oryx and the gazelle could take in food containing an average of 30% water. If they did, then they could meet their water requirements without drinking (Figure 2).

The haired sheep could also come close to meeting its water requirements without having to drink, if it could eat food containing 30% water (Figure 2). Sheep, like other domestic animals, are kept in corrals at night to protect them from predators and thieves. This husbandry procedure would limit sheep to the drier food found during the day and would tie them to the requirement for surface water. It would be extremely interesting to try altering management procedures and find out whether sheep could inhabit these deserts without having to drink if they were grazed at night.

Unlike the sheep, the zebu and Hereford cattle could find less than half of their water requirements in the desert by grazing at night (Figure 2). This seems intuitively obvious for the Hereford, since it is not a desert animal and requires a great deal of water when exposed to desert conditions. The zebu, however, is very frugal in its use of water and is able to reduce its water loss under desert conditions to the same low rates as the oryx and gazelle. The zebu's inability to meet its water requirements by grazing at night, although requiring the same small

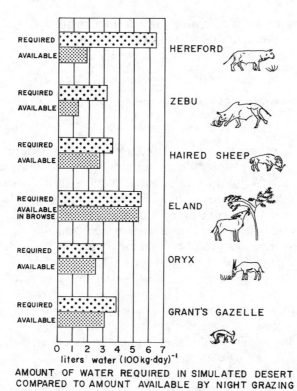

AMOUNT OF WATER REQUIRED IN SIMULATED DESERT
COMPARED TO AMOUNT AVAILABLE BY NIGHT GRAZING

Figure 2 Comparison of water requirements in simulated desert
(see text) and water available to ungulates either browsing on *Acacia*
leaves containing 58% water by weight (the eland) or eating the
desert plant *Disperma* at night when it contained 30% water be
weight. Calculations of water intake were based on the following
assumptions: oxygen consumption was twice that observed for resting animals; 50% digestibility of feed; 4.8 kcal (liters O_2 $)^{-1}$ and 0.54
g of metabolic water produced per gram of dry matter digested. The
caloric value of *Acacia* leaves was found to be about 4.5 kcal · g of
dry matter and the *Disperma* leaves was about 3.14 kcal · g of dry
matter.

amounts of water as oryx and gazelle, is due to the different mechanisms
utilized to achieve the low rates of water loss: primarily a low metabolism by the zebu, and a variable body temperature by the oryx and gazelle.

If an animal depends on its food for all of its water, then to improve
its water balance it must utilize mechanisms which reduce water loss
without reducing food intake. The zebu has achieved its very low water

loss by reducing its metabolism, which also reduces food intake. The variable body temperature of the oryx and gazelle, however, reduces water loss without having an effect on food intake.

Shortage of Food: A Major Problem for Survival of Domestic Ungulates in the Desert?

Of the animals we have considered here, the three wild ungulates utilize a variable body temperature to reduce water loss while the domestic ungulates do not. A possible explanation is that a variable body temperature has evolved in response to shortages of water and that domestic animals have not been confronted with this problem to the same extent as wild animals, since they have been watered regularly. The regular watering, however, has posed a different problem for the domestic animals: a shortage of food during droughts. The food suppliers of the wild ungulates are not limited by the availability of surface water while those of domestic animals are. During droughts as the circle of denuded ground expands around watering points, death from starvation might pose a major threat for domestic animals.

The low metabolic rate of the zebu cattle represents what might be considered a temporal solution to the problem of food shortage. The low metabolic rate effectively shortens the drought or extends the time an animal can survive during the drought on finite energy resources. The fact that water loss could be reduced still further by acquisition of a variable body temperature might be considered as an indication that food rather than water limits the zebu's ability to survive droughts. Also, the zebu does not possess the ability to rehydrate rapidly when supplied with water. These two factors taken together suggest that the low metabolic rate of the zebu has reduced its water requirements to a point where severe dehydration has seldom occurred.

Another solution which domestic animals have used for expanding their food supplies is traveling further between watering. This might be looked on as a spatial solution. The camel (Schmidt-Nielsen, 1956) and the black Bedouin goats (Shkolnik *et al.*, 1972) utilize mechanisms which slow water loss. They withstand severe dehydration and rehydrate quickly when water is available. They can therefore travel further from watering points to obtain food. In a sense this solution is analogous to carrying a canteen. It is interesting to note that the wild desert ungulates which have been studied do not possess the ability to rehydrate quickly, a mechanism which may have evolved in respose to the demands of husbandry procedures.

Summary

The wild desert dwelling ungulates, almost without exception, appear to have adopted a variety of physiological and behavioral adaptations which enable them to survive in hot deserts without drinking, while domestic animals have been tied to water by husbandry procedures. The results suggest some ways in which husbandry procedures might be altered. Night grazing might free some domestic animals, like sheep, from the need for surface water. Lynch (1969), working in Australia, found that a herd of Merino sheep could indeed survive without drinking when the water to their paddocks was accidently cut off for over a year before it was discovered. The results also suggest that the nomadic herdsman who waters his zebu cattle less frequently and leaves them longer at pasture might lose fewer animals during a drought.

It seems safe to conclude that domestication has altered problems which animals face in surviving in the hot desert and that to fully understand the adaptation of domestic animals for this environment we must consider both the problems posed by the environment and those posed by domestication itself.

References

Buxton, P. A. (1924). Heat, moisture and animal life in deserts. *Proc. Roy. Soc. Ser. B* **96**, 123–131.

Fallon, L. E. (1962). "Masai Range Resources: Kajiado District." U.S. Agency for Int. Develop., Mission to East Africa, Nairobi, Kenya.

Lynch, J. J. (1969). The performance of Merino ewes deprived of drinking water. *Austral. J. Sci.* **31**, 369–370.

Maloiy, G. M. O., and Taylor, C. R. (1971). Water requirements of African goats and haired sheep. *J. Agr. Sci.* **77**, 203–208.

Payne, W. J. A. (1963). Water metabolism of cattle in East Africa. I. The problem and the experimental procedure. *J. Agr. Sci.* **61**, 225–266.

Rogerson, A. (1968). Energy utilization by the eland and wildebeest. *Symp. Zool. Soc. London* **21**, 153–161.

Schmidt-Nielsen, K. (1956). Animals and arid conditions: physiological aspects of productivity and management. "The Future of Arid Lands." Amer. Ass. Advan. Sci., Washington, D.C.

Schmidt-Nielsen, K., Schmidt-Nielsen, B., Jarnum, S. A., and Houpt, T. R. (1957). Body temperature of the camel and its relation to water economy. *Amer. J. Physiol.* **188**, 103–112.

Schmidt-Nielsen, K., Crawford, E. C., Jr., Newsome, A. E., Rawson, K. S., and Hammel, H. T. (1967). Metabolic rate of camels: effect of body temperature and dehydration. *Amer. J. Physiol.* **212**, 341–345.

Shkolnik, A., Borut, A., and Choshniak, J. (1972). Water economy of the Beduin goat. *Symp. Zool. Soc. London* **31**, 229–242.

Skinner, J. D. (1971). Productivity of the eland: An appraisal of the last five years' research. *S. Afr. J. Sci.* **67**, 534–539.

Talbot, L. M., Payne, W. J. A., Ledger, H. P., Verdcourt, L. D., and Talbot, M. H. (1965). The meat production potential of wild animals in Africa. A review of the biological knowledge. *Commonw. Bur. Anim. Breed. Genet. Edinburgh Tech. Commun.* No. 16.

Taylor, C. R. (1968a). Hygroscopic food: A source of water for desert antelopes? *Nature London* **219**, 181.

Taylor, C. R. (1968b). The minimum water requirements of some East African bovids. *Symp. Zool. Soc. London* **21**, 195–206.

Taylor, C. R. (1969). The eland and the oryx. *Sci. Amer.* **220**, 88–95.

Taylor, C. R. (1970a). Strategies of temperature regulation: Effect on evaporation in East African ungulates. *Amer. J. Physiol.* **219**, 1131–1135.

Taylor, C. R. (1970b). Dehydration and heat: Effects on temperature regulation on East African ungulates. *Amer. J. Physiol.* **219**, 1136–1139.

Taylor, C. R. (1972). The desert gazelle: A paradox resolved. *Symp. Zool. Soc. London* **31**, 215–227.

Taylor, C. R., and Lyman, C. P. (1967). A comparative study of the environmental physiology of the East African antelope, the eland, and the Hereford steer. *Physiol. Zool.* **40**, 280–295.

Adaptations to Aridity in Amphibians and Reptiles

Vaughan H. Shoemaker

Department of Biology
University of California, Riverside

It is not the intent of this presentation to review categorically and exhaustively the numerous studies bearing on adaptations to aridity in amphibians and reptiles. A number of excellent reviews are available (Dawson and Schmidt-Nielsen, 1964: Bentley, 1966, 1971; Mayhew, 1968; Warburg, 1972; Templeton, 1972). Instead, I will attempt to assess the current "state of the art" in light of some recent findings, and to indicate some promising approaches for future research.

In general it may be said that different adaptive patterns have evolved in the two groups. For amphibians the "strategy" has largely been one of avoidance of the rigors of the arid macroclimate by behavioral means. At the extreme this may involve burrowing to considerable depths within the soil where the animals may wait out long periods of drought in arid regions. Anatomic modifications, such as the development of metatarsal "spades," are present in burrowing frogs in a variety of taxa. Physiological differences between aquatic and terrestrial amphibians are largely related to the ability to withstand, rather than prevent, water loss and the accumulation of nitrogenous wastes. This is accompanied in many amphibians by the ability to restore water and electrolyte balance rapidly when environmental conditions are favorable. Bentley (1966) has characterized these adaptations as "small modifications of the basic physiological pattern." Reptiles, on the other hand, have

evolved toward the ability to remain in balance while active aboveground during dry seasons. Presumably the development of a different
kind of integument which is relatively impermeable to water was of para-
mount importance in the realization of this ability. Indeed, Bentley
(1966) states in regard to amphibians that "the most valuable evolutionary novelty which they could invent to assist their survival (in hot dry
habitats) would be a more impermeable integument. This has not oc-
cured in Amphibia." This reflects the general supposition that reptiles
are better adapted to aridity than are amphibians, and that the latter are
limited in the scope of their adaptation by the general anatomic and physiological characteristics of the group.

Thus at first glance, it appears that amphibians and reptiles represent
such divergent avenues of adaptation to aridity that they could not prof-
itably be discussed together. However, recent discoveries have revealed
that some amphibians have in fact developed water conserving mechanisms similar in effect to those of reptiles. Also, it is becoming increasingly apparent from field studies in arid regions that reptiles may encounter conditions in which they are unable to maintain the steady state
(Bentley, 1959; Bradshaw and Shoemaker, 1967; Nagy, 1972). Thus,
the ability to accumulate and utilize stores of water and energy and to
tolerate and recover rapidly from imbalances is apparently of considerable adaptive significance in both reptiles and amphibians.

The skin of most amphibians offers little, if any, protection from
evaporative water loss. Numerous comparative studies of rates of evaporation from amphibians have been undertaken, but generally these have
not revealed important differences between terrestrial and aquatic species
(Bentley, 1966; Claussen, 1969). Such differences as have been measured probably relate more to body size and shape, conditions of measurement, and activity. Although some differences have been interpreted
as having adaptive significance (Warburg, 1972), these are certainly not
of sufficient magnitude to permit the animal to approach balancing evaporative losses with gains from dietary and metabolic water. Recently,
however, two species of anurans have been shown to possess an integument which greatly restricts evaporation (Loveridge, 1970; Shoemaker
et al., 1972). These animals, *Chiromantis xerampelina* from Africa and
Phyllomedusa sauvagii from South America, show rates of evaporative
loss similar to those of desert reptiles. Rates of water loss for *P. sauvagii*
are compared to a variety of other anurans and to desert lizards in Table
1. The barrier to cutaneous water loss in *P. sauvagii* is apparently a lipid
secretion which coats the skin surface. When the animals are left out of
water, the skin is dry and glossy, and water droplets falling on it remain
beaded. The integument is essentially similar to that of other amphibians

Table 1 Rates of Evaporative Water Loss in *Phyllomedusa sauvagii*, Other Anurans, and Desert Lizards under Comparable Conditions[a]

Species and animal number	Weight (g)	Evaporative water loss (mg · g^{-1} · hr^{-1})
Anurans		
Phyllomedusa sauvagii		
1	22.5	0.68
2	34.5	0.68
3	35.4	0.33
4	25.3	1.61
Bufo cognatus		
1	33.1	12.2
2	40.0	11.8
Scaphiopus couchii		
1	23.8	14.2
2	27.9	13.6
Rana temporaria		
1	32.7	14.2
2	24.4	18.9
Lizards		
Dipsosaurus dorsalis		
1	28.0	0.39
2	21.5	0.36
3	27.3	0.30
Uma scoparia		
1	11.3	0.61
2	29.5	0.42

[a]Conditions: dry air, 26°C, 12 cm · min^{-1}. From Shoemaker *et al.*, 1972.

except for the presence of numerous glands in the stratum spongiosum which stain intensely with a variety of lipid stains.

Two points are noteworthy: (1) *Phyllomedusa* and *Chiromantis* are both arboreal forms and occur in relatively arid regions; and (2) these species represent different families, so that this radical departure from the usual amphibian pattern has apparently arisen at least twice. It will be very interesting to learn the nature of the barrier in *Chiromantis*, but, at least for *Phyllomedusa*, the problem of cutaneous water loss has been solved in a manner quite distinct from that employed by reptiles.

Some fossorial amphibians have been found to form outer coverings (cocoons) which presumably retard water loss during periods of inactivity below ground (Mayhew, 1965; Lee and Mercer, 1967, Reno *et al.*, 1972). Tests of the benefits conferred by such cocoons have been indirect and somewhat difficult to interpret. However, McClanahan *et al.* (in press) have recently investigated cocoon formation in ceratophryd frogs from Argentina. The structure and function of the cocoon of one of these species, *Lepidobatrachus llanensis,* proved relatively easy to study because formation of the cocoon can be readily induced in the laboratory by exposing the animals to dry conditions, either in air or soil. Animals kept without access to water initially have high rates of water loss typical of amphibians, but, within a few days, the parchmentlike cocoon begins to form with a concommitant reduction in water loss (Figure 1). Other individuals were allowed to burrow in moist soil which was then dried and where they remained for 5 months. Upon excavation they were found in good condition and were enclosed in well-developed cocoons which afforded excellent protection from cutaneous water loss. Ultrastructual examination of the cocoon from one of these individuals showed it to consist of about 50 layers of flattened, dry epithelial cells arising from the stratum corneum (Figure 2). Lee and Mercer (1967) describe the cocoon of an Australian frog *(Neobatrachus pictus)* as consisting of a single layer of such cells. Reno *et al.* (1972) describe a multilayered cocoon in a siren *(Siren intermedia)* which they believe to be derived from mucous secretions. It is not known to what extent cocoon formation is typical of fossorial amphibians, but it is apparently not universal. The relatively few examples described to date represent diverse taxa, and the extent to which these structures are similar is presently unclear.

The integument of reptiles is relatively impermeable to water, but

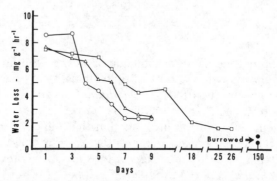

Figure 1   Rates of evaporative water loss in *Lepidobatrachus llanensis* removed from water on day 1. Unfilled symbols represent three individuals kept in open containers. Filled symbols represent two individuals excavated from dry soil. All measurements made in an open flow system (air speed 10 cm·min⁻¹, dry air, 25°C). (From McClanahan *et al.,* in press.)

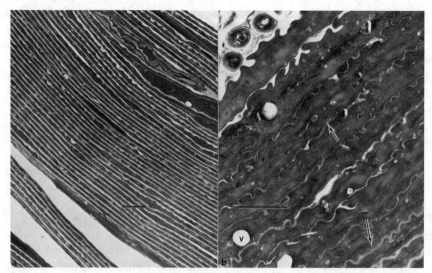

Figure 2 Electron micrographs of cocoon of *Lepidobatrachus llanensis* (scale marks 1 μ). a, Vertical section through entire cocoon showing more than 50 cell layers. Nuclear remnants evident, outer surface of cocoon upper right. b, Greater magnification of outer cell layers. Arrows indicate intercellular substance. Also evident are vesicles (V), desmosomes between cell layers, and bacteria at outer surface at upper left. (From McClanahan *et al.,* in press.)

cutaneous evaporation may be a significant fraction of the total water loss. There is some indication that reduction of water loss by this route is a component of their adaptation to aridity (Bentley and Schmidt-Nielsen, 1966; Dawson *et al.,* 1966; Claussen, 1967). However, there is little information on the nature of the barrier to evaporation in the skin of reptiles, and thus the nature of the adaptation is not known. The epidermis contains several distinct keratinized layers, and it has been suggested that the thickness of a variable portion of the β-keratin layer in the outer epidermis controls this loss (Maderson *et al.,* 1970). The keratinized layers are thinnest in the hinge region under the scales, an observation which has led to speculation that cutaneous evaporation occurs primarily from this area. This now appears unlikely, because Licht and Bennett (1972) found evaporative loss from a scaleless mutant of the gopher snake *(Pituophis melanoleucus)* to be the same as from a normal individual. Histological examination showed the skin of the mutant to resemble the normal hinge region.

The osmotic influx of water across the skin is the primary route of water gain in most amphibians, and, in fact, they have not been observed to drink except when kept in hyperosmotic saline (Bentley, 1966). Thus amphibians may utilize water from moist surfaces and from soil, a fact which reduces their dependence on pools and streams. Cutaneous water uptake may be very rapid in amphibians. Following dehydration, the rate of water uptake in many species is greatly enhanced allowing for very rapid recovery. This increase in the osmotic permeability of the skin is part of a group of responses to dehydration which also includes reduction or cessation of urine production and increased permeability of the bladder to water. The magnitude of this effect, called the water-balance response, can be correlated in a general way with the availability of water (Bentley, 1966; Warburg, 1972). However, rates of water uptake from soil are much lower than those from water (Fair, 1970), and are probably not limited by the permeability of the skin (Hillyard, 1974). Thus the ability to take up water rapidly through the skin may be of greater value to species associated with standing water than in fossorial forms (Bentley et al., 1958). It should be noted that the direction of water movement between amphibians and the soil depends on their relative water potentials. Thus animals in soil may tend to lose water when it becomes sufficiently dry (Ruibal et al., 1969; McClanahan, 1972). It is presumably in this situation that the ability to form a cocoon (see above) is beneficial.

The extent to which it might be advantageous or possible for terrestrial reptiles to be able to absorb water via the skin is not clear. Burrowing reptiles frequently do not have the intimate contact with the soil typical of fossorial amphibians. Nevertheless, there are certainly a variety of situations when reptiles may encounter moisture in forms, such as damp substrate and condensation on the skin (Lasiewski and Bartholomew, 1969), which are not compatible with drinking. An Australian lizard (Moloch horridus) can ingest water collecting on its skin because capillary channels are present which lead to the corners of the mouth (Bentley and Blumer, 1962). The osmotic permeability of reptilian skin tested in vitro can be similar to that of some amphibians, and Uromastix immersed in water gains weight slowly but steadily (Tercafs and Schoffeniels, 1965). In vivo studies with other desert lizards, Phrynosoma m'calli and Sauromalus obesus (Mayhew and Wright, 1971; Bentley, 1971) indicate that they cannot gain appreciable amounts of water via osmotic influx. It seems likely that most desert reptiles must rely on drinking if they are to supplement dietary and metabolic water.

Both amphibians and reptiles are unable to excrete urine that is hyperosmotic to their body fluids. In the absence of other adaptations, this means that considerable amounts of water would be required to eliminate nitrogenous wastes and electrolytes, despite the restrictions on water intake typical of arid environments. In terrestrial reptiles, the problem is partially solved by the excretion of nitrogenous wastes primarily in the form of uric acid and urate salts, although the desert tortoise also produces significant amounts of urea (Dantzler and Schmidt-Nielsen, 1966). Urates are excreted in precipitated form and hence the excretion of nitrogen does not reduce the solute capacity of the urine. The excretion of urate confers an additional advantage because Na^+ and K^+ may be eliminated as insoluble urate salts (Minnich, 1970; Nagy, 1972). Thus, nitrogen and electrolytes can be eliminated via the kidney – cloaca complex with little water expenditure, despite the fact that the kidneys do not have loops of Henle.

Some reptiles possess paired glands in the nasal region which aid in the excretion of salts. The fluid secreted by these glands contains variable ratios of K^+, Na^+, Cl^-, and HCO_3^- and can be greatly hyperosmotic to the plasma (see Bentley, 1971; Templeton, 1972). Additional conservation of water results from the fact that water evaporated from the secretion in the nasal passage reduces the amount of water that would otherwise evaporate from the airways (Murrish and Schmidt-Nielsen, 1970). Available estimates of the excretion of electrolytes via the nasal salt gland indicate this to be roughly equal to that excreted in the urine including urate salts (Minnich, 1970; Nagy, 1972). It would be interesting to know whether lizards lacking salt glands are able to make up the difference by excretion of urate salts. Nagy (1972) indicated that only about half of the excreted urate in the chuckwalla (a species possessing a functional salt gland) is in the form of Na^+ and K^+ salts. In any event, the salt gland confers the additional advantages that electrolyte excretion need not depend on nitrogen excretion and that chloride can be excreted economically with respect to water.

Most amphibians excrete nitrogen as ammonia and urea, with urea predominating in terrestrial forms. Thus nitrogen cannot be excreted economically with respect to water. However, as indicated previously, amphibians deprived of water may cease urine production. The resultant accumulation of urea in the body fluids is appreciable but is apparently without adverse effect up to several hundred millimolar. Fossorial forms, such as *Scaphiopus*, may even use the accumulation of urea to advantage since it lowers the water potential of the body fluids and thereby increases the prospects of obtaining water osmotically from the soil (Shoemaker *et al.*, 1969; McClanahan, 1972). When water is available, high rates of urine production allow rapid elimination of the stored urea.

No amphibian has been found to have extrarenal mechanisms for the excretion of electrolytes. Thus, to remain in salt balance, terrestrial amphibians must obtain enough water both to excrete salts and nitrogen via isoosmotic or hypoosmotic urine and to offset evaporative and fecal water losses. The fact that electrolytes are not excreted during periods of dehydration and renal shutdown is probably advantageous, since this assures that normal electrolyte levels will be restored as soon as the water deficit is removed.

The arboreal frogs *Chiromantis xerampelina* and *Phyllomedusa sauvagii* share the uricotelism of reptiles and presumably reap similar benefits. Comparison of the ability to regulate the composition of the body fluids in *P. sauvagii* and a ureotelic tree frog *(Hyla pulchella)* dramatically illustrates the potential advantage of uricotelism (Shoemaker and McClanahan, in press). Animals of both species were fed mealworms (larval *Tenebrio molitor*) at the rate of 1% of the original body weight per day. No additional water was provided, and the animals were kept in covered containers to minimize evaporative water losses. After about 1 week, the *H. pulchella* were obviously in poor condition at which time they were replaced in water. In contrast the *P. sauvagii* were continued on this regime for a month without apparent ill effects. Total plasma solutes increased by 40 mOsm · day^{-1} in *H. pulchella* and only 3 mOsm · day^{-1} in *P. sauvagii*. This reflects the far greater accumulation of urea and electrolytes in *H. pulchella* (Table 2). No urine was voided by individuals of either species during the feeding trial. At the end of the trial, bladders of *H. pulchella* were empty whereas those of *P. sauvagii* contained an average of 0.12 ml of water and 550 μmoles of nitrogen per gram of body weight. Of this nitrogen, 92% was in the form of urate. Urinary excretion of electrolytes nearly equalled input, and about 30% of the Na$^+$ and 50% of the K$^+$ were urate bound. The urine was isoosmotic with the plasma. When replaced in water, *H. pulchella* excreted the accumulated urea load, along with excess electrolytes, in about 18 hr.

After considering an example of an amphibian with adaptations similar to those more typical of reptiles, it is appropriate to point out that reptiles share with amphibians the capacity to tolerate water losses. Data compiled by Tercafs and Schoffeniels (1965) indicate that members of both groups can withstand the loss of 25–50% of the body weight during dehydration. Observations by Nagy (1972) on a field population of the chuckwalla *(Sauromalus obesus)* are illuminating in this regard. These herbivorous desert lizards are normally active throughout the summer without access to drinking water. Thus their water, electrolyte, and energy budgets are colligated and depend on the characteristics and availability of food. In the spring (April and early May) of 1970, relatively succulent annual vegetation was available to the population studied by Nagy. During this time the animals gained weight rapidly (about 20% of the body weight in a month and a half) and obtained more

Table 2 Changes in Weight and Concentrations of Solutes in Plasma in Frogs with Insect Food as the Only Source of Water

| Species (number) | Weight (g) | Plasma solutes | | | | |
		Na$^+$ (mEq · liter^{-1})	K$^+$ (mEq · liter^{-1})	Cl$^-$ (mEq · liter^{-1})	Urea (mM)	Total solutes (mOsm)
Phyllomedusa sauvagii (5)						
Day 0	21.5	114	2.7	82	4.2	221
Day 31	21.3	146	5.2	116	54	323
Rate of change (mmoles · day^{-1})		1.03	0.08	1.1	1.6	3.3
Hyla pulchella (5)						
Day 0	12.2	108	4.3	77	13	221
Day 8	9.6	168	7.1	139	224	541
Rate of change (mmoles · day^{-1})		7.5	0.35	7.8	26.4	40.0

151

water than required to balance obligatory losses. Because of very low rainfall the preceding winter, vegetation dried rapidly during late May and June. Although the lizards continued to eat during this period, they obtained insufficient water to balance losses and they began to lose weight. For the remainder of the summer the lizards' behavior changed markedly. They stopped feeding, which reduced their rate of weight loss since more water would be lost with the feces than could be obtained with the food. Also, they greatly reduced their activity, remaining in relatively cool rock crevices instead of basking and moving about on the surface during the day. By October, the animals were only 60–80% of their weight in early April. Nevertheless, at least some survived until the following spring when they were 50–65% of their weight a year previous.

The above example points up several characteristics of arid environments which bear importantly on considerations of the adaptations of animals to them. We tend to neglect the fact that conditions in generally arid environments tend to be quite variable, and are on occasion extremely harsh and on other occasions extremely favorable. Thus the ability to quickly and effectively exploit favorable periods is as essential as the ability to withstand adversity. A lizard *(Coleonyx varigatus)* can increase in weight by 50% in 4 days, enough to sustain the animal for 6–9 months (Bustard, 1967). Also, we tend to simplify the enormously complex interactions between the animal and its environment to a few parameters which we assume to be under strong selection pressure. We need now to emphasize the total biology of the organism, rather than assuming *a priori* that a certain adaptation would be beneficial. Why, for example, do many desert amphibians lack an impermeable integument and the ability to excrete uric acid, when we now know these to be within the adaptive capacities of the group?

Having rather superficially discussed "adaptations" in two large and diverse groups of animals, a few words of caution are in order. Many generalizations have been made from examination of relatively few species. Some of these will certainly be shown to be inappropriate. A danger of making such generalizations is that they may inhibit further investigation when, in fact, many important questions remain.

References

Bentley, P. J. (1959). Studies on the water and electrolyte metabolism of the lizard *Trachysaurus rugosus* (Gray). *J. Physiol. London* **145**, 37–47.
Bentley, P. J. (1966). Adaptations of Amphibia to arid environments. *Science* **152**, 619–623.

Bentley, P. J. (1971). "Endocrines and Osmoregulation." Springer-Verlag, New York.

Bentley, P. J., and Blumer, W. F. C. (1962). Uptake of water by the lizard, *Moloch horridus. Nature London* **194,** 699–700.

Bentley, P. J., and Schmidt-Nielsen, K. (1966). Cutaneous water loss in reptiles. *Science* **151,** 1547–1549.

Bentley, P. J., Lee, A. K., and Main, A. R. (1958). Comparison of dehydration and hydration of two genera of frogs *(Heleioporus* and *Neobatrachus)* that live in areas of varying aridity. *J. Exp. Biol.* **35,** 677–684.

Bradshaw, S. D., and Shoemaker, V. H. (1967). Aspects of water and electrolyte changes in a field population of *Amphibolurus* lizards. *Comp. Biochem. Physiol.* **20,** 855–865.

Bustard, R. (1967). Gekkonid lizards adapt fat storage to desert environments. *Science* **158,** 1197.

Claussen, D. L. (1967). Studies of water loss in two species of lizards. *Comp. Biochem. Physiol.* **20,** 115–130.

Claussen, D. L. (1969). Studies on water loss and rehydration in anurans. *Physiol. Zool.* **42,** 1–14.

Dantzler, W. H., and Schmidt-Nielsen, B. (1966). Excretion in the freshwater turtle *(Pseudemys scripta)* and desert tortoise *(Gophrus agassizii). Amer. J. Physiol.* **210,** 198–210.

Dawson, W. R., and Schmidt-Nielsen, K. (1964). Terrestrial animals in dry heat: Desert reptiles. *In* "Handbook of Physiology," (D. B. Dill, ed.), pp. 215–243. Williams & Wilkins, Baltimore, Maryland.

Dawson, W. R., Shoemaker, V. H., and Licht, P. (1966). Evaporative water losses of some small Australian lizards. *Ecology* **47,** 589–594.

Fair, J. W. (1970). Comparative rates of rehydration from soil in two species of toads, *Bufo boreas* and *Bufo punctatus. Comp. Biochem. Physiol.* **34,** 281–287.

Hillyard, S. D. (1974). The role of ADH in the water economy of the spadefoot toad, *Scaphiopus couchi.* Ph.D. Thesis, Univ. Calif., Riverside.

Lasiewski, R. C., and Bartholomew, G. A. (1969). Condensation as a mechanism for water gain in nocturnal desert poikilotherms. *Copeia 1969,* pp. 405–407.

Lee, A. K., and Mercer, E. H. (1967). Cocoon surrounding desert-dwelling frogs. *Science* **157,** 87–88.

Licht, P., and Bennett, A. F. (1972). A scaleless snake: tests of the role of reptilian scales in water loss and heat transfer. *Copeia 1972,* pp. 702–707.

Loveridge, J. P. (1970). Observations on nitrogenous excretion and water relations of *Chiromantis xerampelina* (Amphibia, Anura). *Arnoldia Rhodesia* **5,** 1–6.

Maderson, P. F. A., Mayhew, W. W., and Sprague, G. (1970). Observations on the epidermis of desert-living iguanids. *J. Morphol.* **130,** 25–35.

Mayhew, W. W. (1965). Adaptations of the amphibian, *Scaphiopus couchi,* to desert conditions. *Amer. Midl. Natur.* **74,** 95–109.

Mayhew, W. W. (1968). Biology of desert amphibians and reptiles. *In* "Desert Biology," Vol. 1 (by G. W. Brown, ed.). Academic Press, New York.

Mayhew, W. W., and Wright, S. J. (1971). Water impermeable skin of the lizard *Phrynosoma m'calli. Herpetologica* **27**, 8–11.

McClanahan, L., Jr. (1972). Changes in body fluids of burrowed spadefoot toads as a function of soil water potential. *Copeia 1972,* pp. 209–216.

McClanahan, L. Jr., Shoemaker, V. H., and Ruibal, R. (in press). Structure and function of the cocoon of a leptodactyl frog *Copeia.*

Minnich, J. E. (1970). Water and electrolyte balance of the desert iguana, *Dipsosaurus doraslis,* in its natural habitat. *Comp. Biochem. Physiol.* **35**, 921–933.

Murrish, D. E., and Schmidt-Nielsen, K. (1970). Exhaled air temperatures and water conservation in lizards. *Resp. Physiol.* **10**, 151–158.

Nagy, K. A. (1972). Water and electrolyte budgets of a free-living desert lizard, *Sauromalus obesus. J. Comp. Physiol.* **79**, 39–62.

Reno, H. W., Gehlbach, F. R., and Turner, R. A. (1972). Skin and aestivational cocoon of the aquatic amphibian, *Siren intermedia* LeConte. *Copeia 1972,* pp. 625–631.

Ruibal, R., Tevis, L. Jr., and Roig, V. (1969). The terrestrial ecology of the spadefoot toad *Scaphiopus hammondii. Copeia 1969,* pp. 571–584.

Shoemaker, V. H., and McClanahan, L. L., Jr. (in preparation). Water loss and nitrogen metabolism in phyllomedusid frogs.

Shoemaker, V. H., McClanahan, L. Jr., and Ruibal, R. (1969). Seasonal changes in body fluids in a field population of spadefoot toads. *Copeia 1969,* pp. 585–591.

Shoemaker, V. H., Balding, D., Ruibal, R., and McClanahan, L. Jr. (1972). Uricotelism and low evaporative water loss in a South American frog. *Science* **175**, 1018–1020.

Templeton, J. R. (1972). Salt and water balance in desert lizards. *Symp. Zool. Soc. London.* No. 31, 61–77.

Tercafs, R. R., and Schoffeniels, E. (1965). Phénomenès de permeabilité an niveau de la peau des reptiles. *Ann. Soc. Roy. Zool. Belge* **96**, 9–22.

Warburg, M. R. (1972). Water economy and thermal balance of Israeli and Australian Amphibia from xeric habitats. *Symp. Zool. Soc. London.* No. 31, 79–111.

Part III
Adaptations of Polar-Alpine Organisms

Physiological Ecology of Arctic and Alpine Photosynthesis and Respiration

Larry L. Tieszen and Nancy K. Wieland

Department of Biology
Augustana College
Sioux Falls, South Dakota

Introduction

An analysis of photosynthesis, respiration, and other vital processes necessary to confer success under tundra conditions is imperative for several reasons. It will help provide a basic understanding of the production processes which underlie tundra ecosystem structures and it should aid our understanding of the genetic and physiological mechanisms which account for successful adaptations to conditions which are near the environmental extremes which support life. Furthermore, the impact of recent technological development in polar regions especially in Siberia, Canada, and the United States, and the potential for greater exploitation requires an ability to assess the impact of man on a system which is especially sensitive. An understanding of the basic physiological performances of *native* species in these "cold-dominated" environments is prerequisite to the sound development of ecologically based management policies.

Although arctic and alpine areas have been of special interest to biological scientists for a long time, lack of research facilities and laboratory support has precluded extensive experimental studies of plant responses *in situ*. In the polar regions, however, notable recent advances have been made through the support provided in the United States at the

157

Naval Arctic Research Laboratory at Barrow, Alaska (Johnson and Tieszen, 1974), from the impetus at national and international levels provided by the Tundra Biome portion of the International Biological Program Wielgolaski and Rosswall, 1972; Bliss, 1972; Brown, 1972), and as a result of Antarctic research programs (Llano, 1972; Holdgate, 1970).

This chapter provides a generalized description of tundra and reviews the photosynthetic and respiratory responses of tundra vascular species in the context of whole plant strategies of adaptation to tundra environments. Internal and external control of photosynthesis will be emphasized but the fundamental mechanisms underlying many of the adaptations must await additional research.

Tundra Characterization

Description, Types, and Geographical Extent

"Tundra" is used to refer to either a geographical area or, as in our context, an ecosystem type. Tundra (marshy plain) is the treeless region above timberline on high mountains *(alpine tundra)* and beyond climatic timberline in the north *(arctic tundra)*. It is descriptive of an ecological system characterized by vegetation consisting predominantly of herbs, dwarf shrubs, lichens, and mosses. Tundra systems cover an area of 6–8 million km² or nearly 5% of the earth's land surface (Lieth, 1972) and are located principally north of 60° N latitude.

Although some Europeans define tundra in a more restricted sense to apply to arctic regions underlain by permafrost, here we will use a more generic sense and include alpine areas which possess similar life forms. Thus, in the conterminous United States, alpine tundra includes the relatively isolated areas above timberline in the Mount Washington area, the Rocky Mountains, and the Sierras. Tropical and southern hemisphere alpine tundra areas are somewhat more difficult to delimit due to the absence of montane forests in parts of South America, for example, and due to the inclusion of different life forms such as the giant rosette plants in the African alpine (Hedberg, 1964). However, the generally similar life forms and extreme environmental conditions justify their inclusion as subdivisions of tundra.

Environment

The overriding feature of tundra environments (see reviews by Bliss, 1962; Billings and Mooney, 1968; Lewis and Callaghan, 1975) is the generally low heat budget which imposes (1) a short growing season upon all vascular plants and (2) generally low temperatures even during the 2- to 3-month period when plants are metabolically active. Tundra plants must be able to grow and successfully reproduce in this short growing season at low temperatures. Mean temperatures during the growing season are frequently less than 5°C and even in continental arctic tundra areas mean July maxima are less than 15°C. Diurnal temperature cycles, however, are characteristic in the continuous photoperiod of the Arctic (Tieszen, 1973) but are obviously more pronounced in alpine and especially tropical alpine areas where diurnal temperature ranges may be large.

Another obvious difference between polar tundras and midlatitude or tropical alpine tundras exists because of difference in light intensity and duration. Although the continuous sunlight at Barrow until August 2 provides a continuous photoperiod, a substantial diurnal course of radiation still exists (Tieszen, 1972a, 1973; Figure 1). Due to differences in unit air masses and solar elevation, however, daily maxima rarely ex-

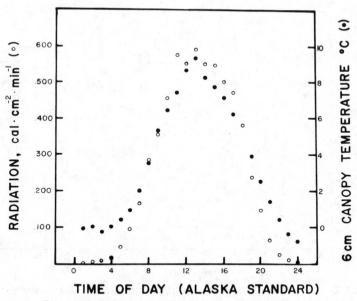

Figure 1 Example of a mean daily course of solar irradiance and 6-cm canopy temperatures at the beginning of August, Barrow, Alaska, 71° N latitude.

ceed 1 cal · cm⁻² · min⁻¹ at 71° N latitude, whereas intensities in alpine areas can frequently exceed the solar constant (Clark and Peterson, 1967). The continuous radiation at Barrow, however, can provide daily totals comparable to or greater than those in the alpine.

One significant effect of the low heat budget and the associated long period of persistent snow cover in high and intermediate latitude tundras is a common delay of the growing season until near the summer solstice (Tieszen, 1972a). The high albedo of the snow cover means that a negative or only slightly positive (Weller and Cubley, 1972) net radiation balance continues well into spring even when downward fluxes are large (Weaver, 1969). This balance changes rapidly during melt-off (Figure 2) and net radiation becomes strongly positive. Subnivean temperatures remain very low, especially in permaforst areas, until meltwater has percolated through the snow blanket; and at Barrow, Alaska, no growth or photosynthesis occurs prior to melt-off. Since the herbaceous canopies cannot begin interception until near the period of the summer solstice, the efficiency of light interception is of necessity low when radiation is

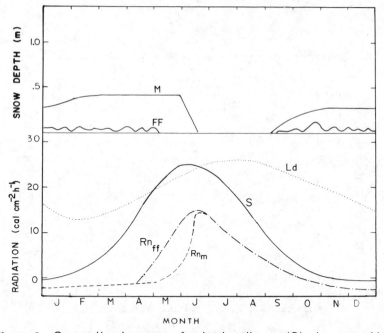

Figure 2 Generalized course of solar irradiance (S), downward long-wave radiation (Ld), and net radiation (Rn) for two tundra sites, a wet meadow (m) and beach ridge or fellfield (ff), with typical patterns of snow cover. (In Lewis and Callaghan, 1975.)

most intense. A developing canopy cannot attain high interception efficiencies until well after the period of maximum irradiance.

Despite the above generalizations about temperatures and radiation, the environmental features in tundra areas vary greatly not only from one region to another but over short distances. For example, the wet tundra system at Barrow (Tieszen, 1972a) stands in sharp contrast to the *Dryas*-dominated beach ridge studied on Devon Island (Mayo *et al.*, 1972). Equally great extremes in moisture and plant and surface temperature regimes are present in each area and exemplify the difficulty of defining adaptations or general adaptive strategies to tundras. In essence the areas included as tundra comprise a mosaic of contrasting environmental extremes. If adaptations exist in tundra plants, they have been selected with respect to these specific environments and not to tundras in the generic sense. As others have indicated, this variation in tundra nearly defies generalizations.

Flora and Evolutionary Heritage

The floras of tundras (see brief review by Bliss, 1971) are considered to be depauparate and the reduction in species numbers (diversity?) with latitude and altitude suggests that the process of natural selection has operated more between the organism and the abiotic environment than it has through biological competition. If this is correct, one could expect that species inhabiting tundra areas might not be as well adapted to these environments as are species where biological competition has been more intense. Evidence for extreme abiotic control of growth is provided by the generally known slow rate of revegetation following tundra disturbances (Bliss and Wein, 1972). On the other hand, reduced biological competition may facilitate establishment of a species over a wider range of habitats and may result in a greater diversity of growth forms and increased intraspecific variation. Certainly, the widespread vegetative reproduction observed in tundras accompanied by high incidences of polyploidy and apomixis could tend to maintain these localized variations. Presumably under at least some conditions these species are adapted only in the sense that they are surviving, but are not necessarily adapted in the sense of performing optimally or possessing a proven capability of successfully withstanding strong biological competition. Populations may, therefore, exhibit marked morphological (e.g., stunting) and physiological (e.g., arthocyanin accumulation) responses, which may represent environmental modifications rather than directly adaptive responses.

Although each tundra area reflects the input from floras in adjacent biomes (see, e.g., Chabot and Billings, 1972; Hedberg, 1964), the species selected share certain features of consequence with respect to photosynthesis and primary production. Perennial herb and dwarf shrub growth forms predominate; and especially in areas of substantial moisture the Gramineae and Cyperaceae not only are represented by a large number of species, but are also responsible for a substantial proportion of the biomass produced (Tieszen, 1972a). This predominant growth form possesses little supporting tissues and one could expect not only an efficient photosynthetic system but also a fairly efficient secondary conversion of biomass from the primary producer level to the herbivores.

Available evidence suggests that the evolutionary heritage of tundra plants provides genetic capabilities for photosynthesis via the C_3 pathway and not the C_4 pathway. As Tieszen and Sigurdson (1973) indicate, the flora of Barrow, Alaska, for example, consists of grasses all of which belong to tribes which are generally considered to be temperate in origin and distribution. In fact, their survey of most species (50) at Barrow showed no plants with a well-developed C_4 pathway of CO_2 fixation. The vascular species of Antarctic tundra also belong to taxonomic groups which are known to photosynthesize only by this C_3 pathway. Tundra floras with desert elements might be expected to include representatives possessing the C_4 pathway. An examination of the flora of the Sierra Nevada as reported by Chabot and Billings (1972) did not produce any species which one would expect to possess the C_4 pathway. It would seem likely that in the tropics the preponderance of C_4 species at lower elevations would have resulted in the migration and adaptation of a few species to the high altitude tundras. Reference to the species described by Hedberg (1964) for East Africa indicates that many of the genera are the same as those in North America and are therefore of the C_3 type. However, some of the African alpine tussocks, e.g., *Andropogon amethystinus*, belong to genera known to photosynthesize by the C_4 pathway and, therefore, may represent the few species of this photosynthetic group which have adapted to tundra regions. These species and some of the dicotyledons in Africa and South America should be studied as soon as possible as an understanding of the adaptations of these C_4 plants to low temperatures could be of fundamental agronomic importance.

The generalization that tundra plants photosynthesize by the C_3 pathway allows us to infer some expected responses and to suggest adaptations (Table 1) to tundras (Tieszen and Sigurdson, 1973). We would expect tundra plants to be characterized by the following: (1) ribulose-1,5-diphosphate (RuDP) carboxylase would be utilized as the principal carboxylating enzyme as opposed to phosphoenolpyruvate (PEP) carboxylase; (2) tundra plants should possess lower temperature requirements for growth and photosynthesis (Cooper and Tainton, 1968;

Table 1 General Characteristics of the Two Principal Photosynthetic Systems

	Calvin system (temperate)	Hatch and Slack system (tropical)
1. Early products	C_3 acids (phosphogly-cerate)	C_4 acids (aspartate, malate)
2. Carboxylation substrate	Ribulose-1,5-diphos-phate (RuDP)	Phosphoenolpyruvate (PEP) + RuDP
3. Carbonic anhydrase	High	Low
4. Apparent photorespiration	Present	Absent
5. O_2 inhibition of photo-synthesis	Present	Absent
6. CO_2 compensation	15–150 ppm (tempera-ture dependent)	<5 ppm
7. CO_2 evolution in light	High	None
8. Maximum photosyn-thetic rate	15–35 mg $CO_2 \cdot dm^{-2} \cdot hr^{-1}$	>35 mg $CO_2 \cdot dm^{-2} \cdot hr^{-1}$
9. Light saturation	Low	High
10. Temperature optima (photosynthesis and growth)	Low to high	High
11. Leaf anatomy	Diffuse mesophyll	Compact around vascular bundles
12. Sheath cells	Poorly developed	Extensively developed
13. Chloroplasts	Granal	Granal and agranal
14. Translocation rate	Slow	Rapid

Charles-Edwards and Charles-Edwards, 1970) than species photosynthesizing by the C_4 pathway; (3) their light-saturated rates would be low (Hesketh and Moss, 1963; Tieszen, 1970) and they would require relatively lower intensities for saturation; (4) photorespiration would be active, in part accounting for the lower rates of photosynthesis (Tieszen, 1973), and would result in temperature-dependent compensation points varying between 15 and 150 ppm; (5) the higher "mesophyll" resistances should result in lower efficiencies of water use (CO_2/H_2O) which could be of special importance on dry windswept tundra areas; (6) the early stable product of carboxylation should be 3-phosphoglycerate which ultimately would be converted to assimilation products which should be translocated at a slower rate than that which characterizes C_4 plants (Hofstra and Nelson, 1969a); and (7) presumably, all chloroplasts will possess photosystems 1 and 2 and therefore should be characterized by lower ratios of chlorophyll a to b.

These generalizations provide a framework within which we can interpret photosynthesis in tundras. They also represent logical hypotheses to be tested; and the extent to which tundra C_3 plants have evolved or adapted with respect to any of the above responses should form our principal goals in an understanding of photosynthetic adaptations.

Life Strategy and CO₂ Balance

A successful species must accumulate sufficient reduced organic material to provide the energy resources necessary for the establishment of its offspring. This truism, however, does not imply that success necessarily demands high productivity. Interception of radiation is obviously a prerequisite for energy transduction, and in tundras the efficiency of this process may be crucially important because of the shortened growing seasons. The conversion of this intercepted radiation to chemical potential is the main subject of this chapter; however, factors other than photosynthesis may be more crucial for adaptation and survival. The photosynthetic process itself can only function following interception; and the allocation of that assimilated material in part dictates the life strategy and may be of more fundamental importance than the actual rates of the photosynthetic process. Although each aspect may be considered independently its ecological significance can only be assessed in the context of the overall strategy.

Perenniality and Radiation Interception

A growing season of limited duration demands an efficient strategy of light interception and presumably the perennial growth habit is an adaptive strategy which allows rapid leaf and canopy development and decreases the necessity for the completion of a life cycle within one season. Annuals are very rare in tundras (Bliss, 1971; Chabot and Billings, 1972) and have evaded the problems of a short season by assuming an extreme dwarf form. In contrast, the typical perennial form is generally a graminoid or leafy dicotyledon with a large belowground biomass (Dennis and Tieszen, 1972; Dennis and Johnson, 1970) usually in roots and/or rhizomes. These perennial storage structures allow a large root absorptive surface to develop, an adaptation perhaps essential in the low soil temperatures. We will distinguish four perennial growth forms which we believe have evolved different strategies associated with specific habitats. The *graminoid* and *nongraminoid herbs* are deciduous (do not retain functional chlorophyll) and are most common where soil moisture is high. *Evergreen dwarf shrubs* tend to characterize areas in which water stress develops during the growing season or where nutrients are limiting. Habitat preferences for *deciduous dwarf shrubs* do not seem as distinct and this growth form decreases with latitude and altitude. The above in some cases have evolved true cushion habits; however little is known concerning their CO_2 exchange.

An important and often overlooked adaptation to increase interception in a number of species characteristic of wet meadows is rapid leaf exsertion and development in graminoids which is facilitated by the existence of partially developed leaves retained in a dormant or quiescent state from the previous fall (Tieszen, 1972a,b). These leaves require several weeks to attain maturity which means that one or more leaves per individual shoot may enter fall freeze-up without having been fully expanded. They characteristically die back (senesce?) only to the older persistent sheaths. After a few days above 0°C, the protected segments within the sheaths can be exserted. These leaves are photosynthetically active although not at full competence (Tieszen, unpublished). Tieszen (1972a) suggests that nongraminoid herbs produced their leaves at a greater rate and with less seasonal replacement than the graminoids. Presumably a greater utilization of belowground reserves occurs in this growth form to develop its canopy rapidly. Although the canopy in these wet sites may develop leaf area indices higher than 1.0 (Tieszen, 1972a; Caldwell *et al.*, 1972), values of this magnitude are not attained until well after the summer solstice. Thus, early development should be beneficial; the simulations of Miller and Tieszen (1972) emphasize the importance of rapid canopy development, for by doubling existing leaf area on June 25 they achieved nearly a doubling of seasonal production. In these arctic regions, where moisture is adequate, relatively complex community structure can develop and appears adaptive by enhancing light interception, absorption, and utilization. Even though canopy height is low, about 10–15 cm in Barrow wet coastal tundra, stratification is evident. The upper "synusium" is composed primarily of grasses and sedges with erectophilic leaves, whereas the understory of mosses and dicotyledonous species have more horizontal leaves. Leaf inclination varies with position of the species within the canopy. *Dupontia fischeri* and *Carex aquatilis* have the most strongly inclined leaves (72° and 62°, respectively), and these two species are positioned with most of the leaf area in the upper portion of the canopy. *Eriophorum angustifolium* occupies a median position in the canopy with a mean leaf inclination of 38°. *Salix pulchra* and *Poa arctica* occupy the 0- to 5-cm level and possess inclinations of 24° and 25°, respectively. Thus, leaf orientation within the canopy is reminiscent of the optimal plant architecture for light utilization proposed for other communities.

Dry beach ridges and fell fields present a contrasting habitat type with different growth forms and strategies. Evergreen dwarf shrubs approaching cushion forms are common and, as in *Dryas* (Mayo *et al.*, 1972), retain functional leaves and thereby achieve a proportionally greater interception early in the season (Figure 2b) at a time when water relations are also more conducive to photosynthesis. Generally high water stress prevents a closed canopy in these areas and high leaf area indices are never attained. Perennial photosynthetic structures may be a general adaptation to shortened growing seasons whether imposed by late season water stress or persistent snow banks.

Pigment Concentration and Distribution

Effective interception of radiation is enhanced by another adaptive feature of tundra plants—the presence of chlorophyllous tissues in most aboveground structures (Tieszen, 1972a). In some species more than 20% of the total plant chlorophyll was contained in nonlaminar structures allowing for considerable photosynthetic contribution by these plant parts (Tieszen and Johnson, in preparation). Again, the simulations of Miller and Tieszen (1972) showed the increasing importance of the photosynthetic capacities of these nonblade structures as their contribution to the total biomass increased. Also, the pigment data support the concept of intracanopy adaptation for at Barrow, as in more temperate canopies, "understory" species possess higher chlorophyll contents and lower chlorophyll a to b ratios, as well as more horizontal leaves.

In an earlier comparative field study, Tieszen (1970) proposed that the suggested latitudinal increase in chlorophyll (Mooney and Billings, 1961; Mooney and Johnson, 1965; Tieszen and Bonde, 1967) was not extensive if in fact it existed at all. He did suggest, however, that arctic plants possessed a greater proportion of chlorophyllous to nonchlorophyllous cells than plants from the alpine, and on this basis he hypothesized higher light requirements for saturated photosynthesis and lower efficiencies of CO_2 uptake at low intensities in the alpine plants. Arctic plants appear (Tieszen, 1970, 1972a; Tieszen and Johnson, 1968) to possess lower chlorophyll a to b ratios; however, the analytic difficulty of these determinations precludes a definitive analysis at this time. If correct, they could imply an enhanced activity of photosystem II, the significance of which is not entirely clear.

Seasonal trends of chlorophyll are similar in various tundra sites (Muc, 1972; Tieszen, 1972a) and show a peak in concentration which precedes the peak standing crop of pigments and dry matter by as much as several weeks. This suggests that individual plant photosynthetic efficiency reaches its maximum before the period of peak standing crop but that maximum community uptake of CO_2 occurs later in the season.

Although dicotyledons may initiate growth a few days after graminoids, they appear to attain maximum chlorophyll concentrations relatively sooner. This may be associated with a more rapid leaf expansion and may indicate different leaf development, maturation, and senescence patterns in dictos than monocots (Tieszen, 1972a). They could possess different seasonal patterns of CO_2 uptake, and we have shown that graminoids require several days to weeks to attain full photosynthetic competency. A similar differentiation in the water relations of monocots and dicots was recently described by Ehleringer (1973).

Photosynthesis and Respiration

External Factors Governing Rates of CO_2 Exchange

The photosynthetic rate expressed by a plant at any given time is dependent upon the interaction of all independent environmental factors with all plant metabolic reactions which ultimately affect the photosynthetic process. Although most photosynthetic experiments are concerned with the importance of a selected independent variable from which interpretations of a causal nature are inferred, it is important to realize that the effect the limiting variable has upon photosynthesis is not independent of other factors. Rather the response to the limiting variable depends upon the remainder of the proximate and ultimate environmental complex. It is the interaction of the recent developmental history and the instantaneous environmental complex operating within a framework of genetic capabilities which determines photosynthetic rates. In tundras the overall effects of such things as low root temperatures, limiting nutrients resulting from slow decomposition, anaerobic soil conditions, high convection, etc., help determine the actual magnitudes of potential photosynthesis.

Maximal Rates. Maximal rates (which in this chapter refer to the approximate level of the upper limit) of photosynthesis for arctic and alpine species range between approximately 2 and 31 mg $CO_2 \cdot dm^{-2} \cdot hr^{-1}$. Tieszen (1973) reports rates between 7 and 31 mg $CO_2 \cdot dm^{-2} \cdot hr^{-1}$ for fully expanded leaves of the major species at Barrow although most species exhibited maximal rates between 10 and 20 mg $CO_2 \cdot dm^{-2} \cdot hr^{-1}$. Rates between 5 and 16 mg $CO_2 \cdot dm^{-2} \cdot hr^{-1}$ are reported for comparable tundra species in the Taimyr region of the USSR. Reported rates for alpine regions are similar and ranged, for example, between 4 and 13 mg $CO_2 \cdot dm^{-2} \cdot hr^{-1}$ in Wyoming (Billings *et al.*, 1966) and between 18 and 27 mg $CO_2 \cdot dm^{-2} \cdot hr^{-1}$ for herbaceous species in the European

Table 2 Estimates of Maximal Photosynthetic Rates under Tundra Field Conditions Arranged by Growth Form and Related to Other Plant Groups

Plant type	CO_2 uptake (mg $CO_2 \cdot hr^{-1}$) per dm² leaf area	per g dry weight	Reference[a]
A. Herbaceous Plants			
1. Cultivated with C_3 pathway	20–35	30–60	—
2. Herbs from sunny habitats	15–60	30–90	—
3. Herbs from shaded habitats	4–16	20	—
4. Tundra graminoids			
Alopecurus alpinus	16	(35)	Tieszen, 1973
	15	33	Shvetsova and Voznessenskii, 1971
Arctagrostis latifolia	14.7	(37)	Tieszen, 1973
Arctophila fulva	19.6	(34)	Tieszen, 1973
	10	27	Shvetsova and Voznessenskii, 1971
Calamagrostis holmii	12.6	(33)	Tieszen, 1973
Carex aquatilis	15.3	(24)	Tieszen, 1973
C. bigelowii		4	Hadley and Bliss, 1964
C. ensifolia	6	9	Shvetsova and Voznessenskii, 1971
Deschampsia caespitosa	—	6	Scott and Billings, 1964
Dupontia fischeri	17.1	(25)	Tieszen, 1973
Eriophorum angustifolium	10	14.5	Shvetsova and Voznessenskii, 1971
	14.1	—	Tieszen, 1975
Elymus arenarius	30.8	(33)	Tieszen, 1973
Hierochlöe alpina	7	(12)	Tieszen, 1973
Juncus trifidus	—	2	Hadley and Bliss, 1964
Poa alpina	—	7	Scott and Billings, 1964
P. arctica	11.5	(14)	Tieszen, 1973
P. malacantha	10.1	—	Tieszen, 1973
5. Tundra nongraminoids			
Allium cepa	18	—	Kostytschew et al., 1930
Arenaria obtusiloba	—	5	Scott and Billings, 1964
Artemisia scopulorum	—	8	Scott and Billings, 1964

Species			Reference
Caltha intraloba	25	—	Phillips and McWilliam, 1971
C. palustris	18	—	Kostytschew et al., 1930
Chrysanthemum alpinum	—	9	Moser, 1973
Doronicum clusii	21	33	Cartellieri, 1940
Geum peckii	—	3	Hadley and Bliss, 1964
G. reptans	—	20–23	Moser, 1969
G. rossii	—	5	Scott and Billings, 1964
G. turbinatum	18	—	Billings et al., 1966
Hedysarum arcticum	9	17	Shvetsova and Voznessenskii, 1971
Oxyria digyna	7	—	Mooney and Billings, 1961
	9	—	Wager, 1941
	10	28	Shvetsova and Voznessenskii, 1971
Petasites frigidus	15	—	Billings et al., 1966
Polygonum bistortoides	9	17	Tieszen, unpublished
Potentilla diversifolia	27	—	Billings et al., 1966
P. tridentata	—	3	Scott and Billings, 1964
	—	2	Hadley and Bliss, 1964
Primula glutinosa	24	30	Cartellieri, 1940
Ranunculus glacialis	27	30	Cartellieri, 1940
	—	30–35	Moser, 1969, 1973
R. nivalis	18	21	Tieszen, unpublished
Rumex acetosella	18	—	Kostytschew et al., 1930
Saxifraga bryoides	—	10	Moser, 1973
S. rhomboidea	15	—	Billings et al., 1966
Sieversia reptans	18	24	Cartellieri, 1940
Trifolium dasyphyllum	—	7	Scott and Billings, 1964
T. parryi	—	9	Moser, 1973
6. C_4 plants	30–70	40–120	—
7. Succulents	4–12	8	—
8. Submerged macrophytes	4–6	—	—
B. Woody Plants			
1. Deciduous broad leaved trees			
Sun leaves	10–25	15–30	—
Shade leaves	6–15	—	—

Table 2 (continued)

Plant type	CO_2 uptake (mg CO_2 · hr^{-1})		Reference[a]
	per dm² leaf area	per g dry weight	
2. Tundra deciduous dwarf shrubs			
Rubus chamaemorus	17	—	Grace and Marks, 1973
	5	—	Johansson et al., 1972
	15	—	Kostytschew et al., 1930
Salix arctica	16	25	Shvetsova and Voznessenskii, 1971
S. herbacea	18	30	Cartellieri, 1940
S. pulchra	25	—	Tieszen, 1975
Vaccinium uliginosum	—	3	Hadley and Bliss, 1964
Betula nana	5	11	Shvetsova and Voznessenskii, 1971
	7	—	Johansson, et al. 1972
3. Tundra evergreen dwarf shrubs			
Calluna vulgaris	4	5	Grace and Marks, 1973; Grace and Woolhouse, 1970
Diapensia lapponica	—	2	Hadley and Bliss, 1964
Dryas integrifolia	—	4.2	Mayo, 1973
D. punctata	9	9	Shvetsova and Voznssenskii, 1971
Empetrum eamesii spp. hermaphroditum	—	2	Hadley and Bliss, 1964
Ledum groenlandicum	—	2	Hadley and Bliss, 1964
Loiseleuria procumbens	—	0.8	Hadley and Bliss, 1964
Rhododendron lapponicum	—	1.3	Hadley and Bliss, 1964
Vaccinium vitis ideae	—	2	Hadley and Bliss, 1964
	5	3	Shvetsova and Voznessenskii, 1971
4. Evergreen broad leaved trees			
Sun leaves	10–16	6–10	
Shade leaves	3–8	—	
5. Semiarid sclerophyllous shrubs	4–12	4–6	
6. Evergreen conifers	4–12	3–15	

[a]Where not cited, data are adapted from Šesták, Jarvis, and Čatský, 1971.

alps (Cartellieri, 1940). Differences are apparent, however, among the life forms we have identified (Table 2).

The plants with the highest rates are generally graminoids where Tieszen (1973) also suggests a positive correlation with aboveground growth rates. Although there are marked species differences, these tundra graminoids are certainly within the range of comparable C_3 herbs. At least some nongraminoids also possess high maximal rates, although the reported values show a greater variability, as for example with *Oxyria*. These two forms may also differ in their seasonal patterns as most of the graminoids are characterized by a rapid leaf turnover – hence a short period within which the maximum for a leaf is even attainable.

Although we have indicated that plants with persistent leaves have an interception advantage early in the season, it appears that these species have had to compensate for maintaining leaves with extended lifetimes by sacrificing high rates of CO_2 uptake. With the possible exceptions of *Calluna* and *Dryas* it appears that the reduction in CO_2 uptake has been greater than in other sclerophyllous shrubs. As Courtin and Mayo (in Part III, this volume) indicate, this reduction is at least accounted for in part by increased leaf resistances which result in lower rates of transpiration and adaptations to moisture stress. These modifications of increased stomatal and cuticular resistances even though conferring lower photosynthetic capacities may be necessary to curb desication injury during the winter, early spring, and especially late summer.

It has been suggested that deciduous shrubs possess lower rates than herbs (Hadley and Bliss, 1964; Shvetsova and Voznessenskii, 1971); however, our data (Tieszen, 1972a, 1975) indicate that at Barrow, rates for *Salix pulchra* (a deciduous shrub) were considerably higher than the photosynthetic rates of the dominant herbaceous monocotyledons, *Dupontia fischeri, Carex aquatilis*, and *Eriophorum angustifolium*. A comparison of the few data available suggests that rates of tundra dwarf shrubs are comparable to other broad-leaved woody plants.

Several investigators (Mooney and Billings, 1961; Billings *et al.*, 1971; Tieszen and Bonde, 1967) who examined responses of arctic and alpine species populations grown under controlled environment conditions have observed higher photosynthetic rates in arctic plants. The differential response was amplified if the representative plants were grown at colder temperatures. Mooney and Johnson (1965) likewise concluded that genetic differentiation in photosynthetic capacity was apparent; however, their data indicated that the alpine population of *Thalictrum alpinum* possessed higher photosynthetic rates than the arctic population when grown under the same conditions. Clear distinctions between maximal rates of arctic and alpine plants are not found although ecotypic and acclimation responses have been established.

Allocation and Patterns of CO$_2$ Uptake. The different patterns of allocation in combination with differing maximal rates could result in strongly different productivities and patterns of seasonal CO$_2$ uptake. We suggest that graminoids rely to a large extent on current photosynthate to provide for leaf turnover whereas nongraminoids presumably mobilize a larger reserve for rapid but perhaps discontinuous leaf production. Therefore, graminoid forms reinvest heavily in leaf allocation and represent very productive communities with high rates of total community CO$_2$ uptake. As Figure 3 indicates maximum biomass is attained well after senescence has developed as indicated by chlorophyll deterioration (Tieszen, 1972a). Shrubs invest more heavily in structural tissue as indicated by the 30% allocation to wood in *Calluna* (Grace and Woolhouse, 1973) and presumably possess lower productivities unless this is overcome by advantages accruing to their being evergreens.

Net photosynthetic rates at any time during the season also vary as a function of leaf elongation, maturation, and senescence with the highest rates generally associated with a fully elongated leaf. Tieszen and Johnson's (in preparation) seasonal patterns in leaf photosynthesis indicate that a developmental senescence is common in the Arctic even though the growing season is short. In both *Alopecurus alpinus* and *Dupontia*

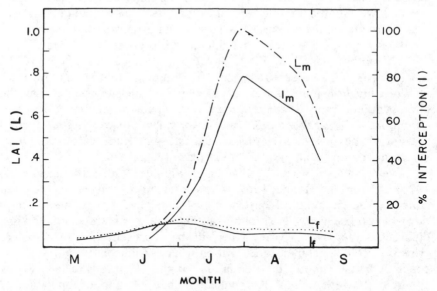

Figure 3 Seasonal development of leaf area index (L), and interception efficiency (I), at Barrow meadow (m) and Devon Island fellfield (f) sites. (Data from Tieszen, 1972a; Svoboda, 1972; in Lewis and Callaghan, 1975).

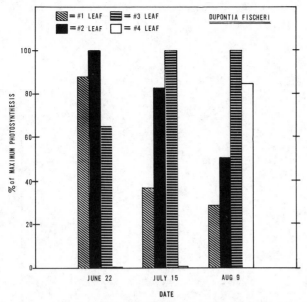

Figure 4 Seasonal trend in photosynthesis of individual leaves of *Dupontia fischeri* under field conditions at Barrow, Alaska.

fischeri, photosynthetic rates were higher in the first two exserted leaves in the season, but leaves produced later assumed higher rates as the season progressed, while in the older leaves photosynthesis decreased (Figure 4). Older portions of the shrubby species *Ledum groenlandicum* and *Vaccinium vitis-idaea* var. *minus* exhibited lower photosynthetic rates than new material (Hadley and Bliss, 1964) and similar results were determined for *Calluna vulgaris* (Grace and Woolhouse, 1970). In these species, however, the leaf period of maximal photosynthesis is extended.

The net effect for Barrow graminoids is that at any time there exists a population of elongating (less than fully competent), mature (photosynthetically competent), and senescent leaves. Thus on a whole plant basis and in a progressively deteriorating environment the predicted daily maxima and totals of photosynthesis decrease through the season (Figure 5). The total community uptake, however, continues to increase due principally to increased interception efficiency (Figure 6) and is responsible for substantial CO_2 uptake even after allocation to leaves has ceased.

The Effect of Light on Photosynthetic Rates of Tundra Plants. The evolution of arctic species under continuous light throughout the major

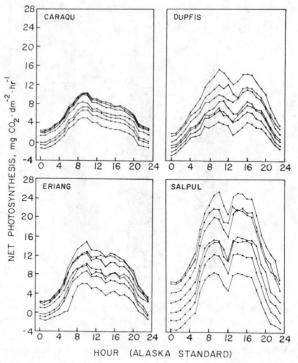

HOUR (ALASKA STANDARD)

Figure 5 The multiple regression simulated seasonal course of daily patterns of whole plant CO_2 exchange in a common arctic wet tundra species, *Carex aquatilis, Dupontia fischeri, Eriophorum angustifolium,* and *Salix pulchra.* Radiation, temperature, time of day, and day of season were all highly significant. Daily courses represent simulated values for 10-day periods from the initiation of the season (top curve) to the end of August (bottom curve).

portion of the growing season is reflected by the ability to photosynthesize and translocate continuously. Net photosynthesis in a number of plants remains positive throughout the 24-hr light period (Pisek, 1960; Billings and Mooney, 1968; Tieszen, 1973, 1975; Mayo *et al.*, 1972), and thus net daily photosynthesis can be substantial despite the characteristic low light intensities. The absolute values of CO_2 uptake vary among arctic species, but in general, responses to light and temperature are similar, and CO_2 uptake appears to be most strongly coupled to radiation intensity (Tieszen, 1973; Shvetsova and Voznessenskii, 1971) as suggested by the *sine* relationship in Figure 5. Thus the highest rates of photosynthesis are observed during the day and lowest near solar midnight. Deviations from this typical wet meadow pattern occur in *Dryas* in which large "midday" depressions in CO_2 uptake may develop

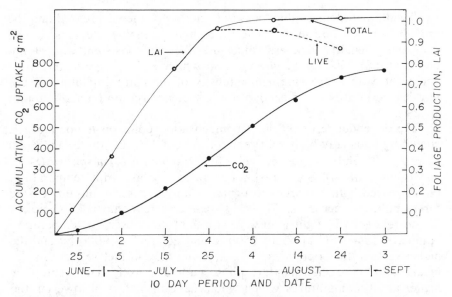

Figure 6 Community accumulation of CO_2 during the growing season and its relationship to live and dead leaf area index. The curve
represents the summation of estimated uptake rates from all vascular plants.

due to heat stress and lower photosynthetic potentials. On cool days,
however, the patterns are similar.

Low light compensation points appear to be advantageous in arctic
species since the range of positive photosynthetic gain is extended.
Compensation points *in situ* were 0.013 J · m^{-2} · min^{-1} for *Carex aquatilis* and *Eriophorum angustifolium*, 0.20 J · m^{-2} · min^{-1} for *Salix pulchra*, 0.024 J · m^{-2} · min^{-1} for *Dupontia fischeri* (Tieszen, 1975) and
less than 0.044 J · m^{-2} · min^{-1} for *Dryas integrifolia* (Mayo *et al.*, 1972).
Since compensation points are low it has been suggested that CO_2 assimilation may take place under snow cover and Mayo *et al.* (1972) cite
data of O'Neil and Gray which showed light intensities as high as 0.06
J · m^{-2} · min^{-1} under 6 cm of snow, or well above reported compensation
points. Mayo *et al.* (1972) suggest such early development and photosynthesis may occur in *Dryas integrifolia;* however, Tieszen has indicated
photosynthetic activity does not take place before snow melt at Barrow.

The low compensation points and low a:b ratios suggest an adaptation to low light intensities as in the case of *Solidago virgaurea*
(Holmgren, 1968). Tieszen's laboratory data (Tieszen and Bonde, 1967)
for alpine and arctic ecotypes of *Deschampsia caespitosa* and *Trisetum
spicatum* support this presumed general adaptations to light intensity.

Leaf width and density thickness (wt · area^{-1}) values decreased and the growth form became more prostrate as light intensities decreased. The decreasing density thickness values are likewise consistent with Holmgren's (1968) data for *S. virgaurea* in which leaf mesophyll thickness decreased with decreasing light intensity of the natural habitats. These physical responses could account for low compensation points in tundra species.

The dependence of the light compensation point on temperature is shown by unusually high light requirements of 130 fc, 700 fc, and 4000 fc at 0°, 20°, and 25°, respectively, for *Deschampsia caespitosa* (Scott and Billings, 1964). Since respiration rates increase with temperature, the increased light requirement is presumably necessary to compensate for respiratory increases. Similarly, temperature compensation points are correlated with light intensity. Moser (1969) observed temperature optima of 15°–19°C at about 6500 fc and 20°–24° at 9000 fc; and the higher temperature optima for alpine plants may in fact reflect this dependence. On the other hand, respiratory rates of arctic plants tend to be higher at all temperatures which would have the effect of lowering the temperature optimum of photosynthesis. Light saturation rates are likewise temperature dependent and perhaps low saturated rates at low temperatures are due to assimilate accumulation.

The light saturation values also reflect the respective light environment differences under which arctic and alpine plant evolution has taken place (Björkman and Holmgren, 1963). Alpine plants typically have higher light saturation values than arctic plants (Cartellieri, 1940; Mooney and Billings, 1961). Maximum photosynthetic rates of six alpine species were observed at the highest experimental intensity of 12,000 fc (Scott and Billings, 1964). Moser (1969) likewise reported *Ranunculus glacialis* and *Geum reptans* increased photosynthesis with increasing intensities up to about 7000 fc. An exception to higher alpine saturation rates appears to occur in Mount Washington species in which saturation values are between 2000 to 3200 fc (Hadley and Bliss, 1964), a range near reported arctic values of about 4000 fc (Tieszen, 1973). The eastern United States alpine region is characterized by frequent periods of low light intensity, and the environmental similarities result in closer affinities to arctic plant responses.

Although the absolute importance of light and temperature as rate-controlling factors is difficult to establish *in situ*, the extensive analyses of temperature and light on photosynthesis rates led Scott and Billings (1964) to the conclusion that light was the major rate determining factor below 25°C in six alpine plants, whereas at higher temperatures the temperature effect was more substantial. Multivariate analysis of rate-deter-

mining factors in production of Barrow plants indicated that a large proportion of the variance in photosynthetic rates (Tieszen, 1975) could be
accounted for by light and temperature. It appears that tundra plants are
sufficiently well adapted to the low thermal environment to optimize for
radiant energy and hence are usually closely coupled to irradiance.

   *The Effect of Temperature on Photosynthetic Rates of Tundra
Plants.*   Low temperatures must impose one of the greatest stresses and
selective pressures on tundra plants, and adaptations reflecting this extreme should be evident in photosynthetic processes. However, as a
result of natural diurnal radiation and temperature patterns most tundra
species experience a wide range of tissue temperatures (Tranquillini,
1964; Mayo *et al.,* 1972; Warren-Wilson, 1957) rather than the consistently low temperatures expressed by mean air temperature data. Furthermore, the low growth stature of tundra plants in combination with
persistent standing dead material reduces convective and advective heat
losses thereby enhancing the maintenance of high leaf temperatures.
Moser (1969) reports leaf temperature variation in alpine populations of
−11° to +33° throughout the growing season and temperatures as great
as 22°C above air temperature have been observed in the Colorado alpine (Salisbury and Spomer, 1964). Mayo *et al.* (1972) measured a value
of 39°C for *Dryas integrifolia* and report that values can frequently be
30°C above ambient. In contrast, grass species in wet meadow sites
appear closely coupled to air temperature and vary by only 2°−3°C.
Warren-Wilson (1957) suggests that leaf orientation for radiation interception is more important in maintaining higher leaf temperatures than
for optimal light absorption for photosynthesis, and the importance of
other structural features which presumably confer "heat trapping" capabilities has been suggested frequently (e.g., Krog, 1955).
   Tundra plants maintain positive photosynthetic rates over a wide
range of temperatures. Net positive photosynthesis has been observed in
Dryas integrifolia at +1°C (Mayo *et al.,* 1972); and Tieszen (1973) reports substantial positive rates in all grasses tested at 0°C. Rates as high
as 23 mg $CO_2 \cdot dm^{-2} \cdot hr^{-1}$ were recorded (Tieszen, 1975) for *Salix
pulchra* at 3°C demonstrating that near maximal photosynthetic rates
can be attained at low temperatures and substantiating Warren-Wilson's
observation that photosynthesis is very temperature dependent near
0°C. Photosynthesis is frequently active as long as the leaf is not frozen.
Lower temperature compensation points for *Geum reptans* and *Ranunculus glacialis* are −3° and −5°C, respectively (Moser, 1969), and Pisek
et al. (1967) report a similar compensation value of −5°C for *Oxyria digyna.* Upper temperature compensation points of 40°C for these same

species have been reported by Moser (1969); and Tieszen's (1973) data confirm those of Zalenskii et al. (1972) and Shvetsova and Voznessenskii (1971) for the Arctic which show positive CO_2 uptake at 35°C (Figure 7) a temperature about 10°C higher than is attained on days of high radiation loads and low convective losses. These leaf data represent higher cardinal temperatures than are obtained with whole plants presumably due to greater respiratory sources from whole plants. Kallio and Kärenlampi (1975) indicate a similarly wide tolerance range for lichens and mosses, and in these groups reactivation following freezing occurs more rapidly.

Temperature optima for photosynthesis range between 10° and 20°C with a tendency for optima of arctic species to be on the lower end of this range, i.e., some 5°–10°C below their alpine counterparts (Billings et al., 1971). Temperature optima for leaves are on the low end of the range for C_3 plants and, as indicated above, in the arctic wet meadows, optima occur at temperatures generally higher than the mean air or leaf maxima (Zalenskii et al., 1972; Tieszen, 1973). Field data on whole plants (Tieszen, 1972c, 1974; Mayo et al., 1972) suggest lower optima than the above leaf-determined optima, and at least where plants are not water stressed optima are lower due to the greater respiratory component.

In addition to wide temperature tolerance there is evidence that widely distributed species have undergone genetic differentiation in response to selection by local environments. Differences in photosynthetic and respiratory responses to temperature in arctic and alpine populations as well as differential acclimation potential among populations appears to be genetically based. Populations of arctic species consistently have lower photosynthetic temperature optima than alpine populations when grown under controlled environmental conditions (Mooney and Billings, 1961; Mooney and Johnson, 1965; Billings et al., 1971), and optima are lower in alpine species than for species from lower elevations (Mooney et al., 1964). Billings et al. (1971) found the differences were accentuated when the plants were grown under "cold acclimation" conditions.

It is still not known if these shifts represent basic adaptive responses in the photosynthetic system or whether they result from the higher respiratory output which would shift the optimum for net CO_2 to lower temperatures. Billings et al. (1971) demonstrated differential acclimatory behavior among populations of Oxyria digyna similar to that reported by Mooney and West (1964). Photosynthetic rates were higher at lower temperatures for arctic populations grown under "arctic" and "alpine" growth regimes; however, rates of arctic plants decreased at higher temperatures under both growth conditions. Alpine plants had lower temperature optima and upper temperature compensation points when grown under "arctic" conditions, but shifted these points to higher temperatures when grown under "alpine" conditions. Thus photosynthetic rates did not decrease with the warm treatment, as in arctic plants. This greater flexibility or adaptability to changing environments is consistent with the more variable environmental conditions of alpine regions.

Metabolic acclimation suggests alterations of enzymatic processes, and it would be reasonable to anticipate enzymatic differentiation fundamental to any ecotypic variation in a major biochemical pathway. In fact, McNaughton (1967) has demonstrated the existence of climatic ecotypes which differ in enzymatic properties. Warm and cool source populations of *Typha latifolia* grown under controlled environment conditions differed in glycolic acid oxidase (GAO) activity. The population adapted to cooler environment had a Q_{10} between 17° and 27°C of 1.4 whereas the population from the warmer site had a Q_{10} of 3.7. Further, the activity of GAO in the warm population continued to increase when temperature was increased to 37°C whereas the enzyme activity decreased with temperature increase above 27°C in the cool site individuals. In a later study (McNaughton, 1969) GAO activity in warm and cool site populations was shown to differ when plants were acclimated in a cool/long-photoperiod versus a warm/shorter-photoperiod regime. The cool-site individuals showed highest activity under longer photoperiodic conditions whereas higher GAO activity was observed for warm site individuals when grown under warm/short-photoperiod conditions.

Even though the GAO response indicates differential protein synthesis in response to temperature environments, very different responses were noted for other enzymes. McNaughton (1966) noted acclimation activity only in malate dehydrogenase (MDH) where the warm site individuals remained relatively unaffected upon 30-min exposure to a temperature of 50°C, whereas approximately 80% inhibition was noted in enzyme extracts from cool-site species for the same treatment. The effect of heat treatment on glutamate oxaloacetate transaminase (GOT) was similar for both populations, and no significant thermolability was observed. Conversely, aldolase activity decreased rapidly and synchronously with almost total inactivation for extracts from both populations occurring within 20 min. These data suggest differential enzyme stabilities and acclimation responses and are significant in demonstrating that enzyme balance can be radically and differentially altered by changes in only one or a few enzymes. It is therefore probable that equilibrium relationships in metabolic pathways could likewise be substantially altered between populations.

The above shifts in temperature optima upon acclimation have been convincingly demonstrated, and several studies suggested that the temperature response of RuDP carboxylase is related to whole leaf photosynthetic responses (Treharne and Cooper, 1969). Phillips and McWilliam (1971) suggested that the alpine *Caltha intraloba* possessed a thermolabile RuDP carboxylase which accounted for loss of photosynthetic capability above 35°C. Tieszen and Sigurdson (1973) showed a lability of the extracted enzyme but a stability *in vivo* to temperatures greater than 40°C. Similarly, reaction optima (Figure 7) were 50° for three arctic species, agreeing with the 45°C optimum reported for *Oxyria* (Chabot *et al.*, 1972). The temperature response curves for photosynthesis are, therefore, not associated with coincident shifts in enzymatic temperature responses and in fact the enzymes appear stable to temperatures substantially higher than those encountered in nature.

The concentration of the carboxylating enzyme is under both genetic and developmental control as shown for *Oxyria* where activity was increased by growth at low temperatures. Alpine populations possessed more plasticity, perhaps a reflection of the greater environmental fluc-

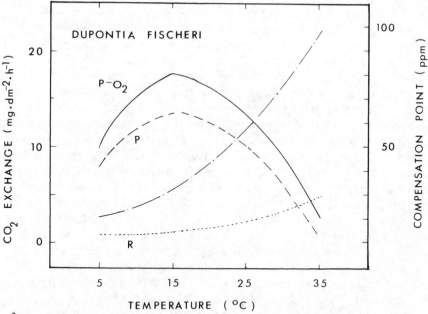

Figure 7a Temperature responses of photosynthetic rates and related processes in *Dupontia fischeri* from Barrow, Alaska. Net photosynthesis (P), photosynthesis near 0% O_2 (P–O_2), dark respiration (R), and CO_2 compensation concentrations (dash-dot line).

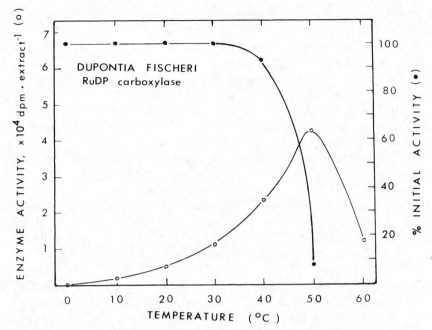

Figure 7b Enzymatic activities (o) and stabilities (●) were determined on young expanded leaves grown under field conditions. Data from Tieszen, 1973, and Tieszen and Sigurdson, 1973. Stability was determined for 30-min exposures of whole leaves.

tuations (Chabot *et al.*, 1972). Phillips and McWilliam (1971) also hypothesized activation energies to be lower for plants from colder climates. However, activation energies for *Oxyria digyna* remained similar in all populations and growth regimes were higher than those reported for *Caltha* (Chabot *et al.*, 1972), and were in the range (13.1 – 14.5 kcal · mole⁻¹) calculated from Tieszen and Sigurdson (1973). It is obvious that more detailed data on *in vivo* and *in vitro* responses of RuDP carboxylase activity are needed.

In addition to differentiation at the enzymatic level, Billings *et al.*, (1971) noted a photoperiodic response in Hill activity and ecotypic differentiation with regard to this response among populations of *Oxyria digyna* similar to that shown for *Typha* (McNaughton, 1966, 1967). Under 14-hr photoperiods, cold acclimation resulted in higher photochemical activity in alpine populations but depressed rates in arctic populations. Warm acclimation, however, resulted in little change in either population. When plants were cultured under a 20-hr photoperiod, however, cold acclimation resulted in enhanced Hill activity in both arctic and alpine populations. Tieszen and Helgager (1968) likewise demonstrated light reaction differences between arctic and alpine ecotypes of *Deschampsia caespitosa*. The temperature optimum for the Hill reaction was 20°C in the arctic population and 25°–30°C in the alpine population. No shift in the temperature optimum for this reaction was noted in arctic individuals in response to three differing growth conditions, whereas alpine plants had a lower optimum when grown at 10°C than when grown either under 22°/10° (16-hr thermoperiod) or 22° (continuous). Again, genetic differentiation is apparent and alpine populations reveal greater acclimation capabilities.

Variations in responses of respiration to temperature appear to be less under genetic than environmental control (Billings *et al.*, 1971) and in general rates tend to increase similarly in arctic and alpine populations in response to increasing temperature. Ecotypic differences between arctic and alpine populations have been suggested by Mooney and Billings (1961) who observed higher respiration rates in arctic populations of *Oxyria digyna* and higher Q_{10} values. Similar data were reported for *Trisetum spicatum* (Clebsch, 1960). However, virtually no differences in temperature response were noted among six Wyoming alpine plants; respiration increased slowly from 0° to 10°C and a slightly greater linear increase from 10° to 30° was observed (Scott and Billings, 1964). Billings *et al.*, (1971) found little variation in respiration rates among 17 populations from differing latitudinal and altitudinal sources and Scholander and Kanwisher (1959) surveyed nine species from northern and southern tundra populations and observed higher rates in only two of the species.

Although there appears to be little variation in respiratory responses among herbaceous tundra species, rates tend to be higher than rates for temperate and tropical species, and thus may be a response to low temperatures. Billings and Mooney (1968) reported that rates for alpine plants were higher than for comparable lowland individuals. Mitochondrial oxidation increased in populations of *Sitanion hystrix* with increasing source elevation (Klikoff, 1966), and Billings *et al.* (1971) observed that mitochondrial oxidative activity increased in both alpine and arctic populations of *Oxyria digyna*, with rates increasing to a somewhat greater extent in the arctic population. Growth temperatures for tundra species affect respiration rates, with higher growth regime temperatures resulting in lower respiration rates (Billings *et al.*, 1971; Tieszen, in preparation). These differences are apparently associated with differences in oxidative activity and not qualitative changes in pathways or enzymes.

Soil temperatures in the Arctic are rarely above 5°C at 15 cm, and decrease to 1°–2° at night when radiation is less intense, although fluctuations in temperature near the surface can be considerably greater. Thus differences between leaf and root temperature can be considerable. Experiments with beans (Brouwer, 1964) and corn (Kleinendorst and Brouwer, 1970) indicated that the difference between growing point and root temperature can influence plant growth responses and that decreasing root temperatures could severely affect plant growth. Effects of low soil temperature on photosynthesis and other growth processes have not as yet been conducted, but could provide informative insights into tundra adaptations, as indicated by McCown (Part III, this volume).

Photosynthesis and Moisture Relations. Soil moisture availability and differential plant sensitivities to moisture conditions are important in species distribution and can determine community patterns in arctic and alpine regions. At Barrow, the most productive areas are correlated with wet sites where almost pure swards of *Dupontia fischeri, Carex aquatilis,* or *Arctophila fulva* develop. Raised polygonal areas and old beach ridges are windswept, and thus evaporative stress may be greater and in part responsible for lower productivity. Recovery to leaf water potentials less negative than −1 bar have been observed in Barrow monocots and recovery patterns do not appear to be much different from open-site temperate species (unpublished data). Thus it appears that water uptake is not severely impaired in arctic plants in cold soils; however, further experimentation is needed to document more conclusively that H_2O uptake occurs efficiently at low soil temperatures.

Differential transpiration responses may imply photosynthetic consequences since increasing leaf resistance, although having a greater effect upon transpiration, can result in a reduction of photosynthesis. Higher transpiration rates have been noted in wet-site alpine species than in drier sites (Mooney et al., 1965). Stomatal sensitivity likewise appeared to be greater in these species since midday transpiration depressions were observed coincident with high radiation load. The plants on scree and rock plateaus showed greater transpiration control since transpiration rates were somewhat lower and depressions were not frequently evident. Tranquillini (1964) likewise found snow bank species (wet site) to have less stomatal control and thus more negative osmotic potentials developed. Scree species again showed greater control, and less negative osmotic potentials were maintained despite the drier site conditions. Similarly, Klikoff's data (1965) showed that photosynthesis declined with decreasing moisture potentials and that this decline in wet-site species was initiated at less negative (higher) water potentials than in dry-site species. It therefore appears that species which have evolved tolerance ranges which include dry sites have also evolved photosynthetic mechanisms which are less sensitive to decreasing water availability as well as a greater stomatal control for the maintenance of water status within tolerance limits.

Photosynthesis and Carbon Dioxide. It has been suggested that the decreasing partial pressure of CO_2 with increasing altitude may be responsible for depressed photosynthetic rates and stunted growth forms of alpine plants. The work of Billings *et al.* (1961) with an arctic sea level population and an alpine population from about 6000 m of *Oxyria digyna* suggested adaptations of alpine plants to reduced CO_2 partial pressures. Throughout the range of CO_2 concentrations investigated alpine populations of *Oxyria digyna* had consistently higher photosynthetic rates and, in addition, showed a lower CO_2 compensation point. At partial pressures corresponding to 3000 m, photosynthesis of the arctic sea level plants was 70% of alpine plant photosynthesis, and at partial pressures corresponding to 12,200 m, arctic plants showed no net assimilation, whereas alpine plants exhibited positive photosynthetic rates. However, several other investigations, notably Decker's (1959) work with *Mimulus* and Mooney *et al.* (1964, 1966) found no adaptations to decreasing CO_2 concentration and, furthermore, indicated that zonation was not correlated with differences in photosynthetic efficiencies of plants in low CO_2 environments. Thus, although there has been a suggestion of more efficient photosynthesis in some alpine species at the lower CO_2 concentrations characteristic of alpine environments the mechanistic basis has not been proposed and the generality of the response is doubtful.

Gale (1972) discussed the availability of CO_2 at high altitudes and suggested that effects of decreasing concentrations could theoretically result in much less photosynthetic inhibition than expected because of the compensating effect of increased diffusivity of CO_2 at lower pressures. The diffusivity change would be reflected primarily in stomatal resistance (r_s) and to a lesser extent in the boundary layer resistance values (r_a). The mesophyll resistance (r_m) would remain unchanged as partial pressure changed, since the effect of this resistance is in the liquid phase and is unaffected by gaseous diffusivity changes. Gale demonstrates the ratio of $(r_a + r_s)/r_m$ would be a decisive factor in the degree to which changing CO_2 partial pressures would affect photosynthetic rates. Species with low r_m, e.g., C_4 species, showed little effect of changing partial pressures. Greater effect would be expected in C_3 species with higher r_m values, although in both cases photosynthetic effects are less dramatic than if one considered the resistances to remain constant and the change in carbon dioxide concentration gradient to be the sole determining factor.

The species characteristic of alpine tundra are C_3 species, and apparently there has not been a selection in favor of species possessing obviously lower compensation values. Thus, factors other than CO_2 partial pressure exert greater selection pressure, and adaptive responses are more evident with regard to light and temperature than to the carbon dioxide environment. Perhaps the same is correct with respect to O_2, since the reduction in partial pressure should not affect mitochondrial respiration; however, photorespiration and oxygen inhibition should be significantly reduced.

Photosynthesis and Mineral Nutrients. The segregation of species into community types (Webber, 1972) indicates adaptations at the species level to changes in moisture conditions but, possibly, also to nutrient and other soil factors. Unfortunately, our understanding of tundra plant – nutrient relationships has not extended far beyond an assessment of responses to nutrient additions. Tundra soils are apparently low in nitrogen (Warren-Wilson, 1957; Callaghan and Lewis, 1971), especially in the nitrate form, and phosphorus (Babb, 1972); and a common response to added nutrients is increased production of at least some species. Preliminary studies at Barrow (McCown and Tieszen, 1972; Miller, 1972) indicate a high degree of tolerance in the photosynthesis mechanism, and it appears that the greatest effect of nutrients on each species is exerted by the control of allocation rather than carboxylation activity. Among species we could expect fundamental differences in the process of photosynthesis related to nutrient status.

Internal Factors Governing Rates of CO_2 Exchange

Boundary Layer and Stomatal Resistances. Photosynthesis can be considered as a net flux which is dependent upon a potential differential across a series of resistances:

$$P_{net} = \frac{CO_{2,\,air} - CO_{2,\,chl}}{r_a + r_s + r_w + r_x}$$

where $CO_{2,\,air}$ = carbon dioxide concentration in air; $CO_{2,\,chl}$ = carbon dioxide concentration at the carboxylation site; r_s = resistance to CO_2 diffusion associated with the stomates; r_a = resistance to CO_2 diffusion associated with the leaf boundary layer; r_w = resistance associated with CO_2 diffusion from the intercellular space through the mesophyll cell to the carboxylation site; and r_x = carboxylation "resistance."

Although only a few measurements are available which allow one to calculate all resistance components, some general inferences can be drawn. Boundary layer resistance (r_a) is basically a function of leaf dimension and wind speed. At Barrow in wet meadows the combination of the high wind and thin narrow leaves results in values of r_a which are on the order of 0,25–0.5 sec · cm^{-1} or quite low relative to other components. In combination with the generally low radiation load, one would expect leaf temperatures to be close to air temperatures. Numerous measurements at Barrow have verified this coupling. In the alpine, plants with similarly low boundary layer resistances may possess higher leaf temperatures due to the increased irradiance. The development of broader leaves would increase r_a and in combination with a cushion habit or other protection from wind could result in substantially higher leaf temperatures as reported by Mayo et al. (1972).

Any modification resulting in decreased diffusion resistances could result in higher photosynthetic rates. Diffusion resistances associated with the stomates and boundary layer ($r_l = r_a + r_s$) for dominant Barrow monocots tend to be low, e.g., between 0.5 and 3 sec · cm^{-1} at saturating light intensities. Values reported for the alpine are of the same order (Ehleringer, 1973) or somewhat higher where greater amounts of material were included. These data suggest that r_l is not the major resistance determining maximal rates of exchange since it is generally smaller than the remaining resistance terms and cannot be reduced to much lower levels. Although the low values of r_l help account for the relatively high rates of photosynthesis, we feel that changes in r_l are more important in governing the actual daily and seasonal courses. The depressions in photosynthesis discussed earlier (Mayo et al., 1972; Tieszen, 1972c; Shvetsova and Voznessenskii, 1971) could result from stomatal closure due to low water potentials which may develop seasonally and daily during times of water stress as indicated by Ehleringer (1973). Depressions of net CO_2 uptake caused by a temperature stimulated dark respiration in the light would be seen as an increase in the residual resistance. The unpublished data from Barrow wet meadows suggest that both resistances increase at high temperatures. Similar data from Mayo's Dryas plants would be very informative.

"Mesophyll" Resistance.   The residual resistance ($r_m = r_w + r_x$) which includes diffusion of CO_2 through the mesophyll cell to the carboxylation site, the "resistance" associated with CO_2 fixation itself, and the effect of respiratory sources of CO_2, is on the order of three to ten times greater than r_l (Tieszen, 1973) and therefore is the most significant component determining rates under optimal conditions. Although there is considerable controversy concerning the components of this resistance, leaf structural features could be important. Shu-Fun Au (1969) noted leaf morphological differences between arctic sea level and alpine populations (approximately 2100 m) of *Oxyria digyna* which appear to correlate with higher photosynthetic rates of the alpine population under lower CO_2 concentrations thereby indicating a greater carboxylation efficiency. Approximately 40% of the cell area was in the paradermal section of leaves from both populations but the number of cells was approximately three times greater in the alpine population. Thus the surface area to volume ratio was greatly increased, resulting in an increase in internal surface area ratio, a response similar to that suggested by Slatyer (1967) for xerophytic plants. Presumably this would facilitate exchange of CO_2 and would be reflected in a reduction of r_m. This enhanced ability to assimilate CO_2 could compensate for higher stomatal resistances and should be adaptive in alpine plants which are exposed to higher radiation loads and thus increased water balance problems. Similarly, at higher elevations where CO_2 partial pressures are lower, any decrease in r_m would reduce the effect of the smaller gradient of CO_2. These speculations, however, require documentation of resistance values in arctic and alpine plants, and to date, these data are unavailable.

It is interesting that similar morphological differences were noted among triploid arctic and diploid arctic and alpine populations of *Thalictrum alpinum* (Mooney and Johnson, 1965). The triploid individuals and alpine individuals had higher photosynthetic rates than individuals from the diploid arctic population. Both the triploid arctic and alpine plants were found to have a greater number of smaller mesophyll cells and smaller stomates. However, stomatal area of the arctic populations was approximately equivalent and it is suggested the enhanced CO_2 exchange was due to a decrease in r_m. Although there has been some controversy over the significance of the increasing incidence of polyploidy in arctic regions, certainly in the case of *Thalictrum alpinum* a potential adaptive advantage of the triploid is demonstrated. However, the generality of this statement cannot be made especially since cell size usually increases rather than decreases with ploidy.

Tieszen's comparison (1970) of arctic and alpine grasses suggested that the arctic plants possessed less structural tissue than similar alpine species. This presumed adaptation or response to low light and temperature would tend to increase photosynthetic efficiency, would decrease the relative dark respiration component and should result in lower light intensity compensation points for arctic plants. The net effect on r_m, however, could be variable.

One of the components of the mesophyll resistance is imposed by the chemical fixation reaction, and although there is considerable controversy concerning the causal relationship between carboxylation enzyme

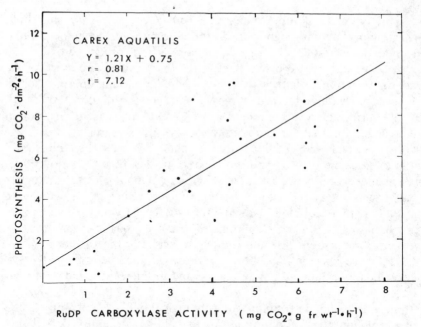

Figure 8 Correlation between the seasonal course of photosynthesis and carboxylation activity in all leaves of *Carex aquatilis*.

concentrations and photosynthetic activity, our data support the contention of Treharne (1972) that RuDP carboxylase constitutes a significant rate-controlling factor in the overall process of assimilation. Among all species tested at Barrow, a high correlation ($r = 0.76$) between photosynthesis and enzymatic activity existed. Also our recent data (Figure 8) indicate that both enzymatic and photosynthetic activity increase with leaf expansion and exsertion, attain maxima at comparable times, and decrease as senescence occurs. These strong seasonal correlations at least suggest that the seasonal course of potential photosynthesis in single leaves is determined by concentrations of carboxylation enzymes. In the absence of established causality, we still cannot conclude that the genetic and acclimatory responses reported for tundra plants (Chabot *et al.*, 1972) confer adaptive significance with respect to CO_2 uptake.

Respiratory Sources. An additional component of the internal resistances is that added by the light and dark respiratory sources. The pattern of photorespiration inferred from Tieszen's data (1973) suggests that the response is not grossly different from that reported for other species. Oxygen inhibition is closely coupled to photosynthesis even at high temperatures which suggests that if photorespiration has a temperature dependence comparable to that of dark respiration the oxygen data must be interpreted to indicate a primary effect on inhibition of photosynthesis rather than on respiration. If CO_2 compensation data are taken as our best measure of respiration in the light, we do show a distinct temperature dependency (Figure 7) of this process. The net effect is rather low (around 15 ppm) compensation concentrations at the low environmental temperatures. Thus, the ability of these plants to continue photosynthesis at very low temperatures is enhanced by an increase in the retention of assimilated CO_2 since light stimulated CO_2 loss is operating at a reduced level.

McNaughton (1969) has suggested that the high rates of photosynthesis in *Typha* result from an adaptation to reduce photorespiratory losses. Additionally, he has shown genetic differences and responses of potential significance in *Typha*. Populations from warm sites showed higher activity of glycolic acid oxidase (GAO) when grown under warm growth conditions, whereas greater activity in species from natural habitats characterized by shorter growing seasons was evident when grown experimentally under long photoperiod/cool temperature conditions (McNaughton, 1969). It is not known whether GAO activity is similarly affected in other species, but if so, could potentially be important in photosynthetic rates because of implications in the photorespiratory pathway (McNaughton and Fullem, 1970).

Carbohydrate Levels and Translocation. Perhaps one of the key adaptations possessed by tundra plants is the ability to photosynthesize under conditions which result in high carbohydrate levels. Agronomic varieties grown as phytometers in polar regions were shown to be markedly temperature sensitive, to contain higher carbohydrate levels at low temperatures, and to possess high respiration and low photosynthesis rates. Warren-Wilson (1966) has also suggested that assimilation is depressed in the tundra due to an accumulation of carbohydrates which occurs because of the greater temperature dependency of respiration than of photosynthesis. Although Neales and Incoll (1968) conclude that a causal relationship has not been established, it is certainly clear that tundra plants possess high levels of carbohydrates (McCown and Tieszen, 1972; Mooney and Billings, 1960) and that a general response to growth under low temperatures is an increased leaf carbohydrate level (Tieszen and Helgager, 1968) which in some cases results in gross physical alterations of the chloroplasts. If this occurred in tundra plants, it should manifest itself as an increase in mesophyll resistance due to interference with CO_2 transfer or feedback inhibition of photosynthesis reactions. Carboxylation activity, however, could remain high.

Even though carbohydrate levels are high, tundra plants can apparently export photosynthate at high rates at low temperatures (Chabot and Billings, 1972; Tieszen, unpublished; Allessio and Tieszen, 1975). Allessio and Tieszen showed efficient translocation within 24 hr and Tieszen and Johnson's (in preparation) measurements of translocation from restricted areas of leaves (Figure 9) indicate export rates at field temperatures only a few degrees above zero which appear equivalent to those of temperate zone C_3 plants at higher temperatures (Hofstra and Nelson, 1969a,b) although lower than C_4 plants reputed to have high rates of photosynthesis. This high export ability at low temperatures may account, in part, for the utilization of the energy provided by the high concomitant respiratory rates in those plants.

This characteristic stimulation of respiration in plants native or acclimated to low temperatures and the acclimatory shift of the temperature response curve is presumed to be an adaptive response providing more energy at low temperatures. The emphasis on CO_2 uptake, however, has tended to lead some investigators to feel that high respiratory rates are inefficient and are not coupled to the condition of "useful work." Respi-

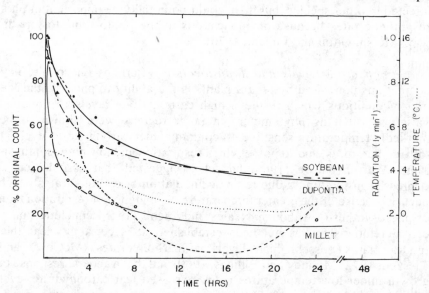

Figure 9 Comparative rates of translocation (export) in a representative temperate zone C_3 plant, a C_4 plant, and in *Dupontia fischeri* in the field at Barrow at the indicated irradiances and temperatures.

ration rates in these plants should generally be considered "useful" even though under stress conditions the energy may be used for cellular repair processes as suggested by Semikhatova (1970). Stressful conditions may simply create new energy requirements. Although Beevers (1970) indicates that an "idling" respiration may exist, he still suggests that respiration is roughly proportional to growth. It has become well established that there are at least two components to mitochondrial respiration, one of which is dependent upon photosynthesis. McCree (1970) indicates that:

$$R = kP + cW$$

where R = respiration rate (mg $CO_2 \cdot m^{-2} \cdot day^{-1}$); P = photosynthesis rate (mg $CO_2 \cdot m^{-2} \cdot day^{-1}$); k = dimensionless constant; c = time^{-1}; and W = plant weight (g $CO_2 \cdot m^{-2}$).

The values for k and c were determined to be 0.25 and 0.015, indicating that 25% of the photosynthate was utilized in respiration. If c is assumed to represent maintenance requirements, the magnitude of this constant should be related to these processes in tundra plants. The magnitude of k may be a direct reflection of loading and unloading photosynthate and the high leaf respiration rates may be a measure of loading costs. It seems of fundamental significance that the magnitude of these constants and their underlying components be determined in tundra plants and acclimatory experiments. Establishment of the functional and adaptive significance of these high respiratory rates at low temperatures should have top priority in further studies.

Summary

1. The floras composing tundra regions consist of species possessing evolutionary characteristics of growth form and physiology which confer certain adaptations and potentials. These species photosynthesize with the C_3 system of carboxylation and thereby reflect selection with respect to low temperatures. Thus, they are characterized by the general responses associated with this pathway. Life forms which stress herbaceous and perennial characteristics also predominate.

2. Although tundras are characterized by a large diversity of environmental extremes, very short growing seasons and generally prevailing low temperatures are characteristic. Adaptations to confer efficient interception are present and include early and rapid leaf exsertion rates by herbaceous plants in wet areas and a tendency to perenniality of photo-

synthetic structures in windblown areas subject to water stress. Most plant parts are chlorophyllous and photosynthetically competent. The dependence of LAI on moisture status indicates canopy adaptations in tundras; and the increase in species with horizontal leaves and high chlorophyll concentrations at the extreme base of the canopy suggests a tendency to maximize light utilization.

3. Tundra species possess maximal rates of photosynthesis under field conditions which are at least comparable to the lower ranges reported for temperate species of a similar life form. Component(s) of the mesophyll resistance are most important in establishing maximal rates and there are positive correlations of CO_2 uptake with the activity of ribulose-1,-5-diphosphate carboxylase. Photosynthesis is active at temperatures higher than tissue freezing points, and at temperatures near 0°C rates may be high. Selection at the carboxylation enzyme level has not been established, although other enzymes and subcellular reactions have shown adaptive capabilities. Adaptations to fairly wide temperature ranges appear common, and the temperature response curve of leaf CO_2 exchange is probably causally related to temperature effects on respiration and water stress.

Polar species have adapted to exploit the continuous irradiation during most of the growing season and therefore accumulate high net daily totals of reduced CO_2. Perhaps a significant and widespread adaptation of polar plants in the ability to translocate efficiently under continuous photoperiods at low temperatures. However, the leaf carbohydrate contents remain high but the potential depression of CO_2 uptake remains to be convincingly established and then mechanistically understood. High rates of mitochondrial respiration are characteristic, and we suggest they represent an adaptive response providing energy for growth and maintenance processes at low temperatures. The specific allocation of this released energy for processes such as phloem loading, growth, and cellular maintenance as well as the efficiency of the energy utilization for these processes at the characteristic low temperature of tundras need to be examined. Although photorespiration is apparent, at the low temperatures its rate appears to be low, thereby providing enhanced efficiency of CO_2 uptake at low temperatures.

4. Four main growth forms and strategies are recognized which possess different patterns of photosynthesis interception and allocation. The established or hypothesized patterns are shown in the following tabulation.

5. Ecotypic differentiation and acclimation responses are well established although field data showing the ultimate significance of seasonal

	Deciduous herbs		Shrubs	
	Graminoid	Nongraminoid	Evergreen	Deciduous
Photosynthetic rates	High	High	Low	Int to high
Leaf resistance	Low	Low	Higher	Low to high
Habitat preference	Wet	Wet to dry	Dry	Wet to dry
Maximum interception	High	Int	Variable	Variable
Seasonality of inter- ception	High	Int	Low	Int
Leaf turnover	High	Int	Low	Int
Aboveground productivity	High	Int	Low	Low
Mobilized reserve	Low	High	Int	High

acclimatization patterns are still needed. There is a tendency for arctic species to possess lower temperature optima and lower light requirements for photosynthesis saturation than for plants from the alpine; and the retention of these characteristics in laboratory studies indicates its genetic basis. Acclimation potential is significant in populations from arctic and alpine areas although it appears to be of greater significance in the more variable alpine environment. This combination of specific genetic potentials and acclimatory abilities has resulted in species which are effective exploiters in tundras and are in some cases unable to compete in more temperate conditions. The underlying mechanisms of these capabilities have not been determined and provide a challenge especially for biochemically and physically oriented ecologists.

6. The overriding adaptation of tundra plants is the ability to integrate growth and metabolic processes even during short periods above freezing. The adapted tundra plant must possess a respiratory and metabolic system capable of efficiently utilizing the products of photosynthesis; and it is the integration of these total reactions in existing tundra environments which must confer adaptive advantage. One of the principal goals in our study of tundra plants should be an understanding of respiratory requirements for growth, maintenance, and allocation processes and the control and feedback of these processes by the photosynthetic system.

Acknowledgments

The research upon which this paper is based has been supported by a number of organizations. We are especially grateful to the Research Corporation (Brown-Hazen Fund) and the Augustana Research-Artist Fund for support early in our studies. More recently the Arctic Institute of North America (ONR-381 and

421) and the N.S.F. (GB-25027 and GV 29343) have materially aided these studies. Some projects were conducted under the auspices of the United States Tundra Biome of the International Biological Program.

References

Allessio, M., and Tieszen, L. L. (1975). Patterns of translocation and allocation of ^{14}C-photoassimilate. *In situ* studies with *Dupontia fischeri* R. Br. Barrow, Alaska. *In* "Primary Production Working Group Meeting," (F. E. Wielgolaski). Dublin, Ireland (in press).

Au, S.-F. (1969). Internal leaf surface and stomatal abundance in arctic and alpine populations of *Oxyria digyna*. *Ecology* **50**, 131–134.

Babb, T. A. (1972). High arctic manipulation and vegetation disturbance studies. pp. 369–391, *In* "Devon Island IBP Project, High Arctic Ecosystem," (Bliss, L. C., ed.). University of Alberta, 413 pp.

Beevers, H. (1970). Respiration in plants and its regulation. *In* "Prediction and Measurement of Photosynthetic Productivity." *Proc. IBP/PP Tech. Meet. Trebon Centre Agri. Publ. Document.* Wageningen, pp. 209–214.

Billings, W. D., and Mooney, H. A. (1968). The ecology of arctic and alpine plants. *Biol. Rev.* **43**, 481–529.

Billings, W. D., Clebsch, E. E. C., and Mooney, H. A. (1961). Effect of low concentrations of carbon dioxide on photosynthesis rates of two races of *Oxyria. Science* **133**, 1834.

Billings, W. D., Clebsch, E. E. C., and Mooney, H. A. (1966). Photosynthesis and respiration rates of Rocky Mountain alpine plants under field conditions. *Amer. Midl. Natur.* **75**, 34–44.

Billings, W. D., Godfrey, P. J., Chabot, B. F., and Bourgue, D. P. (1971). Metabolic acclimation to temperature in arctic and alpine ecotypes of *Oxyria digyna. Arctic Alpine* Res. **3**, 277–289.

Björkman, O., and Holmgren, P. (1963). Adaptability of the photosynthetic apparatus to light intensity in ecotypes from exposed and shaded habitats. *Physiol. Plant.* **16**, 889–914.

Bliss, L. C. (1962). Adaptations of arctic and alpine plants to environmental conditions. *Arctic* **15**, 117–144.

Bliss, L. C. (1971). Arctic and alpine plant life cycles, *Annu. Rev. Ecol. Syst.* **2**, 405–438.

Bliss, L. C. (ed.) (1972). "Devon Island IBP Project, High Arctic Ecosystem." Univ. of Alberta, Edmonton, Alberta, 413 pp.

Bliss, L. C., and Wein, R. W. (1972). Plant community responses to disturbances in the Western Canadian arctic. *Can. J. Bot.* **50**, 1097–1109.

Brouwer, R. (1964). Responses of bean plants to root temperatures. I. Root temperatures and growth in the vegetative stage. *Jaarb.* IBS, 11–22.

Brown, J. (ed.). (1972). *Proc. 1972 Tundra Biome Symp.*, 211 pp.

Caldwell, M., Tieszen, L. L., and Fareed, M. (1972). Comparative Barrow and Niwot Ridge canopy structure. *Proc. 1972 Tundra Biome Symp.* (J. Brown, ed.), pp. 22–28.

Callaghan, T. V., and Lewis, M. C. (1971). Adaptation in the reproductive performance of *Phleum alpinum* L. at a sub-antarctic station. *Brit. Antarctic Surv. Bull.* **26,** 59–75.

Cartellieri, E. (1940). Über transpiration und kohlensäureassimilation an einem hochalpinen standort. *Sitzber Akad. Wiss. Wien Abt.* I **149,** 95–143.

Chabot, B. F., and Billings, W. D. (1972). Origins and ecology the Sierran alpine flora and vegetation. *Ecol. Monogr.* **42,** 163–199.

Chabot, B. F., Chabot, J. F., and Billings, W. D. (1972). Ribulose-1,5-diphosphate carboxylase activity in arctic and alpine populations of *Oxyria digyna*. *Photosynthetica* **6,**(4), 364–369.

Charles-Edwards, D. A., and Charles-Edwards, J. (1970). An analysis of the temperature response curves of CO_2 exchange in the leaves of two temperate and one tropical grass species. *Planta* **94,** 140–151.

Clark, J. M., and Peterson, E. B. (1967). Insolation in relation to cloud characteristics in the Colorado front range. *In* "Arctic and Alpine Environments," (H. E. Wright, Jr., and W. H. Osburn, eds.), pp. 3–11. Indiana Univ. Press, Bloomington, Indiana.

Clebsch, E. E. C. (1960). Comparative morphological and physiological variation in arctic and alpine populations of *Trisetum spicatum*. Ph.D. dissertation, Duke Univ., Durham, North Carolina.

Cooper, J. P., and Tainton, N. M. (1968). Light and temperature requirements for the growth of tropical and temperate grasses. *Herb. Abst.* **38,** 167–176.

Decker, J. P. (1959). Some effects of temperature and carbon dioxide concentration on photosynthesis of *Mimulus*. *Plant Physiol.* **34,** 103–106.

Dennis, J., and Johnson, P. L. (1970). Shoot and rhizome-root standing crops of tundra vegetation at Barrow, Alaska. *Arctic Alpine Res.* **2,** 253–266.

Dennis, J. G., and Tieszen, L. L. (1972). Seasonal course of dry matter and chlorophyll by species at Barrow, Alaska. *Proc. 1972 Tundra Biome Symp.* (J. Brown, ed.) pp. 16–21.

Ehleringer, J. R. (1973). Water relations in the alpine tundra Niwot Ridge, Colorado. M.S. thesis, California State Univ., San Diego, California.

Gale, J. (1972). Availability of carbon dioxide for photosynthesis at high altitudes: theoretical considerations. *Ecology* **53,** 494–497.

Grace, J., and Marks, T. C. (1973). Physiological aspects of bog production at Moor House, *Proc. Brit. Ecol. Soc. Symp. Liverpool.*

Grace, J., and Woolhouse, H. W. (1970). A physiological and mathematical study of the growth and productivity of a *Calluna-Sphagnum* community. *J. Appl. Ecol.* **1,** 363–381.

Grace, J., and Woolhouse, H. W. (1973). A physiological and mathematical study of growth and productivity of a *Calluna-Sphagnum* community. III. Distribution of photosynthate in *Calluna vulgaris* L. Hull. *J. Appl. Ecol.* **10,** 77–91.

Hadley, E. B., and Bliss, L. C. (1964). Energy relationships of alpine plants on Mt. Washington, New Hampshire. *Ecol. Monogr.* **34**, 331–357.

Hedberg, O. (1964). Features of Afroalpine plant ecology. *Acta Phytogeogr. Suecica* **49**, 1–144.

Hesketh, J. D., and Moss, D. N. (1963). Variation in the response of photosynthesis to light. *Crop Sci.* **3**, 107–110.

Hofstra, G., and Nelson, C. D. (1969a). The translocation of photosynthetically assimilated ^{14}C in corn. *Can. J. Bot.* **47**, 1435–1442.

Hofstra, G., and Nelson, C. D. (1969b). A comparative study of translocation of assimilated ^{14}C from leaves of different species. *Planta* **88**, 103–112.

Holdgate, M. W. (ed.). (1970). "Antarctic Ecology," 2 Vols. Academic Press, New York.

Holmgren, P. (1968). Leaf factors affecting light saturated rates in ecotypes of *Solidago virgaurea* from exposed and shaded habitats. *Physiol. Plant* **21**, 676–698.

Johansson, L.-G., Erixon, P., and Linder, S. (1972). The use of labeled CO_2 in field studies of photosynthesis and translocation of assimilates. *In* "Swedish Tundra Biome Project Tech," *Rep. No. 14 Progr. Rep. 1972*, (M. Sonesson, ed.), pp. 78–89.

Johnson, P. L., and Tieszen, L. L. (1974). Vegetation science in arctic Alaska. In "Alaska Arctic Tundra," *Tech. Rep. No. 25 Arctic Inst. N. Amer.*

Kallio, P., and Kärenlampi, L. (1975). Photosynthetic activity of multicellular lower plants (mosses and lichens). *In* "The Functioning of Photosynthetic Systems in Different Environments," (J. P. Cooper, ed.). Cambridge Univ. Press Aberystwyth (in press).

Kleinendorst, A., and Brouwer, R. (1970). The effect of temperature of the root medium and of the growing point of the shoot on growth, water content and sugar content of maize leaves. *Neth. J. Agr. Sci.* **18**, 140–148.

Klikoff, L. G. (1965). Photosynthetic response to temperature and moisture stress of three timberline meadow species. *Ecology* **46**, 516–517.

Klikoff, L. G. (1966). Temperature dependence of the oxidative rates of mitochondria in *Danthonia intermedia*, *Penstemon davidsonii* and *Sitanion hystrix*. *Science* **212**, 529–530.

Kostytschew, S., Tschesnokov, W., and Bazyrina, K. (1930). Untersuchungen über den Tagesverlauf der Photosynthese an der Küste des Eismeeres. *Planta* **11**, 160–168.

Krog, J. (1955). Notes on temperature measurements indicative of special organization in arctic and subarctic plants for utilization of radiated heat from the sun. *Physiol. Plant.* **8**, 836–839.

Lewis, M. C., and Callaghan, T. V. (1975). Tundra. *In* "Climate and Vegetation," (J. Monteith, ed.) Academic Press, New York (in press).

Lieth, H. (1972). The net primary production of the earth with special emphasis on the land areas. *In* "Perspective on Primary Productivity of the Earth," (R. H. Whittaker, ed.). *Symp. AIBS 2nd Nat. Congr. Miami Fla. Oct. 1971.*

Llano, G. A. (1972). "Antarctic Terrestrial Biology," Vol. 20, *Antarctic Res. Ser.* American Geophysical Union, Washington, D.C.

Mayo, J. M., Despain, D. G., and van Zinderen Bakker, E. M., Jr. (1972). CO_2 assimilation studies. *In* "Devon Island IBP Project, High Arctic Ecosystem," (L. C. Bliss, ed.), pp. 217–242. University of Alberta, Edmonton, Alberta.

McCown, B. H., and Tieszen, L. L. (1972). A comparative investigation of periodic trends in carbohydrate and lipid levels in arctic and alpine plants. *Proc. 1972 Tundra Biome Symp.* (J. Brown, ed.), pp. 40–45.

McCree, K. G. (1970). An equation for the rate of respiration of white clover plants grown under controlled conditions. *In* "Prediction and Measurement of Photosynthetic Productivity," *Proc. IBP/PP Tech. Meet. Trebon.* Centre for Agr. Publ. and Documentation, Wageningen, pp. 221–229.

McNaughton, S. J. (1966). Thermal inactivation properties of enzymes from *Typha latifolia* L. ecotypes. *Plant Physiol.* **41,** 1736–1738.

McNaughton, S. J. (1967). Photosynthetic system II: racial differentiation in *Typha latifolia. Science* **156,** 1363.

McNaughton, S. J. (1969). Genetic and environmental control of glycolic acid oxidase activity in ecotypic populations of *Typha latifolia. Amer. J. Bot.* **56,** 37–41.

McNaughton, S. J., and Fullem, L. W. (1970). Photosynthesis and photorespiration in *Typha latifolia. Plant Physiol.* **45,** 703–707.

Miller, P. C. (1972). A model to incorporate minerals into tundra plant production. *Proc. 1972 Tundra Biome Symp.* (J. Brown, ed.), pp. 51–54.

Miller, P. C., and Tieszen, L. L. (1972). A preliminary model of processes affecting primary production in the arctic tundra. *Arctic Alpine Res.* **4,** 1–18.

Mooney, H. A., and Billings, W. D. (1960). The annual carbohydrate cycle of alpine plants as related to growth. *Amer. J. Bot.* **47,** 594–598.

Mooney, H. A., and Billings, W. D. (1961). Comparative physiological ecology of arctic and alpine populations of *Oxyria digyna. Col. Monogr.* **31,** 1–29.

Mooney, H. A., and Johnson, A. W. (1965). Comparative physiological ecology of an arctic and alpine population of *Thalictrum alpinum. Ecology,* **46,** 721–727.

Mooney, H. A., and West, M. (1964). Photosynthetic acclimation of plants of diverse origin. *Amer. J. Bot.* **51,** 825–827.

Mooney, H. A., Wright, R. D., and Strain, B. R. (1964). The gas exchange capacity of plants in relation to vegetation zonation in the White Mountains of California. *Amer. Midl. Natur.* **72,** 281–297.

Mooney, H. A., Hillier, R. D. and Billings, W. D. (1965). Transpiration rates of alpine plants in the Sierra Nevada of California. *Amer. Midl. Natur.* **74,** 374–386.

Mooney, H. A., West, M., and Strain, B. R. (1966). Photosynthetic efficiency at reduced carbon dioxide tensions. *Ecology* **47,** 490–491.

Moser, W. (1969). Die Photosyntheseleistung von Nivalpflanzen. *Ber. Deut. Bot. Ges. Bd. 82, H* **1/2,** 63–64.

Moser, W. (1973). Licht, Temperatur und photosynthese an der Station "Hoher Nebelkogel" (3184 m). (H. Ellenberg ed.), *In* "Sonderdruck aus Okosystemforschung, pp. 203 – 223. Springer Verlag, New York.

Muc, M. (1972). Vascular plant production in the wet meadows of the Truelove Lowland. *In* "Devon Island IBP Project, High Arctic Ecosystem," (L. C. Bliss, ed.), Univ. of Alberta, Edmonton, Alberta.

Neales, T. F., and Incoll, L. D. (1968). The control of leaf photosynthesis rate by the level of assimilate concentration in the leaf: A review of the hypothesis. *Bot. Rev.* **34,** 107 – 125.

Phillips, P. J., and McWilliam, J. R. (1971). Thermal responses of the primary carboxylating enzymes from C_3 and C_4 plants adapted to contrasting temperature environments. *In* "Photosynthesis and Photorespiration," (M. D. Hatch, C. B. Osmond, and R. O. Slatyer eds.), pp. 97 – 104.

Pisek, A. (1960). Die photosynthetischen Leistungen von Pflanzen besonderer Standorte (a) Pflanzen der Arktis und des Hochgebirges. *Handb. Pflanzenphysiol.* **5,** 375 – 414.

Pisek, A., Larcher, W., and Unterholzner, R. (1967). Kardinale Temperaturbereiche der Photosynthese und Grenztemperaturen des Lebens der Blatter verschiedener Spermatophyten. (I. Temperaturminimum der Nettoassimilation, Gefrier-und Frostschadensbereiche der Blatter). *Gra. Abt. B. Bd* **157,** 239 – 264.

Salisbury, F. B., and G. G. Spomer. (1964). Leaf temperatures of alpine plants in the field. *Planta* **60,** 497 – 505.

Scholander, S. I., and Kanwisher, J. T. (1959). Latitudinal effect on respiration in some northern plants. *Plant Physiol.* **34,** 574 – 576.

Scott, D., and Billings, W. D. (1964). Effects of environmental factors on standing crop and productivity of an alpine tundra. *Ecol. Monogr.* **34,** 243 – 270.

Semikhatova, O. A. (1970). Energy efficiency of respiration under unfavorable conditions. *In* "Prediction and Measurement of Photosynthetic Productivity, *Proc. IBP/PP Tech. Meet. Trebon.* Centre for Agr. Publ. and Documentation, Wageningen, pp. 247 – 249.

Šesták, Z., Jarvis, P. G., and Catský, J. (1971). Criteria for the selection of suitable methods. *In* "Plant Photosynthetic Production (Manual of Methods)," (Z. Šesták, J. Čatský, and P. G. Jarvis, eds.), pp. 1 – 48. Dr. W. Junk N. V. Publishers, The Hague.

Shvetsova, V. M., and Voznessenskii, V. L. (1971). Diurnal and seasonal variations in the rate of photosynthesis in some plants of Western Taimyr. *J. Bot.* **55,** 66 – 78. *(Int. Tundra Biome Transl. 2.)*

Slatyer, R. O. (1967). "Plant Water Relationships." Academic Press, New York.

Svoboda, J. (1972). Vascular plant productivity studies of raised beech ridges (semi-polar desert) in the Truelove lowland. *In* "Devon Island IBP Project, High Arctic Ecosystem," (L. C. Bliss, ed.), pp. 146 – 184. Univ. of Alberta, Edmonton, Alberta.

Tieszen, L. L. (1970). Comparisons of chlorophyll content and leaf structure in arctic and alpine grasses. *Amer. Midl. Natur.* **83,** 238 – 253.

Tieszen, L. L. (1972a). The seasonal course of aboveground production and chlorophyll distribution in a wet arctic tundra at Barrow, Alaska. *Arctic Alpine Res.* **4**, 307–324.

Tieszen, L. L. (1972b). Photosynthesis in relation to primary production. *In* "Tundra Biome Proc." *IV. Int. Meet. Biol. Prod. Tundra,* (F. E. Wielgolaski and Th. Rosswall, eds.), pp. 52–62, Leningrad, USSR. Swedish IBP Committee, Wenner-Gren Center.

Tieszen, L. L. (1972c). CO_2 exchange in Alaskan arctic tundra: Measured course of photosynthesis. *Proc. 1972 Tundra Biome Symp.* (J. Brown, ed.), pp. 29–35.

Tieszen, L. L. (1973). Photosynthesis and respiration in arctic tundra grasses: Field light intensity and temperature responses. *Arctic Alpine Res.* **5**, 239–251.

Tieszen, L. L. (1975). CO_2 exchange in the Alaskan arctic tundra: Predicted and measured course of photosynthesis (in preparation).

Tieszen, L. L., and Bonde, E. K. (1967). The influence of light intensity on growth and chlorophyll in arctic, subarctic, and alpine populations of *Deschampsia caespitosa* and *Trisetum spicatum*. *Univ. Colorado Studies Ser. Biol.* **25**, 1–21.

Tieszen, L. L., and Helgager, J. A. (1968). Genetic and physiological adaptation in the Hill reaction of *Deschampsia caespitosa*. *Nature London* **219**, 1066–1067.

Tieszen, L. L., and Johnson, P. L. (1968). Pigment structure of some arctic tundra communities. *Ecology* **49**, 370–373.

Tieszen, L. L., and Sigurdson, D. C. (1973). Effect of temperature on carboxylase activity and stability on some Calvin cycle grasses from the arctic. *Arctic Alpine Res.* **5**, 59–66.

Tranquillini, W. (1964). The physiology of plants at high altitudes. *Annu. Rev. Plant Physiol.* **15**, 345–362.

Treharne, K. J. (1972). Biochemical limitations to photosynthetic rates. *In* "Crop Processes in Controlled Environments," (A. R. Rees, K. E. Cockshull, D. W. Hand, and R. G. Hurd, eds.), pp. 285–303. Academic Press, New York.

Treharne, K. J., and Cooper, J. P. (1969). Effect of temperature on the activity of carboxylase in tropical and temperate Gramineae. *J. Exp. Bot.* **20**, 170–175.

Wager, H. G. (1941). On the respiration and carbon assimilation rates of some arctic plants as related to temperature. *New Phytol.* **40**, 1–19.

Warren-Wilson, J. (1957). Observations on the temperatures of arctic plants and their environment. *J. Ecol.* **45**, 499–531.

Warren-Wilson, J. (1966). An analysis of plant growth and its control in arctic environments. *Ann. Bot.* **24**, 372–381.

Weaver, D. F. (1969). Radiation regime over arctic tundra, 1965. *Sci. Rep. Dep. Atmospheric Sci. Univ. Washington, Seattle.*

Webber, P. J. (1972). Comparative ordination and productivity of tundra vegetation. *Proc. 1972 Tundra Biome Sympo.* (J. Brown, ed.), pp. 55–60.

Weller, G., and Cubley, S. (1972). The microclimates of the arctic tundra. *Proc. 1972 Tundra Biome Symp.* (J. Brown, ed.), pp. 5–12.

Wielgolaski, F. E., and Rosswall, T. (1972). "Tundra Biome Proc." *IV. Int. Meet. Biol. Prod. Tundra.* Leningrad, USSR. Swedish IBP Committee, Wenner-Gren Center.

Zalenskii, O. V., Shvetsova, V. M., and Voznessenskii, V. L. (1972). Photosynthesis in some plants of Western Taimyr. *In* "Tundra Biome," (F. E. Wielgolaski and T. Rosswall, eds.), pp. 182–186.

Arctic and Alpine Plant Water Relations

G. M. Courtin

Biology Department
Laurentian University
Sudbury, Ontario

J. M. Mayo

Botany Department
University of Alberta
Edmonton, Alberta

Introduction

This chapter reviews recent information concerning arctic and alpine plant water relations and compares physiological adaptations to environmental stress where possible. Information which is not recent will be used as needed. A second purpose is to call attention to areas of arctic and alpine plant water relations where more information is desirable. Several good reviews which touch on various aspects of this subject are already available (e.g., Billings and Mooney, 1968; Bliss, 1962, 1971; Savile, 1972; Tranquillini, 1964; and Walter and Kreeb, 1970).

Arctic and Alpine Environments

Even though arctic and alpine tundras have similar vegetation, they differ markedly in climate and the physical environment (Bliss, 1956; Osburn and Wright, 1968). These differences undoubtedly affect the physiological responses of the plants. Savile (1972) characterizes the arctic environment as one of low winter temperatures which may freeze the plants for long periods of time; low summer temperatures; a shallow, cold active layer for root growth; strong winds; low precipitation; low light intensities, but long photoperiod. Alpine environments are characterized as having intense radiation, but a shorter photoperiod; high winds; lower vapor pressure; great diurnal temperature fluctuation; periods of warming during the winter; and greater summer precipitation although periodic drought occurs particularly in the North American alpine (Tranquillini, 1964; Billings and Mooney, 1968; Major and Bamberg, 1967).

Radiation

The radiation environment of arctic plants is considerably different from that of alpine plants. Arctic plants experience continuous day for several months followed by the darkness of winter, whereas alpine plants experience definite light and dark periods.

Total daily radiation during the summer time may not be greatly different in the arctic and alpine areas. Bliss (1962) reports values in the Arctic of $318-510$ J $\cdot$ m^{-2} $\cdot$ day^{-1} and $436-800$ J $\cdot$ m^{-2} $\cdot$ day^{-1} on Mount Washington. He reports values for Umiat, Alaska in June and July of $410-532$ J $\cdot$ m^{-2} $\cdot$ day^{-1} and stated that spot readings in the snowy range of Wyoming indicate higher midday values in the alpine, but only slightly more over a 24-hr period (Bliss, 1956). Courtin (1972) reports values ranging from 176 to 597 J $\cdot$ m^{-2} $\cdot$ day^{-1} during the summers of 1970 and 1971 on Devon Island in the Canadian High Arctic. These are weekly means of daily values; and the maximum daily value was 805 J $\cdot$ m^{-2} $\cdot$ day^{-1}. Previously unpublished data by the same author, for a low arctic site in the Hudson Bay Lowland, show weekly mean values for June and July that range between 487 and 660 J $\cdot$ m^{-2} $\cdot$ day^{-1}. Romanova (1971), for the Taimyr, reports a clear day value of 485.4 J $\cdot$ m^{-2} $\cdot$ day^{-1} in late July. Tranquillini (1963a) reports 550 J $\cdot$ m^{-2} $\cdot$ day^{-1} in midsummer and 100 J $\cdot$ m^{-2} $\cdot$ day^{-1} in midwinter in the Alps. It seems therefore that on a daily basis the total incoming radiation is not greatly different.

The intensity of incoming radiation is considerably different. Tranquillini (1964) quotes data from the Alps indicating incoming radiation can be as great as 2.21 cal $\cdot$ cm^{-2} $\cdot$ min^{-1}. Tranquillini also states that Salisbury and Spomer report values of 170,000 lux in the Rocky Mountains. In 1971 the maximum rate measured on Devon Island, Northwest Territory, was 1.09 J $\cdot$ m^{-2} $\cdot$ min^{-1}, and that occurred only once during the summer (Courtin, 1972). Haag and Bliss's data (1975) for the Mackenzie Delta region in Canada suggest maximum intensities of only slightly more than 1.0 J $\cdot$ m^{-2} $\cdot$ min^{-1}. These results indicate that alpine plants often experience radiation intensities up to twice that experienced by arctic plants. This could have a great influence on transpiration rates.

Radiation is qualitatively different in the Arctic than in the alpine at lower latitudes. Caldwell (1972) states that there is significantly less UV in the biologically active range (280–315 nm) at Barrow, Alaska than can be measured in the mountains at lower latitudes.

The spectral intensity measured by Curl *et al.* (1972) in the California alpine is compared with Devon Island, Northwest Territory data in Figure 1 (Mayo *et al.*, 1972). Even though the times are not exactly the same, and no doubt the sky conditions are somewhat different, it is apparent that the Arctic is considerably richer in the longer wavelengths. Thus arctic plants are subjected to greater amounts of longer wavelengths which, over a 24-hr period, may increase transpiration owing to heating of the leaves.

Wind

Strong wind is characteristic of both alpine and arctic environments (Bliss, 1956) but very high wind speeds seem to be far more frequent in the alpine (Stocker, 1923; Bliss, 1956; Caldwell, 1970a,b; Courtin and Bliss, 1971). Billings and Mooney (1968) compare data for Barrow,

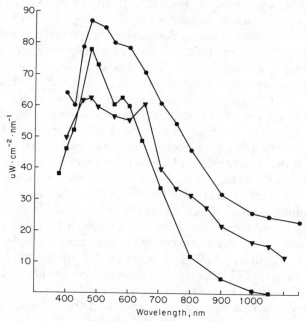

Figure 1 Spectral radiation from Devon Island (high arctic) and Oregon (alpine): ●——● Devon Island, 10 July, 1971, clear day, 1200 EST; ▼——▼ Devon Island, 1 July, 1971, light overcast, 1145 EST; ■——■ Oregon, 8 July, 1969, clear day, 1150 PST.

Alaska and for Niwot Ridge, Colorado, and report annual mean winds of
19.3 km · hr^{-1} for the arctic site and 29.6 km · hr^{-1} for the alpine site.
Mount Washington, New Hampshire has one of the highest recorded
wind regimes on earth with a mean annual wind speed of 59.8 km · hr^{-1}
(Jackman, 1953). The High Arctic on the other hand, seems to experience much lower wind speeds. Mean weekly values on Devon Island
vary between 4.1 and 19.6 km · hr^{-1} (Courtin, 1972), and Belcourt
(personal communication) suggests that the winter pattern is similar.

It is important to note, however, that the above data are from standard weather stations with anemometers at 10 m above the ground. Because profiles of wind speed are logarithmic near the ground (Geiger,
1965; Lowry, 1967; and others), the dwarf tundra plant does not experience winds that are nearly so strong. The highest winds reported by
Courtin (1968) were 6 – 7 m · sec^{-1} at a height of 1 m and these were
reduced to 0.5 – 2 m · sec^{-1} in the zone within 5 cm of the ground surface.

Temperature

Bliss (1956) compared the microclimate at Umiat, Alaska (69°22′ N)
with that found in the Snowy Range in Wyoming (11,000 ft). He found
the diurnal temperature fluctuation to be greater in Wyoming than in
Alaska; but night temperatures at 10 – 30 cm above the ground dropped
below freezing occasionally at both locations.

Soil surface temperatures tend to be higher in the alpine than in the
Arctic. Bliss (1956) measured surface temperatures at the same locations mentioned above. Maximum June soil surface temperatures in
Wyoming were 26° – 31°C, whereas in Alaska they were 18° – 21°C.
Courtin (1972) reports June soil surface maxima of 26° – 28°C on the
raised beach ridge study site at Devon Island and 0.0°C on the meadow
site. The low temperature at the latter site results from snow cover that
persists as much as 2 weeks after the beach ridge melts out.

Soil temperatures at depth present a different picture. In the alpine
Bliss (1956) found the temperature at −4 inches never to be below 4°C
and values of 10° – 12°C were common, whereas in Alaska he reports
2°C consistantly during June, this being caused by the nearness of permafrost. Courtin (1972) reports values for the beach ridges at −10 cm as
high as 12°C in June but only −2°C in the meadows.

It therefore seems that the alpine plants experience greater diurnal
fluctuations in air temperature and soil surface temperature than do the
arctic plants, but the arctic plants may, especially in meadow tundra,
experience lower soil temperatures in the root zone. An arctic plant,
therefore, may be subjected to a greater difference in temperature between root and shoot than plants growing in the alpine. This is especially

true for those plants growing close to the soil surface such as *Dryas integrifolia* or *Salix arctica*.

Müller-Stoll and Lerch (1963) suggest that the temperature gradients which often develop in alpine soils could cause water to move down in the soil in the daytime and up from warmer depths at night. They showed experimentally that rather large temperature differences, up to 30°C, could cause substantial amounts of water to move. These differences forced water to move from warmer to cooler regions regardless of water content. Alpine soils are subjected to fluctuating temperatures owing to the energy flux changing diurnally, whereas Arctic soils are subjected to a steady downward energy flux throughout the growing season. Because of this, through much of the growing season (e.g., mid-June to mid-August on Devon Island) there is a steady downward flux of heat from the warm soil surface to the cold permafrost. Temperature differences can be large; for example on June 20, 1971 on the Devon Island Beach ridge site the temperature at −100 cm was −8°C and at −10 cm it was +7°C, a difference of 15°C. This means that the situation described by Müller-Stoll and Lerch (1963) exists over a long period of time and does not change direction diurnally (i.e., heat flux down during the day and up during the night).

Taylor (1962), using irreversible thermodynamics, has shown the effect of temperature differences upon water movement within soils under conditions similar to those found in the arctic, that is when the temperature gradient causes heat to flow in one direction (i.e., downward) and the isothermal water potential gradient causes water to tend to move in the other direction (i.e., up). According to Taylor when heat and water flow in the soil two equations describe the flow. The expression for water flux is:

$$J_w = -L_{ww} \frac{(\Delta\psi)_T}{T} - L_{wq}(\Delta T/T^2) \tag{1}$$

and the equation for heat flux is:

$$J_q = -L_{qw} \frac{(\Delta\psi)_T}{T} - L_{qq}(\Delta T/T^2) \tag{2}$$

where J_w = water flux; $(\Delta\psi)_T$ = the isothermal water potential difference; T = temperature at the point of interest; ΔT = the difference in temperature between two points in the soil; L_{ww} = the transmission coefficient for water; L_{qq} = the transmission coefficient for heat; and $L_{wq} = L_{qw}$ = the coefficient linking the transfer of water with heat.

If a column of unsaturated soil is subjected to a temperature difference (as in arctic soils), the water will move from the warm to the cold side until a water potential opposing this causes the flux to become zero ($J_w = 0$). Then Eq. (1) becomes:

$$(\Delta\psi)_T/\Delta T = -L_{wq}/L_{ww}T = -Q^*/T \tag{3}$$

where Q^* is the heat of transfer according to Taylor.

This means that there is, depending upon the soil properties for heat and water transfer, an effect of temperature upon water movement as described by Müller-Stoll and Lerch (1963). Taylor reports that when this type of study was carried out on a silt loam soil at -19 J $\cdot$ kg^{-1} water potential, the $\Delta\psi/\Delta T$ was 18.7 bars $\cdot$ deg^{-1} which means that a one degree temperature difference which opposes the water potential difference causes a reduction of 18.7 bars. Temperature differences of 15°C between the root zone and the active layer–permafrost interface have been measured on a dry beach ridge on Devon Island (Courtin, 1972). This creates a very real driving force for water to move to greater depths as the active layer increases and could cause the soil to be quite dry. The phenomenon, coupled with the low precipitation in the Arctic, created desertlike conditions. Hence the term polar desert is quite correct; not only climatically and physiognomically, but also physiologically. Knowledge of the $(\Delta\psi)_T/\Delta T$ is needed for the arctic soils where the active layer is deep enough such that the soil is not saturated. Where the active layer is not too deep and the root zone remains saturated (e.g., meadows) this phenomenon would not be of any significance according to Taylor and Cavazza (1954).

Elevation

Gale (1972) has shown, theoretically at least, that decreasing air pressure with elevation can enhance transpiration by increasing the leaf to air vapor gradient and increasing the diffusivity of water vapor in air. Thus alpine plants may be subjected to greater moisture stress because of elevation.

The foregoing, while not a complete review of arctic and alpine environment differences, serves to emphasize that although both environments are harsh and often produce the same adaptations (e.g., the pulvinate form); they are by no means the same.

Water Relations of Arctic and Alpine Plants

Water Potential and Component Potentials

Water potential and its components could perhaps be the most meaningful measurements in evaluating how well plants are adapted to their environment. It needs to be stressed that to assess any given situation, a knowledge of all factors in the water potential equation [Eq. (4)] need to be evaluated.

$$\psi = \psi_P + \psi_\pi + \psi_\tau \qquad (4)$$

where ψ = water potential; ψ_P = turgor; ψ_π = osmotic potential; and ψ_τ = matric potential.

Slatyer (1967) stated this a few years ago: "since both water movement and water metabolism are of importance in cell and tissue physiology, measurements of both ψ and π are needed, preferably combined with estimates or measurements of the nature and magnitude of other component potentials when they exist." More attention needs to be paid to this recommendation. It is evident in the literature that much of the early work, particularly European, concentrated on osmotic potentials (ψ_π) and that more recent work has been centered upon the total water potential (ψ). There is no information on matric potentials (ψ_τ) and very little has been done on combined matric and osmotic potentials.

Osmotic potentials vary on a diurnal as well as seasonal basis. Since water potential varies diurnally and seasonally as well; it is of the greatest interest to know what is happening to all potentials. We do not know in most cases; nevertheless, some inferences may be drawn. Maximum plant water potentials observed under conditions of high soil water potential are of particular interest. Water potentials under these conditions are shown in Table 1.

The interesting suggestion in these data is that the alpine plant water potentials tend to be high, near zero under conditions of high soil water potential, whereas the arctic plants with the exception of the Barrow data seem to have fairly negative water potentials even when the plants are standing in water. This suggests a high resistance to water movement somewhere within these plants and, in particular, it suggests that the arctic plants are perhaps not as well adapted to the cold soil (and water) as might be expected and that this is the reason for the low leaf water potentials under conditions when it would not be expected.

Pulvinate plants such as *Dryas octopetala*, *Dryas integrifolia*, and *Silene acaulis* grow on very dry sites both in the alpine and the Arctic. Since these sites often have low soil water potentials it is to be expected that leaf water potentials would be low as well. Addison (1973) reported that ψ_{leaf} for *Dryas integrifolia* varied from −10 bars to approximately −35 bars in 1971 on Devon Island. Teeri (1973) shows no water potentials greater than −10 bars for *Saxifraga oppositifolia* on Devon Island in 1970 and 1971. He reported values of −25 to −35 bars during periods of high radiation, and found that leaf wilting did not occur until −55 bars.

Table 1 Maximum Leaf Water Potentials of Arctic and Alpine Plants under Conditions of High Soil Water Potential

Species	$\psi_{leaf\ max.}$	Location	Source
Epilobium lateum	−1 bar	Alpine	Kuramoto and Bliss (1970)
Arctogrostis latifolia	0.0 to −2.1 bars	Arctic—Barrow Alaska	Dennis (1969)
Kobresia	~0.0	Alpine—Colorado	Bell (1973)
Dupontia fischeri	~0.0	Arctic—Barrow Alaska	Tieszen (1973)
Eriophorum russeolum	−35 bars	Arctic—Mackenzie delta	Haag (1972)
Carex rariflora	−25 bars	Arctic—Mackenzie delta	Haag (1972)
Carex stans	−8 bars	Arctic—Devon Island	Addison (1973)
Carex stans	−4 bars	Arctic—Devon Island	Hartgerink (1973)
Arctogrostic sp.	−12 bars	Arctic—Mackenzie delta	Younkin (1973)
Diapensia lapponica[a]	−53 bars	Mt. Washington, N.H.	Courtin (1968)
Carex bigelowii[a]	−23 bars	Mt. Washington, N.H.	Courtin (1968)

[a]Field measurements under broken skies following a long period of very heavy rain. These measurements are probably not maxima and are included solely for perspective.

He further reported that net positive assimilation did not decline to zero until about −25 bars in growth chamber experiments. Hartgerink (1973) has followed net assimilation and water potential of *Dryas integrifolia* plants, collected on Devon Island, under growth chamber conditions. She has found net assimilation rates at −16 bars leaf water potential to be as great or greater than field values (Thompson and Mayo, 1973). She has measured water potential and its components at various development stages (Table 2).

These results, while preliminary, are of interest. The water potential of plants under no moisture stress was not higher than −15 atm. An attempt was made to provide conditions for complete water potential recovery and the values would not rise above −15 atm. Plants that were maintained under conditions of no stress as they entered dormancy had decreasing water potential and matric and osmotic potentials. The dormant plants had very low potentials with no detectable turgor. Either turgor is practically zero or the liquid nitrogen used to freeze the samples for $\psi_\pi + \psi_\tau$ determination was not cold enough (−196° C). These data are interesting for two reasons: (1) the decreasing water potential and combined potentials ($\psi_\pi + \psi_\tau$) associated with dormancy occurred under conditions which should not have placed any moisture stress on the plant; and (2) it was impossible even when the plant was under no moisture stress, to measure high water potentials.

This seems to indicate that the plant physiologically prevents high water potentials perhaps owing to high root resistance and that the lowered osmotic and matric potential develop physiologically and are

Table 2 Water Potential and Component Potentials for *Dryas integrifolia*[a]

Development stage	Water potential (ψ) bars	Combined osmotic and matric potentials bars	Treatment
Dormant	−60.5	−60.5	Plants dormant 5 months in dark at −10°C
Active growth	−15	−17	In growth chamber at 10°C; RH ~65%; continuous light
Active growth	−15	−17	In growth chamber 10°C saturated atmosphere well-watered soil; continuous light
Beginning to enter dormancy	−33	−35	In growth chamber at 10°C; saturated atmosphere; well-watered soil

[a]Hartgerink, 1973.

not a consequence of frozen soil. The change in the combined osmotic and matric components may be due to a matric component change, rather than osmotic, since Svoboda (1972) found less total carbohydrates in the shoot in August on Devon Island than earlier. Hence carbohydrates did not increase later in the season and the monosaccharide content was extremely low. This suggests the lowered $\psi_\pi + \psi_\tau$ may be due to matrix changes. Pisek *et al.* (1935) reported osmotic potentials for *Dryas octopetala* and *Silene acaulis* in the alpine. They found that *Dryas* had an osmotic potential of −18.3 atm when the plant was in good condition in the field. This compares with −17 atm for *Dryas integrifolia* from Devon Island. When they placed the plants in a saturated atmosphere for 24 hr the ψ_π rose to −13.3 atm indicating a considerable change which was not observed in the Devon Island *Dryas* over a period of 20 days. This may be a species difference or may indicate a difference between arctic and alpine plants. Pisek (1956) reports winter ψ_π values of −31 atm and summer values of −20 atm for various conifers and ericaceous shrubs. These differences are not as great as those found in *Dryas* from Devon Island (Table 3).

There has been a considerable interest in tree species found at or near timberline and because of this they are included even though they are not considered true arctic–alpine plants. Water potential and component potentials from several sources are shown in Table 3.

Lindsay (1971) followed water potentials of spruce, *Picea engelmanii*, through the winter at two elevations and different winter exposure. He found considerably lower water potentials in wind-exposed needles caused by several factors, such as wind and frozen soil. His data show high water potentials no higher than −10 bars at anytime of the year in any needle age class, elevation, or exposure, indicating that these plants must tolerate a certain degree of stress year round. Walter and Kreeb (1970) quote earlier data of Goldsmith and Smith from Colorado on the variation in osmotic potential of spruce at nearly the same elevations as Lindsay. These data (Table 3) show minimum osmotic potentials occurred during May which is attributed to high solar radiation with frozen soils. Lindsay's data for exposed needles agree with this, but not from protected sites. Values for May are increasing and are not the minimum. Levitt and Scarth (1936) report higher summer osmotic potentials as do Pisek *et al.* (1935). An unanswered question is how much of the yearly fluctuation in osmotic and water potential is due to desiccation and subsequent concentration of cell sap and how much is due to cellular changes which would occur without desiccation. Lindsay's comparison of exposed and nonexposed needles indicates that winter desiccation is

Table 3 Tree Water Potential and Component Potentials from Various Arctic and Alpine Regions

Measurement	Potential					Source and species
	Feb.	May	July	Sept.	Nov.	
ψ_{leaf} bars	−28	−28	−17	−25	−27	Lindsay (1971) *Picea engelmannii* 3300 m; exposed needles
ψ_{leaf} bars	−17	−17	−	−18	−17	Lindsay (1971) *Picea engelmannii* 3300 m; protected needles
ψ_{leaf} bars	−20	−16	−13	−15	−18	Lindsay (1971) *Picea engelmannii* 2900 m; mature needles
ψ_π atm	−	−48	−25	−22	−30	Walter and Kreeb (1970) *Picea engelmannii* 3800 m
ψ_π atm	−	−33	−26	−25	−30	Walter and Kreeb (1970) *Picea engelmannii* 3750 m
ψ_π atm	−	−28	−24	−22	−27	Walter and Kreeb (1970) *Picea engelmannii* 2700 m
ψ_π atm	−27	−18	−15	−18	−28	Levitt and Scarth (1936) *Picea pungens* (Cortex)
ψ_π atm	−30	−23	−	−	−	Pisek *et al.* (1935) *Pinus cembra*
ψ_{leaf} atm	−54	−30.1	−13.8	−	−24	van Zinderen Bakker (1973) *Picea mariana*
$\psi_\pi + \psi_\tau$ atm	−56	−34.0	−15.6	−	−	Boreal forest

certainly a major cause. Levitt and Scarth (1936) followed *Picea pungens* osmotic potential through the year. Their data agree with those of previous workers. When they brought a plant in winter condition indoors the osmotic potential changed from −21.2 atm to −18.0 to −13.7 atm in 0, 11, and 31 days, respectively. The slowness of recovery indicates that the desiccation may be more than just the inability of cold frozen soil to supply moisture. Van Zinderen Bakker (1973) has measured water potentials as low as −54 atm when black spruce breaks dormancy and begins positive net assimilation indicating that the restoration of higher ψ values is not necessary for the onset of activity in the spring. Michaelis (1934) measured osmotic potentials as low as −65.7 atm in spruce under winter alpine conditions. More information is needed about water potential and its components before we can say by what mechanism low values develop and the manner of spring recovery.

Transpiration

Mention was made earlier that water absorption could be influenced by cold soils. Whether or not roots grow in cold soils and thus follow the retreating ice and the liquid water above it is of interest. Larcher (1963) reports that *Loiseleuria* absorbs water from surface melt water via adventitious roots when most of the soil mass is still frozen; *Diapensia* on Mount Washington appears to behave in the same way (Courtin, 1968). How well roots penetrate cold arctic soils and at what rate is not well known, Bliss (1962) stated that roots in tundra were mostly confined to the warmer better-drained layers above the permafrost. However he quotes Dadykin (1954) as saying that *Calamagrostis* and *Rosa acicularis* roots are found near the frozen layer at 0°C and that *Carex globularis* and *Equisetum silvaticum* from frozen soils are alive with cell division taking place. Bliss (1956) reported *Carex elynoides* and *Geum turbinatum* roots to 0.8 m in the alpine, whereas not all plants have roots that follow the melting permafrost down in arctic situations. A few grasses and sedges do this, but the dwarf heath seldom penetrates the soil more than 10 cm. Species which have the ability to produce roots at a rate fast enough to follow the receding permafrost and absorb water clearly are better adapted. Two such species are *Arctogrostis latifolia* and *Eriophorum vaginatum*. Bliss (1962) reported finding roots of these two species within $0.5 - 1.5$ cm of the retreating frost which was between 0° and 1°C.

Little can be said about stomatal mechanisms. Net assimilation studies (Mayo *et al.* 1972; Tiezen, 1973) indicate that the stomata of arctic plants can remain open during the 24-hr day. Polunin (1955) reports that diurnal rhythms with incomplete closure occur in the Arctic. Ketellapper (1963) cites Kuiper as saying that stomatal movement is inhibited below 10°C, and Scarth (1927) reported that low temperatures tend to prevent stomatal opening in the light. Thus, low temperatures may be limiting water loss in both arctic and alpine plants by depressing the degree of stomatal opening. More information is needed. Schulze *et al.* (1972) have shown that the stomata of desert plants respond to relative humidity rather than water content of the leaves. Stomata tend to close with low RH and open with high RH. If this is so for arctic and alpine plants then the low water potentials often reported do not necessarily indicate that the stomata are closed. Tranquillini (1963b) has shown CO_2 assimilation of conifers to be reduced by low relative humidities even with saturated soils. This tends to agree with Schulze's results. Caldwell (1970a,b) has compared the effects of wind on transpiration and net CO_2 assimilation of *Rhododendron ferrugineum*, a plant which grows in protected areas, with *Pinus cembra* which grows on windy sites near ridge tops. High winds cause immediate stomatal closure in the *Rhododendron*, but not *Pinus*, thus indicating that the alpine plant is adapted to the windy habitat. Cushion plants avoid high winds altogether because of their growth form which places the leaf canopy essentially at the ground–air interface where wind speed is at a minimum (Courtin, 1968). Whether grasses and sedges of intermediate stature have any such adaptation is not known. Leaf resistances vary considerably between species and this may play a role in the adaptation of plants to their environment (Miller and Gates, 1967).

The resistances of several plant species in Table 4 indicate the range of some of the plants of interest. Courtin (1968) reports considerable difference between the leaf resistance of *Diapensia* and *Carex*, indicating a real adaptation on the part of *Diapensia* to the dry habitat in which it grows. Hartgerink (1973) has measured quite high leaf resistance in *Dryas*. It is particularly interesting to see the very great differences in leaf resistance between the three species of *Picea*. This could represent an adaptation of black spruce to its environment. There are periods, particularly in the spring, when incident radiation is high and the soil is frozen. High leaf resistances under these conditions could greatly reduce water loss.

In the case of tundra plants not only leaf resistance but also boundary and canopy resistance can play a role in preventing water loss. This is especially true in the pulvinate or cushion form of plant where the plant canopy is essentially contiguous with the ground surface. The cushion acts as if it was a large flat leaf rather than the sum of many small, narrow leaves. Since boundary layer thickness, and hence resistance, increases with increase in leaf width the growth form leads to the maximum boundary layer resistance possible. Furthermore, the cushion, because of its position, is sheltered from the wind, an important considera-

Table 4   Leaf Resistance to Water Loss

Species	Resistance (sec · cm^{-1})	Conditions	Source
Dryas integrifolia	~58	Well-watered plant detached leaf	Hartgerink (1973)
Diapensia lapponica	2.37	Leaf resistance	Courtin (1968)
Carex bigelowii	0.63	Leaf resistance	Courtin (1968)
Picea sitchensis	7	Bottom of canopy	Beardsell *et al.* (1972)
Picea sitchensis	1.5	Top of canopy	Beardsell *et al.* (1972)
Picea mariana	45	Potometer	Miller and Gates (1967)
Thuja occidentalis	70–200	Potometer	Miller and Gates (1967)
Picea engelmannii	63	Well-watered plant	Kaufmann (1973)

tion since boundary layer thickness is very sensitive to wind speed (Gates, 1962).

The tight packing of the many small leaves to form a cushion leads to high resistance to water loss because of the increase in vapor path length. However, this also constitutes an increased resistance to heat loss since the same physical principles are operating and together with the boundary layer resistance, gives rise to a very high leaf temperature when the radiant heat load is high.

Maximum transpiration rates of several arctic and alpine plants are shown in Table 5. Although the units used for reporting transpiration are not all comparable, several conclusions are inferred. Bliss (1960) compared transpiration rates of alpine shrubs on Mount Washington, New Hampshire, with alpine shrubs in Wyoming and arctic shrubs in Alaska, and concluded that transpiration was highest on Mount Washington and lowest in Wyoming. These rates are much lower than those reported by Courtin (1968) for *Carex bigelowii* and *Diapensia lapponica* on Mount Washington. The latter results were obtained using entire plants in small lysimeters (Courtin and Bliss, 1971) and sod blocks (Courtin, 1968), whereas in earlier work potometers were used. Alpine plants studied in Europe appear to have very low transpiration rates compared to those studied in the Sierra Nevada. This is not surprising since the alpine in Europe is less severe than in the Sierra Nevada. The transpiration rate of *Carex stans* on Devon Island is only one-tenth as great as that of *Carex bigelowii* on Mount Washington. This, coupled with the always low leaf water potential of *Carex stans*, perhaps indicates the lack of adaptation to the very cold soils encountered in the high arctic. *Dryas integrifolia* had a transpiration rate only a fraction of that for *Diapensia lapponica* indicating that the arctic cushion plants do not transpire as much as those in the alpine. Gale (1972) has shown theoretically that alpine plants can transpire more than arctic plants due to elevation and the data of Courtin and Addison tend to support this. However, Whitfield (1932) reported that *Mertensia alpina* transpiration increased with decreasing elevation in Colorado, and Mooney *et al.* (1965) found that *Polygonum bistortoides* did the same in the Sierra Nevada.

The effect of wind on transpiration appears to be a reduction in water loss with increasing wind speed until approximately $3.5 \text{ m} \cdot \text{sec}^{-1}$ is attained. This has been shown theoretically (Knoerr, 1965) and the same phenomenon has been documented in the field (Bliss, 1960; Courtin, 1968). Increasing wind speed causes an increase in convective transfer of heat away from the leaf, lowering leaf temperature and, hence, the vapor pressure of water within the leaf. This reduces the vapor pressure gradient between leaf and air, and transpiration is reduced. Conversely,

Table 5 Maximum Transpiration Rates of Several Arctic and Alpine Plants

Species	Maximum transpiration rate	Location	Source
Alnus crispa	0.04[a]	Umiat, Alaska	Bliss (1960)
Betula nana	0.075[a]	Umiat, Alaska	Bliss (1960)
Salix brachycarpa	0.010[a]	Wyoming, 11,000 ft.	Bliss (1960)
Salix planifolia	0.010[a]	Wyoming, 11,000 ft	Bliss (1960)
Betula minor	0.082[a]	Mt. Washington, N.H.	Bliss (1960)
Salix planifolia	0.050[a]	Mt. Washington, N.H.	Bliss (1960)
Rumex scutatus	12.3[b]	Alpine scree slope	Tranquillini (1964)
Pinus silvestris	0.004[c]	Alpine–Europe	Pisek (1956)
Loiseleuria	0.005[c]	Alpine–Europe	Pisek (1956)
Betula verrucosa	0.018[c]	Alpine–Europe	Pisek (1956)
Lupinus lyallii	1.03[d]	Sierra Nevada 9100 ft. plateau plants	Mooney, Billings and Hillier (1965)
Eriophyllum lanatum	0.033[d]		
Oxyria digyna	0.74[d]	Sierra Nevada 9100 ft. scree plants	Mooney, Billings and Hillier (1965)
Senecio fremontii	0.26[d]		
Caltha howellii	0.63[d]	Sierra Nevada 9100 ft. spring plants	Mooney, Billings and Hillier (1965)
Polygonum bistortoides	0.50[d]		
Caltha howellii	1.73[e]	Sierra Nevada 9100 ft. spring plants	Mooney, Billings and Hillier (1965)
Polygonum bistortoides	3.23[e]		
Helianthus annuus	3.0[e]	Pikes Peak, Colorado	Whitfield (1932)
Carex bigelowii	2.31[f]	Mt. Washington, N.H.	Courtin (1968)
Diapensia	1.73[f]	Mt. Washington, N.H.	Courtin (1968)
Carex stans	0.23[f]	Devon Island, N.W.T.	Addison (1973)
Dryas integrifolia	0.30[f]	Devon Island, N.W.T.	Addison (1973)
Dupontia fischeri	1.4[f]	Barrow, Alaska	Tieszen (1973)

[a] Data in cm³ · dm⁻² · hr⁻¹.
[b] Data in g · (gram fr wt)⁻¹ · day⁻¹.
[c] Data in g · (gram fr wt)⁻¹ · hr⁻¹.
[d] Data in g · (gram fr wt)⁻¹ · hr⁻¹.
[e] Data in g · dm⁻² leaf hr⁻¹.
[f] Data in g · dm⁻² · hr⁻¹.

Table 6 Energy Budgets for Arctic and Alpine Regions During Periods of Maximum Evapotranspiration[a]

Energy budget (cal · cm⁻² · min⁻¹)				Percent of Rn as:			Location and plant community	Source
Rn	LE	G	H	LE	G	H		
0.63	0.29	0.084	0.26	46	13	41	*Diapensia* community; Mt. Washington, N.H.: 1100–1200 h; 1650 m	Courtin (1968)
0.41	0.28	0.030	0.10	68	7	24	*Carex bigelowii* community; Mt. Washington, N.H.; 1400–1500 h; 1845 m	Courtin (1968)
1.25	0.75	0.20	0.30	60	16	24	White mountains, Calif.; 3580 m; grass and sedge sod; 1200 h	Werner *et al.* (1969)
0.70	0.06	0.03	0.61	9	4	87	*Dryas* microsite on beach ridge; approx sea level; 1200–1300 h; Devon Island, N.W.T.	Addison (1973)
0.90	0.08	0.03	0.79	9	3	88	*Carex* microsite; meadow; approx sea level; 1200–1300 h; Devon Island, N.W.T.	Addison (1973)
0.42	0.20	0.12	0.14	42	29	33	Dwarf shrub-heath tundra; 1200 h; Tuktoyaktuk, N.W.T.	Haag and Bliss (1975)
0.26	0.19	0.02	0.05	73	9	18	*Dupontia fischeri*; Barrow, Alaska	Weller and Cubley (1972)
—	—	—	—	40	30	30	Taimyr, U.S.S.R.	Romanova (1971)

[a]Rn = net radiation; L = latent heat of vaporization; E = rate of evaporation; G = soil heat flux; H = sensible heat flux.

wind across the surface of the leaf sweeps away the vapor shells that form outside each stoma. This tends to increase the gradient and hence to increase transpiration. Under high radiant heat load, however, the latter effect is overshadowed by the cooling effect of wind upon the leaf and thus the internal water vapor pressure. To what extent stomata close under these conditions will depend on the transpiration rate, the length of time for which it is maintained, and whether or not the resistances from soil to leaf are sufficiently low for an adequate transport of water to be maintained.

In recent years there has been considerable interest in energy budgets in plants (Gates, 1968; Gates and Papian, 1971). Energy budgets from several arctic and alpine sites are shown in Table 6. The very low energy exchange by latent heat on the Devon Island communities is strikingly different from the other communities. These two communities appear to exchange energy by convective heat to a far greater degree than the other communities. This type of energy exchange suggests that leaf temperatures would necessarily be fairly high. This has been confirmed by Addison (1973) who measured sustained *Dryas* leaf temperatures of 46°C. Warren-Wilson (1957) measured leaf temperatures significantly greater than ambient among plants on Cornwallis Island, Northwest Territory, and Mayo *et al.* (1972) measured *Dryas* leaf temperatures of 39°C (25° > ambient). The plants in the high Arctic Islands do seem to be exchanging considerable amounts of energy as sensible heat rather than latent heat.

Summary

Environment

Arctic and alpine regions are noted for their vegetational similarity. However, the environments of these two regions are different in several notable ways. In addition to the obvious differences in day length; there may be significant differences in radiation quality. The apparent enrichment of longer wavelengths (Figure 1), particularly between 700 and 800 nm, may be important. The effect of this enrichment particularly on the red–far red phytochrome system may be significant. The influence of greater ultraviolet radiation in the alpine has been studied by Caldwell (1968) who found *Trifolium dasyphyllum* flowering to be enhanced by shielding from UV. Whether these differences (UV and longwave) have any effect upon the water relations of these plants is not known. The greater radiation intensities to which alpine plants are subjected undoubtedly cause greater transpiration rates, at least over short periods of time. The effect of permafrost upon water movement within the soil and upon root resistances to water flux needs further study.

Adaptation of Cushion Plants

Arctic cushion plants such as *Dryas* appear to be well adapted to their environment. Addison (1973) has shown that energy exchange is largely by convective transfer (Table 6), they do not exhibit high rates of transpiration, and water potentials are generally quite low in these plants (Teeri, 1973; Hartgerink, 1973; Addison, 1973). Even with low water potentials, net assimilation continues to be positive (Teeri, 1973; Hartgerink, 1973). It has been shown, at least with *Dryas,* that high water potentials do not occur under favorable moisture conditions (Table 2) and that with the onset of dormancy the osmotic potential decreases, even though the plant is not stressed. It appears then that cushion plants may have a high internal resistance to water flux which prevents water potential from ever being very high. This would in effect keep these plants hardened (Levitt, 1941). They appear to be physiologically adapted to the dry, often cold, yet sometimes very warm environment in which they grow.

Spomer (1964) studied the effects of wind, radiation, and temperature upon stem elongation of cushion plants and found that reducing wind and light had little influence, and that there was little difference between a wet and dry year. The substantially greater longwave radiation 0.7 – 1 μm in the Arctic (Figure 1) does not stimulate elongation as might be expected (Wassink, 1953). The low water potential and subsequent low turgor value would reduce the rate of stem elongation and thus help to maintain the compact growth habit because turgor is necessary for cell elongation (Cleland, 1967).

Since these plants appear to be physiologically adapted to low water potentials within the leaves, the question arises as to what constitutes a genuine moisture stress. They can fix carbon and grow with tissue water potentials that would be lethal to many plants.

Carbon fixation tends to be slow, however, at least in *Diapensia* (Hadley and Bliss, 1964) because of the high resistance to gaseous flow (Courtin, 1968). It is suggested that the slow rate may be compensated for, in part, by a long growing season. Because the plant essentially forms part of the ground surface, absorbed radiation is high and tissue temperatures are frequently several degrees higher than those of the surrounding air. This means that physiological processes such as photosynthesis may proceed even though air temperatures dictate the opposite.

The leaves of the pulvinate growth form are usually persistent and turn red or purple during the winter owing to degradation of chlorophyll and the presence of anthocyanin. Furthermore, the exposed sites that this growth form inhabits are mostly blown free of snow, or at best are lightly covered, during the winter (Tiffney, 1972).

Courtin (1968) has observed that in late winter or early spring, thaw is accelerated within the canopy of the dark-colored cushions while the surrounding ice and snow, and the ground beneath, remains frozen. Nevertheless, this phenomenon may help to increase the length of the growing season. Desiccation of the thawed tissue does not seem to occur owing, it is presumed, to the occurrence of adventitious roots below the terminal rosette of leaves that have been observed by Larcher (1963) for *Loiseleuria procumbens* and by Courtin (1968) for *Diapensia lapponica.*

Although *Diapensia* is partially or fully exposed in winter to both wind and cold, Sakai and Otsuka (1970) report that after winter hardening it could survive temperatures of −196°C. Although no water potential data are available for *Diapensia* in the dormant condition, one should stress that Hartgerink's (1973) value of −60.5 bars for a dormant *Dryas* plant may indicate the mechanism whereby such winter hardiness is achieved.

Adaptation of Grasses and Grasslike Plants

The situation with grasses and sedges does not seem as clear cut (Table 1). High water potentials in *Kobresia* occur under conditions in which the root system is immersed in cold water (Bell, 1973). Bell (1973) reports that *Kobresia* has maintained leaf water potential near zero for 12 consecutive days during May during snow melt. More information on other alpine grasses would be desireable. *Epilobium,* though not a grass, appears to respond in a similar manner. These are alpine situations. Dennis (1969) reports high water potentials in plants at Barrow, Alaska, whereas data from the Canadian Arctic suggest quite low water potentials which seems to suggest some sort of resistance to water movement as is the case with *Dryas.* Addison's (1973) data from Devon Island (Table 6) indicate that *Carex stans* exchanges energy largely as heat much the same as *Dryas.* High leaf temperatures have also been measured. This again suggests high root resistances; however, since water potential and its components have not been followed under more favorable conditions it is not possible to suggest whether this is a characteristic of these plants or just a response to the environment. Kramer (1940) found that root resistance in temperate region plants is greatly reduced at low temperatures and it is conceivable that this is the cause for the low water potentials. If this is the case it argues for a lack of real adaptation for these plants. If, however, at higher root temperatures and favorable moisture conditions the situation does not change, then this would not be the case. There appears to be a real difference between the high and low arctic (e.g., Devon Island and Barrow, Alaska). There appear to be substantial differences in energy budgets, water potentials, and transpiration rates between the two areas. The greater dissipation of energy by latent heat at Barrow suggests a greater degree of adaptation to the environment than at Devon Island.

Tree Adaptations

Trees at timberline are of interest if for no other reason than for comparison with the true tundra plants adjacent to them. There seems little doubt that exposure coupled with frozen soil causes desiccation which may be a major factor in limiting the range of trees. However, the ability to break dormancy and fix carbon at low needle water potentials and the slowness for recovery of water potential under favorable conditions suggests that the effect of severe cold, as found in arctic regions or the alpine may have effects other than desiccation. The high leaf resistances of arctic and alpine trees suggests adaptation to reduce water loss, particularly under conditions of high incident radiation and frozen soils.

References

Addison, P. A. (1973). Studies on evapotranspiration and energy budget in the High Arctic: A comparison of hydric and xeric microenvironments on Devon Island, N.W.T. M.Sc. thesis, Laurentian Univ., Sudbury, Ontario.

Beardsell, M. F., Jarvis, P. G., and Davidson, B. (1972). A null-balance diffusion porometer suitable for use with leaves of many shapes. *J. Appl. Ecol.* **9** (3), 677–690.

Bell, K. (1973). Ph.D. thesis, Univ. of Alberta, Edmonton, Alberta.

Billings, W. D., and Mooney, H. A. (1968). The ecology of arctic and alpine plants. *Biol. Rev.* **43**, 481–529.

Bliss, L. C. (1956). A comparison of plant development in microenvironments of arctic and alpine tundras. *Ecol. Monogr.* **26**, 303–337.

Bliss, L. C. (1960). Transpiration rates of arctic and alpine shrubs. *Ecology* **41**, 386–389.

Bliss, L. C. (1962). Adaptations of arctic and alpine plants to environmental conditions. *Arctic* **15**, 117–144.

Bliss, L. C. (1971). Arctic and Alpine plant life cycles. *Annu. Rev. Ecol. Syst.* **2**, 405–438.

Caldwell, M. M. (1968). Solar U.V. radiation and plant processes on alpine tundra. Ph.D. thesis (1967), Duke Univ., Durham, North Carolina.

Caldwell, M. (1970a). The wind regime at the surface of the vegetation layer above timberline in the central Alps. *Cent. Gesmate Fortwesen.*

Caldwell, M. (1970b). Plant gas exchange at high wind speeds. *Plant Physiol.* **46**, 535 – 537.

Caldwell, M. (1972). Biologically effective solar ultraviolet irradiation in the arctic. *Arctic Alpine Res.* **4**(1), 39 – 43.

Cleland, R. (1967). A dual role of turgor pressure in auxin induced cell elongation in *Avena* coleoptiles. *Planta* **77**, 182 – 191.

Courtin, G. M. (1968). Evapotranspiration and energy budgets of two alpine microenvironments, Mt. Washington, N.H. Ph.D. thesis, Univ. of Illinois, Urbana, Illinois.

Courtin, G. M. (1972). Micrometeorological studies of the Truelove lowland. *Devon Island I.B.P. Proj. Rep. 1970 – 71.*

Courtin, G. M., and Bliss, L. C. (1971). A hydrostatic lysimeter to measure evapotranspiration under remote field conditions. *Arctic Alpine Res.* **3**(1), 81 – 89.

Curl, H., Jr., Hardy, J. T., and Ellermeier, R. (1972). Spectral absorption of solar radiation in alpine snowfields. *Ecology* **53**, 1189 – 1194.

Dadykin, V. P. (1954). Pecularities of plant behavior in cold soils. *Vopt. Bot.* **2**, 455 – 472.

Dennis, J. (1969). Growth of tundra vegetation in relation to arctic microenvironments at Barrow, Alaska. Ph.D. thesis, Duke Univ., Durham, North Carolina.

Gale, J. (1972). Elevation and transpiration: some theoretical considerations with special reference to mediterranean-type Climate. *J. Appl. Ecol.* **913**, 691 – 701.

Gates, D. M. (1962). Energy Exchange in the Biosphere. *Biol. Monogr.*

Gates, D. M. (1968). Transpiration and leaf temperature. *ARPP* **19**, 211 – 238.

Gates, D., and Papian, L. E. (1971). "Atlas of Energy Budgets of Plant Leaves," Academic Press, New York.

Geiger, R. (1965). "The Climate near the Ground." Harvard Univ. Press, Cambridge, Massachusetts.

Haag, R. W. (1972). Mineral nutrition and primary production in native tundra communities of the Mackenzie delta region, N.W.T. M.Sc. thesis, Univ. of Alberta, Edmonton, Alberta.

Haag, R. W. and Bliss, L. C. (1975). Energy budget changes following surface disturbance to upland tundra. *J. Ecol.* (in Press).

Hadley, E. B. and Bliss, L. C. (1964). Energy Relationships of Alpine Plants on Mt. Washington, New Hampshire. *Ecol. Monogr.* **34**, 331 – 357.

Hartgerink, A. (1973). Personal communication. (Dept. of Botany, Univ. of Alberta, Edonton, Alberta).

Jackman, A. H. (1953). "Handbook of Mt. Washington Environment." *Natick QM Res. Develop. Lab. Rep. No. 218.* Research and Development Division, Office of the Quartermaster General, Natick, Massachusetts.

Kaufmann, M. R. (1973). Design, calibration, and use of a porometer for conifers. *Plant Physiol.* **51** (Suppl.), 8.

Kettellapper, H. J. (1963). Stomatal physiology. *Annu. Rev. Plant Physiol.* **14**, 249 – 270.

Knoerr, K. R. (1965). Contrasts in Energy Balances between individual leaves and vegetated surfaces. *Inst. Environ. Sci. Proc.* **1965,** 615–624.

Kramer, P. J. (1940). Root resistance as a cause of decreased water absorption by plants at low temperatures. *Plant Physiol.* **15,** 63–79.

Kuramoto, R. T., and Bliss, L. C. (1970). Ecology of subalpine meadows. *Ecol. Monogr.* **40**(3), 317–347.

Larcher, W. (1963). Zur spätwinterlichen Erschwerung der Wasserbilanz von Holzpflanzen au der Waldgrenze. *Ber. Natur. Med. Ver. Innsbruck* **53,** 125–137.

Levitt, J. (1941). "Frost Killing and Hardiness of Plants." Burgess Publ. Co., Minneapolis, Minnesota.

Levitt, J. and Scarth, G. W. (1936). Frost hardening studies with living cells. *Can. J. Res. Sec. C. Bot. Sci.* **14,** 267–284.

Lindsay, J. H. (1971). Annual cycle of leaf water potential in *Picea engelmanii* and *Abies lasiocarpa* at timberline in Wyoming. *Arctic Alpine Res.* **3**(2), 131–138.

Lowry, W. P. (1967). "Weather and Life." Academic Press, New York.

Major, J., and Bamberg, S. A. (1967). Comparison of some North American and Eurasian alpine ecosystems, *In "Arctic and Alpine Environments,"* (H. E. Wright, Jr., and W. H. Osburn, eds.), pp. 89–118. Indiana Univ. Press,

Mayo, J. M., Despain, D. G., and van Zinderen Bakker, E. M., Jr. (1972). CO_2 assimilation studies. *Devon Island I.B.P. Proj. Rep. 1970–71.* (L. C. Bliss, ed.), pp. 217–251.

Michaelis, P. (1934). Zur kenntnis des Winterlichen Wasserhaushaltes. *Jahrb. Wiss. Bot.* **80,** 169–243.

Miller, P. C. and Gates, D. M. (1967). Transpiration resistance of leaves. *Amer. Midl. Natur.* **77,** 77–85.

Mooney, H. A., Billings, W. D. and Hillier, R. D. (1965). Transpiration rates of alpine plants in the Sierra Nevada of California. *Amer. Midl. Natur.* **74,** 374–386.

Müller-Stoll, W. R., and Lerch, G. (1963). Model tests on the ecological effect of vapour movement and condensation in soil due to temperature gradients. *In* "The Water Relations of Plants," (A. J. Rutter and F. W. Whitehead, eds.), Wiley, New York.

Osburn, W. S. and Wright H. E. (eds.) (1968). "Arctic and Alpine Environments," *V 10 Proc. VII Congr. Int. Ass. Quatern. Res. U.S. Nat. Acad. Sci.* Indiana Univ. Press, Bloomington, Indiana.

Pisek, A. (1956). Der Wasserhaushalt der Meso-und Hygrophyten. *In* "Handbuch der Pflanzen Physiologie," Vol III, pp. 826–853. Springer-Verlag, Berlin and New York.

Pisek, A., Sohm, H., and Cartellieri, E. (1935). Untersuchungen uber osmotischen Wert und Wassergehalt von Pflanzen und Pflanzengesellschaften der Alpinen. *Beih. Bot. Zentr. Abt. B* **52,** 63–675.

Polunin, N. (1955). Aspects of arctic botany. *Amer. Sci.* **43,** 307–322.

Romanova, E. N. (1971). Microclimate of tundras in the vicinity of the Taimyr Station. "Biocenoses of Taimyr Tundra and their Productivity," (B. A. Tikhomirov, ed.), pp. 35–44. Publ. House Nauka, Leningrad. (Translation: P. Kuchar, Univ. of Alberta, Edmonton, Alberta.)

Sakai, A., and Otsuka, K. (1970). Freezing resistance of alpine plants. *Ecology* **51**, 665–671.

Savile, D. B. O. (1972). Arctic adaptations in plants. *Plant Res. Inst. Ottawa Monogr. 6.*

Scarth, G. W. (1927). Stomatal movement: Its regulation and regulatory role. A review. *Protoplasma* **2**, 498–511.

Schulze, E. D., Lange, O. L., Buschbom, U., Kappen, L., and Evenari, M. (1972). Stomatal responses to changes in humidity in plants growing in the desert. *Planta* **108**(3), 259–270.

Slatyer, R. O. (1967). Terminology for cell and tissue water relations. *Z. Pflanzenphysiol.* **56**, 95–97.

Spomer, G. G. (1964). Physiological ecology studies of alpine cushion plants. *Physiol. Plant.* **17**, 717–724.

Stocker, O. (1923). Kimamessungen auf Kleinstem Raum an Wisenwald-und Heidepflanzen. *Ber. Deut. Bot. Ges.* **41**, 145–50.

Svoboda, J. (1972). Vascular plant productivity studies of raised beach ridges (semi-polar desert) in the Truelove lowland. *Devon Island. I.B.P. Proj. Rep. 1970–71.* (L. C. Bliss, ed.), pp. 146–184.

Taylor, S. A. (1962). The influence of temperature upon the transfer of water in soil systems. Overdruk uit de Mededelingen van de Landbouwhogeschool en de Opzoekingsstations van de Staat Te Gent Deel XXVII 2.

Taylor, S. A., and Cavazza, L. (1954). The movement of soil moisture in response to temperature gradients. *Proc. Soil Sci. Soc. Amer.* **18**, 351–358.

Teeri, J. A. (1973). Desert adaptations of a high arctic plant species. *Science* **179**, 496–497.

Thompson, R., and Mayo, J. M. (1973). *Devon Island* 1972 report.

Tieszen, L. L. (1973). Personal communication.

Tiffney, W. N., Jr. (1972). Snow cover and the *Diapensia lapponica* habitat in the White Mountains, New Hampshire. *Rhodora* **74**, 358–377.

Tranquillini, W. (1963a). Abhangigkeit der Kohlensaureassimilation junger Larchen, Fichten und Zirben von der Luft und Boden feuchte. *Planta* **60**, 70–94.

Tranquillini, W. (1963b). Climate and water relations of plants in the subalpine region. *In* "The Water Relations of Plants," (A. J. Rutter and F. H. Whitehead, eds.), pp. 153–167. Blackwell, London.

Tranquillini, W. (1964). The physiology of plants at high altitudes. *Annu. Rev. Plant Physiol.* **15**, 345–363.

van Zinderen Bakker, Jr., E. (1973). Personal communication. (Dept. of Botany, Univ. of Alberta, Edmonton, Alberta.)

Walter, H., and Kreeb, K. (1970). "Die Hydration and Hydrature des Protoplasmas der Pflanzen und ihre Oko-Physiologishe Bedeutung." Protoplasmatol. Band II. Springer-Verlag, Berlin.

Warren-Wilson, J. (1957). Temperatures of arctic plants and their environment. *J. Ecol.* **45**, 499–531.

Wassink, E. C. (1953). Specification of radiant flux and radiant flux density in irradiation of plants with artificial light. Report of the Dutch Committee on plant irradiation. *J. Hort. Soc.* **28,** 177–184.

Weller, G., and Cubley, S. (1972). The microclimates of the arctic tundra. *Proc. 1972 Tundra Biome Symp.* (S. Bowen, ed.), U.S. I.B.P. pp. 5–12.

Werner, H. T., Rickert, R. N., Potter, G. L., and Swarts, S. W. (1969). Energy and moisture balance of an alpine tundra in mid-July. *Arctic Alpine Res.* 1(4), 247–266.

Whitfield, C. J. (1932). The vegetation of the Pikes peak region. *Ecol. Monogr.* **3,** 75–105.

Younkin, W. (1973). Personal communication. (Dept. of Botany, Univ. of Alberta, Edmonton, Alberta.)

Physiological Responses of Root Systems to Stress Conditions

Brent H. McCown

*Institute for Environmental Studies and
Department of Horticulture
The University of Wisconsin
Madison, Wisconsin*

With the hope of stimulating such research, this chapter will review some aspects of the response of root systems to the environmental extremes in arctic and alpine conditions. The intention was not to present an exhaustive exposé of all facets of this topic, for this would do little but reveal the paucity of information available. Instead, by developing some especially pertinent aspects of the topic, it is hoped that the relative value of such research may be realized. To this end, it is necessary to draw on studies conducted in temperate regions for applicable data that may be unavailable about arctic and alpine communities.

The belowground plant system can be viewed as a complex of organs and tissues which may consist of considerably more than just roots. For this reason, the "belowground root–stem complex" or simply the "root–stem complex" will be used in this chapter and can be considered to consist of some or all of the following tissue systems: (1) root system; (2) rhizomes (underground horizontal stems and shoot axes); (3) crowns (stem–root juncture with associated offshoots and divisions); and (4) specialized storage structures (bulbs, corms, tubers, fleshy roots). Any such division into parts will necessarily be accompanied by some ambiguity; however, these tissue systems are usually under direct influence of edaphic conditions and therefore will experience similar stresses.

Since selection may act in general to maintain those few gene combinations that enable the root–stem complex to function more effectively under arctic and alpine environments, realization of the diverse functions that these tissues serve is essential. In addition to the obvious functions of anchorage, water and mineral uptake, and translocation, the functions of storage, perennation, and vegetative reproduction may be fulfilled by the root–stem complex. The importance of the storage of organic nutrients, principally carbohydrates, in the root–stem complex of herbaceous plants has been detailed in both alpine and arctic species (Russell, 1940; Billings and Bliss, 1959; Mooney and Billings, 1960) and in temperate species (Brown, 1943; McCarty and Price, 1942). In the alpine species *Polygonum bistortoides,* which stores large amounts of carbohydrates in rhizomes, nearly one-half of the reserves were utilized within a week during spring growth (Mooney and Billings, 1960). Whether similar activities occur in alpine and arctic woody species or whether storage of water and/or minerals may also occur has yet to be investigated. The storage and rapid utilization of such reserves enables arctic and alpine plants to capitalize on early warm periods to produce sexual reproductive structures and a substantial leaf area early in the short growing season.

The root–stem complex serves as the perennating organ for the grasses and herbs. Although being in or near the soil tempers the extremes in environment considerably, a degree of cold hardiness is necessary to survive the minimum soil temperatures (to $-20°$). Failure of some plants in temperate zones to survive winter has been attributed to a lack of hardiness of the root–stem complex (Smith, 1964; Tumanov, 1967; Mityga and Lanphear, 1971). Frost hardiness of aboveground tissues of alpine and arctic plants seems highly developed (Bliss, 1962), and survival of overwintering flower buds is common (Sørensen, 1941; Hodgson, 1966). Arctic and alpine plant roots are known to be able to function at temperatures near $0°$ (Dadykin, 1954; Bliss, 1956; Chapin, 1973), but the extent to which root resistance to freezing temperatures acts as a selective pressure is unknown.

Probably because of a combination of a severe aerial environment and limiting edaphic factors, arctic and alpine plant communities maintain an extensive biomass under the soil surface. Whereas estimates of the ratio of above- to belowground biomass in temperate climates generally may range from $1:1$ to $1:2$ (Brouwer, 1966; Rogers and Head, 1968), estimates of $1:2$ to $1:11$ (Aleksandrova, 1958; Billings and Mooney, 1968; Dennis and Johnson, 1970; Dennis and Tieszen, 1972) have been made in arctic and alpine environments. Indeed, many of the plant species, particularly the predominant herbs and grasses, may be viewed as underground organisms with annual aerial appendages.

Realizing this rather lopsided distribution in allocation, one may at first find it rather incongruent that the activity of the underground tissues of far-northern plants still remains unfamiliar to the plant scientist. However, a survey of the plant sciences reveals that this lack of understanding is not limited to cold-dominated ecosystems. Root – belowground stem systems are perhaps most studied in the agronomic sciences, but relatively little attention has been given them in the ecological sciences. This information void is the result of a combination of factors including the relative unimportance of root crops in general and the immense difficulties in working with belowground tissues. With the increased sophistication and availability of controlled environmental facilities, a rapidly expanding interest in the physiology and ecology of root systems can be anticipated. Specifically, as regards adaptation of belowground plant systems, arctic and alpine regions may be well-suited study areas; not only are belowground organs and tissues extensive and of importance in the seasonality of growth and survival (Bliss, 1962; Billings and Mooney, 1968), but the environmental extremes encountered may dictate similar extremes in adaptation.

Vegetative reproduction occurs primarily through the activity of the root – stem complex by horizontal growth of rhizomes, tiller development, and crown divisions. Growth of the rhizome may be particularly important, especially with the graminoids, because such activity can permit the invasion of new ground in an environment hostile to seedling establishment (Bliss, 1962; Billings and Mooney, 1968). More will be said about this factor later in this chapter.

A number of soil conditions typically observed under arctic and alpine environments may be particularly selective. Arctic-alpine soils have low minimum temperatures (Billings and Mooney, 1968), almost twice as low as in temperate climates. However, the temperatures are relatively stable as compared to temperate regions. In addition, annual mean soil temperatures are low with summer temperatures in the Arctic averaging less than 3° (at 15 cm depth). The soils may be water saturated most of the season on permafrost plains; such high moisture conditions are commonly accompanied with an anaerobic soil atmosphere. Where permafrost or bedrock forms a limit to the depth of the soil profile, rooting depth may be restricted to 20 – 30 cm (Billings and Mooney, 1968), thus severely limiting the volume of available soil. Finally, of special importance in arctic regions is the stress imposed during winter and spring by frost-heaving activity (Brown and Johnson, 1965).

Of these soil conditions, recent work has noted the importance of the low mean soil temperature during the growth season to plant production, survival, and distribution in cold-dominated environments. The marked differences in community structure between north- and south-facing slopes may at least in part be a function of the differences in seasonal soil temperatures. Soil temperature has been indicated as a factor distinguishing alpine and subalpine vegetation in the Venezuelan Andes as well as in the delineation of timber line (Walter and Medina, 1969). In areas where the usual soil temperature is abnormally elevated, e.g., near warm springs and over heated, buried, manmade structures, marked differences in the structure and functioning of the affected plant communities can be observed. The northern extent of some plant species in Alaska may be closely associated with the occurrence of warm springs (unpublished observations of the author). In experiments utilizing a buried, heated pipeline where soil temperatures were maintained $5°-25°$ above normal, advanced phenology, increases in aboveground annual biomass production of $300-500\%$, and changes in the physiological state of the affected plants have been recorded (McCown, 1973a).

Any adaptation must occur within the limits of genetic variation. Studies on temperate and subtropical plants have shown that considerable variation exists as regards tolerance of low soil temperatures. Mitchell (1956) demonstrated that the festucoid grasses grow well at low temperatures $(7°-20°)$ but poorly at temperatures stimulating to nonfestucoid grasses $(25°-35°)$. Soil temperatures entirely appropriate for the festucoid grasses $(15°$ or lower) may be highly inhibitory to the growth of the nonfestucoid grasses (Evans *et al.,* 1964). At the species level, Kramer (1942) effectively showed that plants adapted to warm soil regimes are more affected by cold soils than are similar species adapted to cooler soil regimes. Variation within a closely related population has been shown with inbred lines of corn (Jones and Mederski, 1963).

Complex interactions obviously occur between soil temperatures and almost all other soil environmental factors. Soil temperature – mineral nutrient interactions may be of particular importance as a selection pressure in arctic-alpine communities for both factors may occur generally at below optimum levels during the growing season. Of special importance may be nitrogen nutrition since this element has been cited as limiting plant growth in arctic conditions (Russell, 1940; Bliss and Wein, 1972), and nitrogen utilization is markedly influenced by low soil temperatures, especially below $10°$ (Shtrausberg, 1955). In a comparison of a native Alaskan north slope grass, *Dupontia fischeri,* with a northern grass, manchar brome, that in general was successful in Alaska except in cold soil areas, marked differences between the ability of these two grasses to utilize soil nitrogen under arctic temperatures were found (McCown, 1973b). Although the growth of the arctic grass was still inhibited by soil temperatures of 5°, both above and belowground growth were substantial (Figure 1). More importantly, this arctic grass in contrast to the brome grass, was able to capitalize on increased levels of soil nitrogen in the cold soils and produce greater biomass. A further analysis of the components of this production, individual tiller growth (leaf growth rate) and total number of tillers (stem density), showed that both the difference between species and the increased production with higher nutrition were primarily the result of increases in stem density (Figure 2). Thus it appeared that the arctic grass had adjusted to its native cold soil conditions by adaptations allowing rhizome growth and subsequent tiller production at low soil temperatures.

The ability of arctic grasses to respond to increased levels of soil nutrition principally by increasing stem densities in contrast to increasing individual tiller growth rates may be an adaptive advantage in northern regions. Greater stem densities would allow increased leaf area indices without producing a taller canopy that would be subject to greater internal shading (important under the low light, low sun angle conditions of the Arctic) as well as greater aerial environmental stresses. Such a strategy would also promote the invasion of new territory and thus the expansion of the total soil volume explored. Mitchell (1956) noted that, in general, festucoid grasses respond to changes in temperature principally through changes in tillering rates, the growth rate per tiller remaining relatively constant. In nonfestucoid grasses, the effect of temperature was more marked on the individual tiller growth rate. Therefore, this phenomenon may also represent a general response of northern grasses in which allocations are made preferentially to belowground structures (e.g., rhizomes), thus insuring an abundant supply of perennating organs.

The physiological basis of the temperature – soil nutrient interactions is as yet unknown. Studies in temperate regions indicate that the main effect may be inhibition of translocation rather than absorption (Humphries, 1951; Shtrausberg, 1955; Nielsen, et al., 1960; Power et al., 1970; Frota and Tucker, 1972). With nitrogen nutrition in arctic and alpine soils, a potentially important factor is that the principal form of available nitrogen is ammonium (Gersper, 1972; VanCleve, 1971). In order to prevent the toxic effect of high ammonium levels in roots, ammonium is generally incorporated into an organic molecule, usually an amino acid or glutamine before translocation (Folkes, 1959; Sims et al., 1969). This requirement dictates that before translocation of the nitrogen to the shoot, not only must a biochemical reaction be performed in the root (which may be at temperatures near 0° in the Arctic) but an

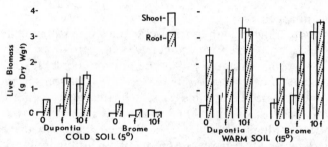

Figure 1 The influence of soil temperature and soil ammonium concentration on the biomass production of a native arctic grass, *Dupontia fischeri,* and an introduced grass, manchar brome. Nutrient levels: 0 = no ammonium added to medium; F = ammonium concentration approximately equal to arctic field concentrations (0.05 mg NH^+_4 per gram media) and 10 F (0.5 mg NH^+_4 per gram media). Data presented with ± 1 standard error of the mean.

organic skeleton (usually α-ketoglutaric acid or glutamic acid) must be supplied. Thus greater demands are placed on translocation of organics from the shoots or centers of storage, and adaptations allowing high rates of translocation of organics at low soil temperatures would be highly advantageous. There are some indications that both the assimilation of nitrogen into organic compounds and the translocation of carbohydrates from shoots may be limiting at low soil temperatures (Dadykin,

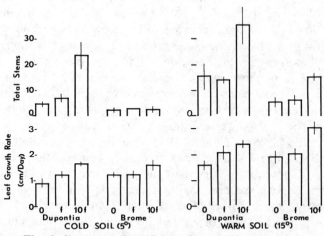

Figure 2 The influence of soil temperature and soil ammonium on tiller growth and vegetative reproduction of a native arctic grass, *Dupontia fischeri,* and an introduced grass, manchar brome. Nutrient levels as in Figure 1.

1954; Nielsen and Cunningham, 1964). Specific adaptations in these processes in arctic and alpine plants have yet to be thoroughly documented.

Adaptations within an Alaskan species to the soil temperature–mineral nutrient environment of the Arctic have been shown by the recent work of Chapin (1973). In a comparison of the phosphate absorption capacity of two clones of the sedge *Carex aquatilis,* the clone from a warm soil area of a hot spring had considerably lower V_{max} than the arctic clone, while both clones had approximately the same apparent K_m in any one environment (Table 1). The physiological basis for the higher rates of phosphate absorption in the arctic selections was hypothesized to be differences in the rates of synthesis of carrier complexes. The warm-adapted species also showed a greater temperature sensitivity and acclimation potential, a trend evident in comparisons between Alaskan and Californian species of graminoids. Acclimation to low temperature as evidenced by a change in the apparent K_m for phosphate absorption, occurred in all the species and selections studied but was more pronounced in the temperate selections. Acclimation may be a method by which organisms compensate for fluctuations in the environment; the difference in acclimation potential for phosphate absorption between temperate and arctic plants supports the proposition that selection for a higher acclimation potential will occur in the more fluctuating environments, e.g., temperate climates (Chapin, 1973; see Prosser and Mooney, this volume).

In a study of the potential value of various native grass species for revegetation of far-northern regions, Younkin (1973) found that *Arctagrostis* was more capable of growing in cold, nutrient-rich soils than

Table 1 A Comparison of The Phosphate Absorption Characteristics of Two Alaskan Selections of The Sedge, *Carex aquatilis*[a]

Characteristic	Selection from a warm spring[b]		Arctic selection from Barrow[c]	
	5°[d]	20°[d]	5°[d]	20°[d]
Apparent K_m (μm P_i/liter)	2.80	2.01	3.00	2.95
V_{max} [μm · hr^{-1} · (g fr. wt.)$^{-1}$]	0.12	0.07	0.48	0.61
Q_{15}[e]	3.65	4.60	1.93	2.32
Acclimation potential[e]	6.20	4.91	1.82	1.51

[a]From Chapin (1973).
[b]July mean soil temperature of 18°.
[c]July mean soil temperature of 7°.
[d]Root temperature for growth and measurement.
[e]At nonsaturating levels of phosphorus.

Calamagrostis. In these growth chamber experiments, *Arctagrostis* allocated a greater percentage of its resources to belowground structures in both cold and warm soils than did *Calamagrostis*.

Since the ability of roots to absorb nutrients depends at least in part on their ability to extend into new soil, adaptations in root growth and morphology may play an important part in a plant's response to soil stresses. Brouwer and Hoogland (1964) noted that roots exposed to temperatures higher or lower than their optimum respond with a reduction of the distance between the root tip and the region where differentiation is completed. In addition, suberization of the endodermal cell walls was more prevalent at the temperature extremes. Bowen and Rovira (1971) emphasized the importance of lateral roots in nutrient uptake and showed that low soil temperatures greatly decreased the number of laterals of wheat roots. The combination of the changes in individual root morphology and the reduction in lateral root formation may have important ramifications by reducing the total root surface area while also limiting the ability to explore new soils.

There are limited indications that the roots of arctic plants have adapted morphologically. Roots of arctic species grown in low soil temperatures in growth chambers remain white and succulent and display a rather uniform absorption pattern along a considerable root length (Chapin, 1973). Such roots also maintain a smaller diameter than temperate species under similar conditions. In addition to individual root characteristics, differences in root system structure have been noted in arctic and alpine plants. In general, roots in arctic permafrost soils are confined to the warmer and better drained upper soil layers (Bliss, 1956; Chapin, 1973). However, root tips of some species follow the retreating permafrost during summer and are thus exposed to temperatures near 0°. Billings and Shaver (1972) noted that the three predominant monocots at Barrow, Alaska had different rooting strategies; *Carex aquatilis* had few and shallow roots, *Eriophorum angustifolium* had plentiful and deep roots, and *Dupontia fischeri* was intermediate. Thus, it appears that there may be a number of adaptive strategies for root system structure in cold, arctic soils, which vary from avoidance of the low temperature, high moisture conditions to capitalizing on the possible nutrient fluxes near the retreating permafrost boundary.

A perennial root habit may have certain advantages in not requiring a complete annual regeneration of the root system in what may be unfavorable soil conditions. Little information is available on this subject, although the perennial habit of both woody and herbaceous roots in temperate regions has been established (Stuckey, 1941; Evans *et al.*, 1964; Rogers and Head, 1968). In some northern graminoids, roots have been observed to survive at least one season (Stuckey, 1941); however, limited evidence on arctic graminoids indicates that perennial roots are lacking (Chapin, 1973). Whether this is the result of seasonal senescence or loss through a lack of winter hardiness is unknown.

The interrelationships of root and shoot have long been a topic of considerable discussion (Brouwer, 1966; Luckwill, 1960; Leonard, 1962). A possible adaptive feature of arctic and alpine plants may be a greater allocation of plant resources to belowground structures to facilitate nutrient absorption (Chapin, 1973; Younkin, 1973) and the establishment of perennating and storage structures. However, as was shown in Figure 1, this response of high root/shoot ratios in cold, nutrient-poor soils is not limited to arctic and alpine plants or to plants especially adapted to such conditions. The inverse relationship between root development and nitrogen supply is well known in temperate regions (Bosemark, 1954) and may help to explain the generally high root/shoot ratios encountered in the nitrogen-poor arctic and alpine sites. The low soil temperature conditions can enhance this response, especially with unadapted species, by reducing nutrient utilization and thus promoting high root/shoot ratios (Nightingale, 1933). The lack of nitrogen in the tissues can limit carbohydrate utilization, especially protein synthesis, and thus help to account for the high carbohydrate levels common in arctic and alpine plants (McCown and Tieszen, 1972). As to what degree these responses are truly adaptive cannot as yet be determined.

The complexity of the interrelationships between tissues, organs, and above/belowground systems as well as between components of an ecosystem is both bewildering and intellectually challenging. The main limitation in thoroughly developing such an understanding, especially as regards adaptation phenomena, is that our descriptions have been necessarily static with time. Recent work in the Tundra Biome (Figure 3) has shown the value of modeling as a tool to develop a more dynamic realization of plant above/belowground relationships. In addition, and probably as important, the modeling efforts have helped to pinpoint those areas where research is especially desirable in expanding our information base.

Many factors that may be involved in the overall response of arctic and alpine root–stem complexes have not been discussed. The anaerobic condition in the water-saturated arctic soils may require oxygen transfer from aerial parts to the roots and rhizomes (Greenwood, 1968). Stem growth factors in addition to water and minerals may be synthesized in and supplied by roots and such synthesis may require relatively high oxygen levels (Luckwill, 1960). Changes in the viscosity and permeability of the protoplasm and membranes of root cells must also oc-

PLANT NUTRIENT INTERRELATIONSHIPS

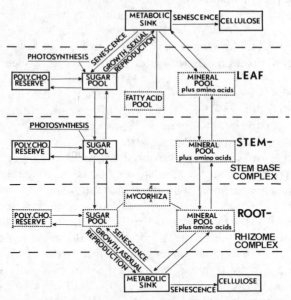

Figure 3 A schematic representation of possible plant nutrient in-interrelationships adapted from Barrow data. Boxes with dashed lines are hypothetical; arrows refer to translocation pathways. The dominating feature is the multiple pathways for allocation of photosynthate to prevent excess accumulations at the site of synthesis which might inhibit photosynthesis, especially under inorganic mineral deficiencies (from McCown and Tieszen, 1972).

cur, and such changes undoubtedly involve fatty-acid metabolism. A soil temperature – water utilization interaction also occurs (Kramer, 1942), and such changes in permeability may be especially important here. A myriad of root – soil organism associations can exist and materially influence the capacities of root systems (Bowen and Rovira, 1968). Adaptation in all of these processes may be significant to arctic and alpine plants and research on such topics, along with the integration as supplied by modeling efforts, should yield exciting results.

Acknowledgments

The author's work cited in this paper was conducted under programs with the Cold Regions Research and Engineering Laboratory, Hanover, New Hampshire; the Tundra Biome, International Biological Program; and the Institute of Arctic Biology, University of Alaska, Fairbanks, while serving a visiting Assistant Professorship of Plant Physiology at the University of Alaska.

References

Aleksandrova, V. D. (1958). An attempt to measure the over- and underground mass of tundra plants. *Bot. Zh. SSSR,* **43,** 1748–1761 (in Russian)

Billings, W. D., and Bliss, L. C. (1959). An alpine snowbank environment and its effects on vegetation, plant development, and productivity. *Ecology* **40,** 388–397.

Billings, W. D., and Mooney, H. A. (1968). The ecology of arctic and alpine plants. *Biol. Rev.* **43,** 481–529.

Billings, W. D., and Shaver, G. (1972). Root growth and root respiration in tundra soils as affected by temperature. *U.S. Tundra Biome Data Rep.* 73–3, pp. 4–5, Fairbanks, Alaska.

Bliss, L. C. (1956). A comparison of plant development in microenvironments of arctic and alpine tundras. *Ecol. Monogr.* **26,** 303–337.

Bliss, L. C. (1962). Adaptations of arctic and alpine plants to environmental conditions. *Arctic* **15,** 117–144.

Bliss, L. C., and Wein, R. W. (1972). Plant community response to disturbance in the western Canadian arctic. *Can. J. Bot* **50,** 1097–1109.

Bosemark, N. O. (1954). Influence of N on root development. *Physiol. Plant.* **7,** 497.

Bowen, G. D., and Rovira, A. D. (1968). The influence of microorganisms on growth and metabolism of plant roots. In "Root Growth," (W. J. Whittington, ed.), pp. 170–199. Butterworths, London.

Bowen, G. D., and Rovira, A. D. (1971). Relationship between root morphology and nutrient uptake. *Recent Advan. Plant Nutr.* (R. M. Samish, ed.) **1,** 293–303.

Brouwer, R. (1966). Root growth of grasses and cereals. *In* "The Growth of Cereals and Grasses," (F. L. Milthorpe and J. D. Ivins, eds.), pp. 153–166. Butterworths, London.

Brouwer, R., and Hoogland, A. (1964). Responses of bean plants to root temperatures. II. Anatomical aspects. *Meded. Inst. Biol. Scheick.* 235/256, 23–31.

Brown, E. M. (1943). Seasonal variation in the growth and chemical composition of Kentucky bluegrass. *Mo. Agr. Exp. Sta. Res. Bull.* **360,** 1–56.

Brown, J., and Johnson, P. L. (1965). Pedo-ecological investigations, Barrow, Alaska. *Tech. Rep. Cold Regions Res. and Engin. Lab.* Hanover, New Hampshire, No. 159.

Chapin, F. S., III. (1973). Morphological and physiological mechanisms of temperature compensation in phosphate absorption along a latitudinal gradient. Ph.D. thesis, Stanford Univ., California.

Dadykin, V. P. (1954). Peculiarities of plant behavior in cold soils (in Russian). *Vop. Bot.* **2,** 455–472.

Dennis, J. G., and Johnson, P. L. (1970). Shoot and rhizome-root standing crops at Barrow, Alaska. *Arctic Alpine Res.* **2,** 253–266.

Dennis, J. G., and Tieszen, L. L. (1972). Seasonal course of dry matter and chlorophyll by species at Barrow, Alaska. *1972 Tundra Biome Symp. Proc.,* pp. 16–21. U. S. Tundra Biome, Fairbanks, Alaska.

Evans, L. T., Wardlaw, I. F., and Williams, C. N. (1964). Environmental control of growth. *In* "Grasses and Grasslands," (C. Barnard, ed.) pp. 102–125. Macmillan, New York.

Folkes, B. F. (1959). The position of amino acids in the assimilation of nitrogen and the synthesis of proteins in plants. *Symp. Soc. Exp. Biol.* **13**, 126–147.

Frota, J. N. E., and Tucker, T. C. (1972). Temperature influence on ammonium and nitrate absorption by lettuce. *Soil Sci. Soc. Amer. Proc.* **36**, 97–100.

Gersper, P. L. (1972). Chemical and physical soil properties and their seasonal dynamics at the Barrow intensive site. *1972 Tundra Biome Symp. Proc.,* pp. 91–93. U. S. Tundra Biome, Fairbanks, Alaska.

Greenwood, D. J. (1968). Effect of oxygen distribution in the soil on plant growth. *In* "Root Growth," (W. J. Whittington, ed.), pp. 202–221. Butterworths, London.

Hodgson, H. J. (1966). Floral initiation in Alaskan Gramineae. *Bot. Gaz.* **127**, 64–70.

Humphries, E. C. (1951). The absorption of ions by excised root systems. II. Observations on roots of barley grown in solutions deficient in phosphorus, nitrogen or potassium. *J. Exp. Bot.* **2**, 344–379.

Jones, J. B., Jr., and Mederski, H. J. (1963). Effect of soil temperature on corn plant development and yield. II. Studies with six inbred lines. *Soil Sci. Soc. Amer. Proc.* **27**, 189–192.

Kramer, P. J. (1942). Species differences with respect to water absorption at low soil temperatures. *Amer. J. Bot.* **29**, 828–832.

Leonard, E. R. (1962). Interrelations of vegetative and reproductive growth with special reference to indeterminent plants. *Bot. Rev.* **28**, 353.

Luckwill, L. C. (1960). The physiological relationships of root and shoot. *Sci. Hort.* **14**, 22–26.

McCarty, E. C., and Price, R. (1942). Growth and carbohydrate content of important mountain forage plants in Central Utah as affected by clipping and grazing. *U.S. Dep. Agr. Tech. Bull.* **818**, 1–51.

McCown, B. H. (1973a). The influence of soil temperatures on plant growth and survival in Alaska. *Proc. Symp. Oil Resource Develop. Impact North. Plant Commun.* (B. H. McCown and D. R. Simpson, eds.). Univer. of Alaska.

McCown, B. H. (1973b). Growth and survival of northern plants at low soil temperatures: Growth response, organic nutrients, and ammonium utilization. *USACRREL Spec. Rep. 186.*

McCown, B. H., and Tieszen, L. L. (1972). A comparative investigation of periodic trends in carbohydrate and lipid levels in arctic and alpine plants. *1972 Tundra Biome Symp. Proc.,* pp. 40–45. Fairbanks, Alaska.

Mitchell, K. J. (1956). Growth of pasture species under controlled environment. I. Growth at various levels of constant temperature. *N.Z.J. Sci. Technol.* **38A**, 203–215.

Mityga, H. G., and Lanphear, F. O. (1971). Factors influencing the cold hardiness of *Taxus cuspidata* roots. *J. Amer. Hort. Sci* **96**, 83–87.

Mooney, H. A., and Billings, W. D. (1960). The annual carbohydrate cycle of alpine plants as related to growth. *Amer. J. Bot.* **47**, 594–598.

Nielsen, D. F., and Cunningham, R. K. (1964). The effects of soil temperature, form, level of N on growth and chemical composition of Italian ryegrass. *Soil Sci. Soc. Amer. Proc.* **28**, 213–218.

Nielsen, K. R., Halstead, R. L., MacLean, A. J., Holmes, R. M., and Bourget, S. J. (1960). Effects of soil temperature on the growth and chemical composition of lucerne. *Proc. 8th Int. Grassl. Congr.,* pp. 287–292.

Nightingale, G. T. (1933). Effects of temperature on metabolism in tomato. *Bot. Gaz.* **95**, 35–58.

Power, J. F., Grunes, D. L., Reichman, G. A., and Willes, W. O. (1970). Effect of soil temperature on rate of barley development and nutrition. *Agron. J.* **62**, 567–571.

Rogers, W. S., and Head, G. C. (1968). Factors affecting distribution and growth of roots of perennial woody species. *In* "Root Growth," (W. J. Whittington, ed.), pp. 280–293. Butterworths, London.

Russell, R. S. (1940). Physiological and ecological studies on an arctic vegetation. II. The development of vegetation in relation to nitrogen supply and soil micro-organisms on Jan Mayen Island. *J. Ecol.* **28**, 269–288.

Shtrausberg, D. Y. (1955). Effect of soil temperature on the utilization of various nutrient elements by plants *Mech. Atom. Issled, Pitan. Rast. Primen. Udobr.,* pp. 157–165 (in Russian).

Sims, A. P., Folkes, B. F., and Bussey, A. H. (1969). Mechanisms involved in the regulation of nitrogen assimilation in micro-organisms and plants. *Recent Aspects Nitrogen Metab. Plants,* (E. J. Hewitt and C. V. Cuttings, eds.), pp. 91–114. Academic Press, New York.

Smith, D. (1964). Winter injury and survival of forage plants. *Herb. Abs.* **34**, 203–209.

Sørensen, T. (1941). Temperature relations and phenology of the northeast Greenland flowering plants. *Medd. Groenland* **125**, 1–305.

Stuckey, I. H. (1941). Seasonal growth of grass roots. *Amer. J. Bot.* **28**, 468–491.

Tumanov, I. I. (1967). Causes of poor cold resistance in roots of fruit trees. *Fiziol. Rast.* **14**, 763–770.

VanCleve, K. (1971). Nitrogen cycling in tundra and taiga soils as influenced by temperature and moisture. *In* "The Structure and Function of the Tundra Ecosystem," *U. S. Tundra Biome Prog. Rep.,* Vol. 1, pp. 169–171. Fairbanks, Alaska.

Walter, H., and Medina, E. (1969). Soil temperature as the differentiating factor between subalpine and alpine vegetation in the Venezuelan Andes. *Ber. Deut. Bot. Ges.* **82**, 275–281 (in German).

Younkin, W. (1973). Autecological studies of native species potentially useful for revegetation, Tuktoyktuk Region N. W. T. *In* "Botanical Studies of Natural and Man Modified Habitats in the Mackenzie Valley, Eastern Mackenzie Delta Region, and Its Arctic Islands," (L. C. Bliss, ed.), pp. 50–96. ALUR 72-73. Dept. Indian Affairs and North. Dev., Ottawa, Canada.

Some Aspects of Nutritional Adaptations of Arctic Herbivorous Mammals

Robert G. White

Institute of Arctic Biology
University of Alaska
Fairbanks, Alaska

Introduction

The arctic tundra is inhabited by both endemic and widespread arctic and subarctic species of herbivorous mammals. The endemic species include the brown and collared lemming (*Lemmus trimucronatus* and *Dicrostonyx groenlandicus* respectively), the caribou and wild reindeer (*Rangifer tarandus* subsp.), muskoxen (*Ovibos moschatus* subsp.), the arctic hare *(Lepus arcticus* and *L. timidus)* and the willow ptarmigan *(Lagopus lagopus)*. Others, including some species of *Microtus* and at least two hibernators, the marmot *(Marmota caligata)* and arctic ground squirrel *(Spermophilus undulatus),* also inhabit polar and alpine environments on a year-round basis (Morrison, 1964; Batzli, 1973a). Since these species survive the Arctic, they have presumably adjusted to the marked seasonality in the environment which includes changes in ambient temperature, photoperiod, precipitation, and nutrition. Thus, these species may have evolved adaptations involving unique behavioral, nutritional, metabolic, thermoregulatory, and biochemical responses. However, as outlined by Prosser (this volume), the criteria used to identify adaptive processes under genetic control are strict, requiring a critical evaluation of the response in question, whereas transient physiological adaptations may be less strictly defined. Many of the arctic herbivores have not been studied in sufficient detail to determine the nature of the adaptive features of these species. Therefore, in this review I am speculative in indicating characteristics of nutrition and associated intermediary metabolism which may be adaptive.

Batzli (1973a) has recently discussed some aspects of the nutrition in his review of the role of small mammals in arctic ecosystems. Klein (1967, 1970a,b) has reviewed the nutrition of large herbivores, particularly caribou. Other reviews (Palmer, 1934; Courtright, 1959; Zhigunov, 1961; Kelsall, 1962; Tener, 1965; Skoog, 1968; Skjenneberg and Slagsvold, 1968) have discussed the general ecology of large herbivores. Thus far, specific adaptive mechanisms of mammals in the Arctic have been reviewed with more emphasis on thermoregulation and metabolism than on nutrition. The adaptations of small mammals to arctic conditions has been reviewed by Morrison (1964, 1966) and Hart (1971) and both large and small mammals as well as arctic birds have been discussed by Irving (1964a,b, 1972) and West and Norton (this volume). Since nutrition includes phagia and digestive function, reference must be made to spatial and temporal variations in the quality, structure, and biomass of vegetation on the one hand and of physiological and metabolic factors which dictate the animal's nutrient requirements on the other. In this paper more emphasis will be placed on recent findings for large than on those for small mammals, and an attempt will be made to integrate these components of nutrition.

It is convenient to divide polar herbivores into four groups depending on their response to the onset of winter. These are (a) latitudinal long distance migratory species which leave for more temperate climates; (b) resident hibernators; (c) resident subnivian dwellers; and (d) resident surface dwellers. Members of the first three groups exhibit an adaptive behavioral response to the onset of winter. The possible behavioral, nutritional, physiological, and biochemical adaptations which allow for migration are under investigation but are of marginal interest in this discussion of mammals since these adaptations occur only in birds, and have less to do with cold and more to do with the preparation for, and the execution of, sustained flight (West and Norton, this volume).

The unique metabolic pattern and adaptations of hibernators have been reviewed frequently (Lyman and Dawe, 1960; Hoffman, 1964; Suomalainen, 1964; Fisher et al., 1967; South et al., 1972) and is not discussed in this chapter. Emphasis is placed on the subnivian and surface dwellers which must obtain food and thermoregulate under seemingly extreme adverse conditions in winter. Discussion is confined to an example of a subnivian dweller, the brown lemming, and a surface dweller, the caribou. Caribou are migratory, since they frequently have distinctly separated summer and winter habitats. But since the extreme southern boundaries of migration of the major Alaskan and Canadian arctic herds are within the subarctic (Kelsall, 1962; Hemming, 1971; Jakimchuk, 1975; LeResche, 1975), they will be treated as resident. The muskox is another important large herbivore of the arctic. Although the physiology and metabolism is less well known than that of the caribou, the general nutrition, population dynamics, and ecology have been studied by Tener (1965) and new aspects are ·becoming available from studies at Devon Island, Canada (Bliss et al., 1973) and at Nunivak Island, Alaska (Lent, 1973).

Thompson (1955), Pitelka (1957; 1972), and Schultz (1964, 1969) have documented the temporal changes in relative population size of the brown lemming. It has been concluded that the reproductive response of the lemming population increases with herbage availability and quality and is not confined to the summer. In fact, it has been calculated that most of the final increase to peak numbers prior to a population "crash" occurs in winter. Thus, the microenvironment, as described by Morrison (1966), and the nutrient content of herbage in the subnivian space of the lemming apparently allow for intensive reproduction, and winter herbage availability could possibly set the upper limit in population size. It has also been hypothesized that the carrying capacity of the winter range governs the upper size limit of caribou populations (Klein, 1967); the carrying capacity of summer range determines the physical condition of individual caribou (Klein, 1967) and may indirectly influence population size by modifying winter mortality (Klein, 1970a). Hence, some comparisons will be made between the winter nutrition of caribou and lemming. The theme will be developed that the phagic behavior of these species in winter has led to different forms of exploitation of the habitats based on the mode of acclimatization to cold.

The following interrelated sections provide a framework which allows the investigator to evaluate the adaptive features of the various nutritional processes in the caribou and lemming: (a) phagic responses; (b) interrelationships between components of nutrition and cold acclimatization in caribou and reindeer; and (c) comparisons of caribou and lemming.

Phagic Responses

Habitat choice and plant species selection depend on inherent (or evolved) and adventitious characteristics of the species. The phagic and grazing behavior of the lemming and caribou may differ qualitatively in response to body size and the sizes of home range of the species. By virtue of their mobility, caribou have the choice of many plant communities. Except for the reports of mass emigration of *Lemmus* following periodic high population numbers (for critical discussion see Batzli, 1973b), the lemming may be considered to utilize only one plant community. The habitat of the brown lemming, which consists of the low, grass-sedge marsh of the arctic tundra, has been described in detail by Thompson (1955), Pitelka (1957), and more recently in the intensive study of the IBP-U.S. Tundra Biome Program (Bowen, 1971, 1972). The brown lemming habitat may also overlap with that of the collared lemming but the latter prefer the dryer environment of raised polygons and ridges. The diet of collared lemming may be more varied than that for the brown lemming (Batzli, 1973b) and from this standpoint is of interest for comparison with the caribou. However, since information on the collared lemming is minimal, this paper will emphasize comparisons of the brown lemming and caribou.

Winter Diets

Constituents of the winter diet of lemming are not well known. Recent evidence (Batzli, 1973a) suggests that grasses *(Dupontia fischeri)* and sedge *(Eriophorum angustifolium* and *Carex aquatilis)* are present and that mosses may constitute up to 40% of the winter diet. The above-mentioned monocotyledonous vegetation and the mosses constitute the dominant plant groups in the lemming habitat. No preference has been noted for particular plant species found as minor constituents of the herbage. However, selection of green stem bases of monocotyledonous plants undoubtedly enables the lemming to maintain a higher nutrient intake than would occur if food items from the habitat were ingested with no selection. The ability of the lemming to digest the mosses has yet to be determined.

Lichen is well documented as a major component of the winter food of caribou and reindeer (see reviews by Palmer, 1934; Banfield, 1954; Courtright, 1959; Kelsall, 1962; Hale, 1967; Skoog, 1968; Pegau, 1968; Skjenneberg and Slagsvold, 1968). Though a matter of speculation (see for example, Bergerud and Nolan, 1970), it is suggested by herders and animal scientists (e.g., Palmer, 1934) that caribou and reindeer can detect a lichen beneath the snow. Few if any other animal species have a preference for lichens; perhaps most species have only a limited ability to digest them (see Courtright, 1959; Westerling, 1975). It may be significant that lichens contain bacteriostatic agents (Hale, 1967) and that adaptation to them by ruminants, and animals with well-developed ceca, may involve establishment of specific microbial populations in their fermentation organs (Courtright, 1959; Westerling, 1975; Dehority, 1975a,b). Mosses are generally not important components of the diet of caribou although they have been noted in rumen contents of North American and USSR caribou and reindeer in winter (Kelsall, 1962; Bergerud and Russell, 1964; Scotter, 1967; Skoog, 1968; D. Miller, personal communication). Skjenneberg *et al.* (1975) suggest that mosses may be ingested inadvertently with lichen where lichens are intertwined in the moss carpet (Figure 1). The reported frequency of occurrence of mosses in rumen contents may also be in error due to sampling techniques (Bergerud and Nolan, 1970) and due to their easy recognition in relation to other plant fragments (Courtright, 1959; Deardon *et al.*, 1975). Moreover, recent *in vivo* and *in vitro* microdigestion studies in our laboratory show that reindeer have a very poor ability to ferment mosses (Pegau *et al.*, 1973) (Table 1).

Whether the brown lemming and caribou are showing a specific euphagia, that is, selecting for specific nutrients within their winter diet, is not known. Certainly, the low nitrogen (N) content of the main lichens

Table 1 Comparison of Apparent Dry Matter Digestibilities (%) of Plant Species by Brown Lemming and Caribou[a]

	% Digested[b]	
Food injested	Lemming	Caribou/Reindeer
Carex aqualitis	27[c]	56–73
Dupontia fischeri	35–37[c]	69–80
Arctophila fulva	–	56
Eriophorum angustifolium	–	48–57
Salix arctica	–	48–71
S. pulchra	–	54
S. reticulata	–	38
S. ovalifolia	–	35–38
Dryas integrifolia	–	33
Cetraria cuculata	–	71–73
Cladonia alpestris	–	12–49
Mosses	–	6–18
Reindeer E. F. samples	–	44–50
Alfalfa pellets	55[c]	–
Purina cattle starter #1	–	63[(58 ± 2)[d]]

[a]Estimates for lemming were made *in vivo*; those for caribou were made with an *in vitro* microdigestion technique.
[b]Unless otherwise noted, data are from Person, White, and Luick, (unpublished observation).
[c]Batzli (1973a).
[d]Cameron (1972) (estimated *in vivo*).
[e]Melchior (1972).

selected by reindeer and caribou (*Cladonia* spp., *Cetraria* spp., and *Stereocaulon* spp.) suggests that selective processes may be against,rather than for, protein. A comparison of the frequency of occurrence of plant groups in herbage and in esophageal egesta of a summer and winter range, indicate that reindeer select for lichen in winter (Figure 1). These findings confirm earlier reports based on comparisons of range with rumen contents and feeding craters (Courtright, 1959; Kelsall, 1962; D. Miller, personal communication).

Rarely do lichens constitute the sole winter diet of caribou and their actual contribution varies markedly with time of year and location (Courtright, 1959; Skoog, 1968). Thus, the other constituents of the diet may also be under active selection processes. As discussed below, this may be of particular importance to the lemming in winter when food intake is apparently high.

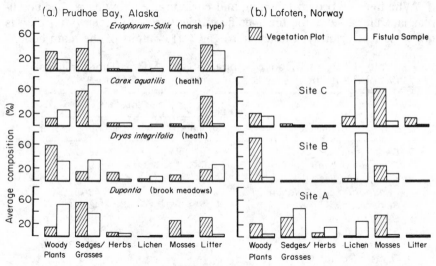

Figure 1 Evidence for selection of plant groups from comparisons of botanical composition of vegetation plots and esophageal fistula samples from reindeer. Values shown in the figure are taken from Prudhoe Bay (Skogland, 1975a,b) for summer vegetation (a) and from Lofoten, Norway (Skjenneberg *et al.*, 1975), for early winter (b). For summer vegetation a strong selection against mosses in all communities can be noted and lichen is unimportant in the diet. In early winter a strong selection for lichen on sites of low (Site A) and high (Site B) lichen biomass is evident. Average composition of herbage is expressed as percent ground cover and of esophageal fistula samples, as percent of 200 point identifications.

Summer Diets

The summer nutrition of the lemming and caribou is markedly different from that in winter. The quality and quantity of food changes abruptly with spring growth at melt-off. Previous studies (e.g., Pitelka, 1957; Schultz, 1964) point to the importance of *D. fischeri, E. angustifolium,* and *C. aquatilis* in the summer diet. In recent studies involving microscopic examination of stomach contents, *D. fisheri* has been identified as the single most important plant species, and sedges, particularly *C. aquatilis,* may also be important components of their diets in drier habitats (Batzli, 1973a,b). Melchior (1972) suggests that the brown lemming selects against naturally occurring dicotyledonous plants. However, as the season progresses, and perhaps as the nutritive value and availability of *D. fischeri* declines, mosses become increasingly important, making up to 20% of the diet by late August.

In comparison, the mobility of caribou allows them to make use of many plant species and communities during the summer. At the U.S. Tundra Biome site at Prudhoe Bay, five plant communities have been identified. Table 2 lists the approximate relative distribution of each community in the study area in relation to relative use made of them by caribou. Although statistical significance is lacking, the data provide evidence that caribou selectively graze the *Dryas integrifolia* dry heath community immediately after melt-off and the *D. fischeri* wet meadows at other times. Although some preference is shown for the above communities, the dominant community utilized by caribou is the *E. angusti-*

Table 2 Relative Distribution of Caribou on Plant Communities with Respect to The Relative Availability of Communities at Prudhoe Bay[a]

Plant community		Relative caribou usage	
Type	Availability[b]	Grazing[c]	All activities[d]
Eriophorum type	51	46	43
Carex aquatilis type	31	13	1
Dryas integrifolia dry heath	5	15	25
Dupontia fischeri wet meadow	4	13	12
Salix ovalifolia sand dunes	—	12	18

[a]Adapted from Skogland, 1975a. Studies were made during July 1972.
[b]Relative occurrence of the communities based on line transects in the study area. The transects did not include the sand dune habitat.
[c]Percentage of all caribou which were grazing.
[d]Percentage of all animal encounters for the study period. This estimates also includes an indication of the use made of the communities as refuges from insect harassment (e.g., sand dune habitat).

folium polygon marsh type. Analysis of rumen samples taken from caribou and esophageal fistulae samples from domestic reindeer grazing these sites, show that on a species basis, *E. angustifolium* plus sedges of similar appearance constitute approximately 37% of the diet. *Dupontia fischeri* and *C. aquatilis,* respectively, constituted 2% and 4% of the diet. The four dominant willows, *Salix ovalifolia, S. arctica, S. rotundifolia,* and *S. scirpoidea* together constitute approximately 24% of the diet.

Thus, both the brown lemming and caribou consume mainly the abundant higher plant species in their respective summer habitats. Although moss is a dominant component of the summer habitats of both the lemming and caribou, in no instance did mosses constitute more than 1–2% of the diet of caribou (Figure 1) and it is only important in the lemming diet from late August through May.

Current emphasis in studies of both brown lemming and caribou in the U.S. Tundra Biome Program is to find if there is selection for chemical nutrients within the habitats. Selection by the brown lemming for rapidly growing plant parts would lead to high soluble carbohydrate, protein, and phosphorus, and to low calcium and lignin components of the diet. Although such a strategy should lead to maximizing apparent digestibility and hence to high digestible energy intake and energy retention (see below), it could also lead to an extremely low Ca:P ratio (Bunnell, 1973). Caribou cannot differentiate between plant parts to the same extent as the lemming and the diet may be qualitatively lower in nutrient content than that of the lemming. Caribou movement patterns not associated with insect harassment can be correlated with the successional patterns in the maturity of plant communities (Lent, 1966; Skogland, 1975a,b). Except for the possibility of high water content and toxicity of plants in the very early growth stages, in most herbages the nutritive value to animals (as judged by palatability, nutrient content, and digestibility) tends to be highest when the plants are growing rapidly (McDonald, 1968; Klein, 1970a,b; Jones, 1972). A marked increase in lignification of arctic grasses and sedges takes place when growth is curtailed or flowering is initiated (McCown and Tieszen, 1972; P. Flanagan, personal communication); the decline in quality has been associated with translocation of nutrients to belowground carbohydrate and phosphate reserves (Mooney and Billings, 1960; McCown and Tieszen, 1972). Thus, by eating rapidly growing plant species, groups, or communities in the ecosystem, caribou ensure a high quality to their diet. This observation agrees with previous observations of Klein (1968) that caribou select for soluble carbohydrate, N, and P. Whether this is a specific euphagia as defined by McClymont (1967) has not been determined.

Regulation of Food Intake

Recent work by Baumgardt (1970) suggests that principles governing the control of food intake are similar in ruminants and nonruminants. In general, the amount of food ingested by an animal increases with the nutritive value [i.e., the dry matter digestibility (DMD) or digestible energy (DE) content] of the food to a maximum intake (Figure 2). In sheep and cattle, gut distension probably signals the end of a feeding period for DMD up to 66–70% (Blaxter, 1962; Conrad et al., 1964). However for foods of DMD in excess of 70%, voluntary intake is apparently regulated by chemostatic factors including plasma glucose and lipid concentrations and heat production in nonruminants, plus ruminal volatile fatty acid (VFA) levels in ruminants (Baile and Mayer, 1970). Food intake may be regulated by short- and long-term components (see Blaxter, 1962; Mayer, 1967); however, the existence of separate components is a matter of conjecture (Kennedy, 1967; Baumgardt, 1970).

Baumgardt (1970) has clearly shown an adaptation in the relationship between voluntary food intake and the DE content of the diet in rats. Figure 3 shows that in lactating rats, where there is a high demand for energy and protein, a marked increase in voluntary intake is noted at most levels of DE content of the food. In this example adaptation involves both the distension and chemostatic mechanisms. Similar relationships presumably exist for ruminants as alimentary hypertrophy, which presumably allows for an increased food intake, has been shown for lactating sheep (Head, 1953; Fell et al., 1964).

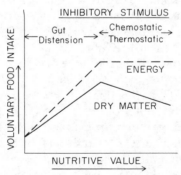

Figure 2 Graphic representation of stimuli controlling the relationship between voluntary food or energy intake and nutritive value of food. Nutritive value can be expressed as apparent dry matter or energy digestibility (Blaxter, 1962) or the digestible energy content of the food (Baumgardt, 1970). This relationship is taken from Montgomery and Baumgardt (1965).

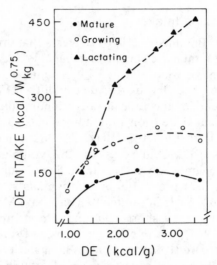

Figure 3 An example of an adaptive increase in voluntary food intake in response to an increased total energy demand due to growth or lactation in the rat. Relationships were taken from Baumgardt (1970). (DE = digestible energy.)

The interrelationships between factors controlling food intake are many. McClymont (1967) has outlined a conceptual model of regulation which involves the central nervous system. The model is based on phagic behavior being manifested when summated facilitatory stimuli exceed summated inhibitory stimuli (Figure 4). Energy balance is the regulated component of this concept. A more detailed description of the feedback, or inhibitory stimuli, and actuating signals, or facilitatory stimuli, has been described by Baumgardt (Church *et al.,* 1971) and the physiological mechanisms are under intensive investigation in field and laboratory experiments (Longhurst *et al.,* 1968; Arnold, 1970; Baumgardt, 1970; Baile and Mayer, 1970). In this context, Figure 2 represents the changeover from one inherent inhibitory stimulus (gastrointestinal distension) to another (energy intake) with an increase in food quality. Adaptation to lactation, shown in Figure 3, is presumably brought about by an increase in the total demand for energy, an inherent facilitatory stimulus, which when coupled with an increase in alimentary volume could also affect the rumen distension stimulus. Observations on activity patterns of caribou and reindeer show that grazing can be a synchronized group activity (Thomson, 1971, in preparation) which suggests the possibility of social facilitation in the control of phagic behavior.

In our search for principals of phagic behavior in arctic herbivores,

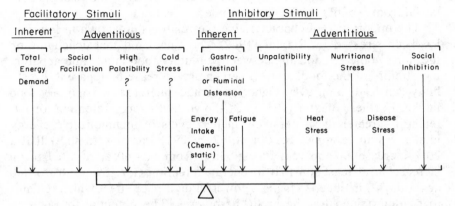

CENTRAL NERVOUS SYSTEM SUMMATION and BALANCING

in the CONTROL of PHAGIC BEHAVIOR of HERBIVORES

Figure 4 A conceptual model, from McClymont (1967), depicting the role of the central nervous system in summating and balancing facilitatory and inhibitory stimuli for the manifestation of phagic behavior. Daily food intake is the product of the time during which phagic behavior is manifested and the level of intake during this time. It is hypothesized that cold acclimatization of arctic herbivores brings about a change in the threshold of the facilitatory stimuli; for small herbivores it is raised, for large herbivores it is lowered. The change in threshold probably acts through total energy demand; a specific adventitious facilitatory stimulus elicited by cold stress cannot be discounted. A more detailed description of the relationships of the inherent, physical, and chemical stimuli, with setpoints, has been proposed by Baumgardt (see Church *et al.*, 1971).

relationships between voluntary food intake and forage quality, for typical forages, must be determined. Further, the responses of the various cohort groups (e.g., the subadult, adult male and nonpregnant, pregnant, and lactating females) should also be characterized. If the DMD or DE content of foods are known for the species under consideration, it can be determined if the animal is regulating its appetite under the distension or chemostatic mechanism. Clearly, the characterization of alimentary fill and emptying rates in the laboratory in order to predict food intake under field conditions, will have limited biological significance if the animal's food intake is regulated chemostatically.

Cessation of eating may be governed by gut distension in arctic herbivores such as the brown lemming and the caribou. This conclusion is based on the observations of Melchior (1971) and Batzli (1973a,b) who have noted DMD of 34–37% for a diet of *D. fischeri* in the brown lemming and for work at Prudhoe Bay with caribou (Person, White, and Luick, unpublished observation), that shows *in vitro* digestibilities (Tilley and Terry, 1963) of between 42 and 48% for plant samples obtained from esophageal fistulated reindeer.

The importance of characterizing the relationship shown in Figure 2 has been stressed by Blaxter (1962) who calculated that depending on the slope of the relationship between voluntary food intake and apparent digestibility of the food, a given percentage increase in apparent digestibility can lead to an even higher percentage increase in voluntary food intake. Further, Blaxter (1962) has shown that energy retention for fattening is greater at successively higher levels of metabolizable energy intake. As an example, Blaxter (1962, p. 291) was able to show that a 20% increase in apparent digestibility, from 50–60%, resulted in an increase of at least fourfold in energy retention (i.e., from 140 to 640 kcal · day^{-1}) in sheep. This is a powerful multiplier effect which remains to be determined for the arctic herbivores. The potential for such an effect can be seen in Table 2 which shows estimates of *in vitro* digestibilities for hand-picked samples of the main plant species available to caribou at Prudhoe Bay. There is a range of *in vitro* digestibilities from as high as 80% for immature *D. fischeri* to as low as 6% for some mosses. The main components of the summer diet are *E. angustifolium* and *Salix* spp., *in vitro* digestibilities are between 35 and 71%, which is a sufficient range to account for an increase in voluntary food intake of over 150% from the lower to higher DMD.

The comparison of apparent digestibility of *D. fischeri* in lemming (35–37%, Melchior, 1972; 34%, Batzli, 1973a) and caribou, indicates a considerable advantage (20 digestibility units) to the caribou over the lemming. However, the comparisons should be made with caution since the forages given the lemming may have been different in chemical composition from those consumed by caribou. Also, the DMD estimate for caribou was made by the *in vitro* microdigestion technique (Tilley and Terry, 1963) and may be an overestimate (Person *et al.*, 1975. Perhaps a more realistic comparison with the *in vivo* DMD of *D. fischeri* in lemming is the *in vitro* DMD of a mixed forage (44–50%, Table 1), obtained from esophageal fistulated reindeer. This comparison suggests an advantage of approximately 10 digestibility units in ruminant over monogastric digestion. The effects of such a difference in digestibility could be compensated for by an increase in the rate of passage of food. Melchior (1971) has determined the maximum capacity of the stomach of the subadult male lemming (approximately 60 gm body weight) at 10% of body weight using Holling's experimental component analysis (Holling, 1966). Food consumption to satiation was determined following fasting periods of various durations. Melchior (1972) calculates that at maintenance, members of the same cohort group would ingest food at approximately 169% of their body weight daily. Thus, the stomach is filled 170/10 or 17 times per day giving a turnover time of 24/17 or 1.4 hr. In comparison, experimentally determined rumen turnover times for reindeer grazing a wet meadow tundra are 9 – 12 hr. Thus, at first approximation, the rate of passage of food in the lemming would be almost five times that of reindeer. However, rates of turnover of body components must be adjusted for body size. Kleiber (1961) shows that for animals behaving isokinetically the ratio of turnover of body pools should be related to body weight (W, kg) in the ratio of $W^{1/4}$. For a lemming weighing 60 g (0.06 kg) and a caribou weighing 100 kg, the respective $W^{1/4}$ values are 0.495 and 3.16 kg, a ratio of approximately 1:6.5. Thus, the increase in rate of passage of food for the lemming (2.8 hr $\cdot$ kg$^{-1/4}$) is in fact similar to that of the experimental reindeer (3.3 hr $\cdot$ kg$^{-1/4}$). Taking into account the difference in digestive efficiency of 10 units gives an advantage to the caribou. These preliminary estimates should be validated by experimentation.

Before the relative production efficiencies of lemming and caribou can be calculated, an estimate must be made of the metabolizability of the diet and of the nonproductive energy expenditure of both species. Values have been reported for the lemming (Batzli, 1973b) but are not currently available for caribou. At this time it must be assumed that on an individual, as opposed to a population basis, the lemming is slightly less efficient than the caribou as a grazer.

Finally, in comparing the phagic responses of the lemming and caribou the relationship between voluntary food intake and density of herbage should be considered. Eating rates for reindeer have been estimated at 6 g dry weight $\cdot$ min^{-1} for herbage dry matter availability of approximately 70 g $\cdot$ m^{-2}. At herbage availabilities of 25 g $\cdot$ m^{-2} dry matter intakes are as low as 3 g $\cdot$ min^{-1} (White, Russell, and Holleman, unpublished observations). In these studies on reindeer the herbage dry matter availability was 40 – 50 g $\cdot$ m^{-2} and a peak eating rate of 5 g $\cdot$ min^{-1} would be expected. A similar relationship between eating rates and herbage availability is not yet available for the lemming, also the herbage biomass in the studies of Melchior (1971, 1972) was not given. Hence, the apparently similar grazing efficiencies which were deduced above must be interpreted with caution until all components governing the phagic behavior of both species have been formulated.

Interrelationships Between Components of Nutrition and Cold Acclimatization in Caribou and Reindeer

Energy Metabolism

Body weight growth of caribou and reindeer is virtually zero in winter, even when the animals are offered food *ad libitum* (McEwan, 1968). Also, Segal (1962) suggests that energy metabolism of reindeer is approximately 30% lower in winter than summer. Similar lowered growth and metabolic phenomena are common in other deer species (Wood *et al.*, 1962; Silver *et al.*, 1969). The daily fasting metabolic rate of caribou in winter (91–102 kcal · kg$^{-3/4}$; McEwan, 1970) is 20–30% greater than the interspecies line of 70 kcal · kg$^{-3/4}$ (Kleiber, 1961), and is similar to estimates of fasting metabolism for other wild ungulates (McEwan, 1970). Luick, White, and Reimers (1971) indicate that growth cessation may be regulated by phagic behavior, for when given food of high (18%), medium (12%), or low (7%) crude protein, weaned reindeer calves tend to regulate at a constant dry matter intake. Based on the hypothesis that phagic behavior of grazers is a summation and balancing of above threshold facilitatory and inhibitory stimuli (Figure 4), it can be suggested that in response to a lowered total energy demand in winter an inhibitory stimulus acts on the inherent facilitatory stimulus or, a new lowered set-point in the facilitatory stimulus, is somehow achieved.

In view of a lack of stimulus for winter growth and a virtual absence of lactation, it can be concluded that winter requirements for production are less than those for summer. This conclusion should be revised as estimates become available of the energy costs of thermoregulation, gestation, and of foraging in winter. Energy expended in thermoregulation may be minimized by an increased insulation of caribou hair coat (Hammel *et al.*, 1962).

Whether the winter diet of caribou and reindeer is capable of meeting the maintenance energy requirements is a matter of conjecture. Though there are conflicting reports (see Courtright, 1959), current evidence suggests that lichen as a sole food source cannot be eaten in sufficient amounts to balance the maintenance energy requirements of reindeer; a decline in both body weight (Cameron, 1972; Jacobsen and Skjenneberg, 1975) and body solids (Cameron, 1972; White, Holleman, and Luick, unpublished observations) has been noted. The intake of lichen can be increased by supplementation with various forages and additives (Jacobson and Skjenneberg, 1975; Person, Pegau, White, and Luick, unpublished observations) and the complex lichen-carbohydrates are rapidly fermented (White and Gau, 1975). In spite of this facilitatory phagic response, it seldom results in a significant increase in body weight

(Jacobson and Skjenneberg, 1975; Person *et al.*, unpublished observations).

Nitrogen Metabolism

McEwan and Whitehead (1970) have determined that the digestible N requirement of reindeer and caribou for equilibrium in winter (0.46 g · $kg^{-3/4}$ · day^{-1}) is similar to that for domestic sheep. The N intake of reindeer given forages which simulate winter nutrition is frequently less than this value. Under situations of low N intake, ruminants and cecalids conserve N by a decrease in N excretion and a return of N, mainly as urea, to the rumen and cecum for reuse by the microbiota (McDonald, 1952, 1968; Houpt, 1959, 1963; Cocimano and Leng, 1967; Houpt and Houpt, 1971). This is known as urea or N recycling and its quantification and control has been studied intensively in domestic species. Conditions in the rumen must be favorable for microbial synthesis in order to incorporate N, from saliva and plasma urea, into microbial protein. It is critical that a readily fermentable supply of carbohydrate be available as an energy source. From this standpoint, diets high in lichen are fermented by reindeer (White and Gau, 1975) indicating the lichen-carbohydrates are readily utilized as an energy source by the specifically adapted rumen microorganisms (Giesecke, 1970; Dehority, 1975a,b). Recently, Wales *et al.* (1975) compared the rates of urea N synthesis and recycling in caribou given diets low and high in protein with those for sheep and beef cattle given diets of similar low N content. Table 3 is a summary of this work and shows that urea N resynthesis is generally less in summer than winter for caribou. Also, of the urea synthesized on a low protein diet, 58% was recycled to the alimentary tract (rumen and cecum) in the caribou and 43% and 48% was recycled in the sheep and cattle respectively. Thus, caribou appear particularly well adapted to low protein nu-

Table 3 Comparison of Seasonal Adaptation to Low Protein Nutrition by Urea N Recycling to the Alimentary Tracts in Caribou, Sheep, and Beef Bulls[a]

Species	Season	N intake (g · day^{-1} · $kg^{-3/4}$)	Urea-N recycled (g · day^{-1} · $kg^{-3/4}$)	Percent[b]
Caribou	Summer	1.50	0.37	46.8
Caribou	Winter	0.96	0.65	57.9
Sheep	Winter	0.80	0.55	42.6
Beef bulls	Winter	0.97	0.32	47.8

[a]Adapted from Wales *et al.*, 1975.
[b]Urea N recycled as a percentage of urea N synthesized. All animals were nonpregnant and nonlactating.

trition, an attribute consistent with the low N content of their natural winter herbage.

Glucose Metabolism

Except for specially prepared diets high in digestible carbohydrates, the diet of grazing ruminants supplies little, if any, glucose *per se* for alimentary absorption (Armstrong, 1965; Ballard *et al.*, 1968; Leng, 1970). Therefore, the glucose requirements of ruminants must be synthesized *de novo* by gluconeogenesis from absorbed dietary precursors such as some ruminal volatile fatty acids (mainly propionic acid), glucogenic amino acids from microbial and plant protein, and protozoal carbohydrates (see reviews by Armstrong, 1965; Ballard *et al.*, 1968; Leng, 1970; Lindsay, 1970). Luick *et al.* (1973) have shown that for comparative states of nutrition, the *de novo* or net rates of glucose synthesis in reindeer are similar to those of sheep. Luick *et al.* (1973) also noted that during late winter and under severe food shortage, reindeer had an enhanced ability to conserve glucose carbon (Table 4). Thus, total and net glucose synthesis was considerably reduced in winter over summer rates, and during winter, 70% of all glucose carbon synthesized was resynthesized from intermediates of glucose metabolism (e.g., lactate, pyruvate, and glycerol) presumably to meet the total requirements of the animal. In feeding ruminants, between 11 and 30% of the net synthesis of glucose is derived from glucogenic amino acids abosrbed from the alimentary tract (Leng, 1970; Reilly and Ford, 1971; Wolff and Bergman, 1972). Thus, the parallel decline in N intake and glucose synthesis and the concomitant increase in urea N and glucose carbon recycling may be more than fortuitous. Both effects are in phase with a lowered overall metabolism.

Table 4 Seasonal Changes in Metabolism and Conservation of Glucose in Grazing Reindeer Cows[a]

Season	Synthesis ($mg \cdot min^{-1} \cdot kg^{-3/4}$)		Glucose resynthesis	
	Total	Net	$mg \cdot min^{-1} \cdot kg^{-3/4}$	%[b]
Grazing				
Winter (January)	5.58 ± 0.39	1.70 ± 0.27	3.88	70
Summer (August)	9.99 ± 0.42	5.47 ± 0.11	4.52	45
Pen-fed				
Winter (January)	6.65 ± 1.19	4.26 ± 0.75	2.39	36

[a]Comparisons are made with pen-fed controls at maintenance. Adapted from Luick *et al.*, 1973.
[b]Glucose resynthesis as a percentage of total synthesis. All animals were nonpregnant and nonlactating.

Water Metabolism

The water requirement of arctic herbivores are met by ingestion of free water, as liquid, snow, ice in herbage, plus metabolic water. The amount of energy required to thaw and warm free water to deep body temperature depends on the temperature of the free water and the amount consumed. Cameron and Luick (1972) have shown that the water flux of grazing reindeer in winter (30–60 ml · kg^{-1} · day^{-1}) is 25–35% of the peak rates in spring and summer. The metabolic cost of melting ice or snow at a temperature of −30°C and ingested at a rate of 50 ml · kg · day^{-1} would be 50 × 0.133* or 6.65 kcal · kg^{-1} · day^{-1} which is approximately 21% of resting metabolism. From snow profiles for interior Alaska (Johnson, 1957; Morrison, 1966) it can be calculated that temperatures of ingested snow and forage may generally be from 0 to −15°C. Thus, these estimates of energy cost of warming free water should be considered as maximal. To this metabolic cost should be added that of warming ingested dry matter. The specific heat of typical forages is not known, but based on a specific heat of 0.32 cal · g · °C^{-1} for cellulose (*Chemical Engineering Handbook,* 1950) and a lichen dry matter intake of 4.1 kg · day^{-1} (Hanson *et al.,* 1975) an energy cost of 90–150 kcal · day^{-1} (3–5 kcal · kg$^{-3/4}$ · day^{-1}) can be calculated (White, Cameron, and Luick, unpublished observations). The maximum metabolic cost of ingesting cold food and water may be 20–25% of fasting metabolism (taken as 100 kcal · kg$^{-3/4}$ · day^{-1}).

The decline in water flux of reindeer in winter (Cameron and Luick, 1972) was brought about by a five- to sevenfold increase in the biological half-time of the total body water pool. In the same animals an increase was noted in the size of the body water pool and Cameron (1972) suggested that this pool may serve as a thermal buffer. The increase in pool size was attributed to a gradual replacement of fat reserves by water (Cameron and Luick, 1972) plus an expansion in alimentary water (Cameron *et al.,* 1975). The increase in biological half-time was related to cold acclimatization (Cameron and Luick, 1972) and to a decline in food intake. The main influence of diet on water flux was through a decline in the intake of dietary protein rather than dry matter (Figure 5) or energy (Cameron, White, and Luick, unpublished observations).

*Specific heat of warming ice from −30 to −1°C is approximately 0.48 cal · g^{-1} · °C^{-1} (mean of 0.449 at −30°C and 0.502 at −1°C). Heat of fusion of water is 79.7 cal · g^{-1}. Specific heat of warming water to 39°C is approximately 1 cal · g^{-1} · °C^{-1}. Calorific value = 30 × 0.48 + 79.7 + 39 × 1 = 133.1 cal · g^{-1}.

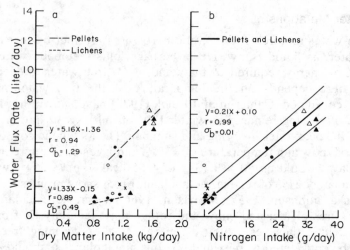

Figure 5 Relationship between water flux and dry matter (a) or nitrogen intake (b) in reindeer held at −5° or −20°C in a winter photoperiod and given diets of commercial pellets (12% CP) or lichen (3% CP) (Cameron, 1972). These data suggest water flux of reindeer in winter may be controlled more by protein than dry matter intake. (Filled symbols, water given as snow; unfilled symbols, water given as liquid; △, ▲, ambient temperature −5°C; ○, ●, ambient temperature −20°C.)

Substitution of Regulative Heat Production

Classic theory dictates that "heat produced by activity substitutes for regulatory heat production in the cold" (Hart, 1971). Since caribou are migratory in nature and dig for food beneath the snow, such a function would seem advantageous to the species. However, a review of the literature produced no evidence which either confirms or refutes the theory of heat substitution in arctic and subarctic ungulates.

In ruminants the possibility that heat of fermentation may also substitute for regulatory heat production has been suggested by Griffin *et al.* (1951) and its potential contribution in reindeer was estimated by Hammel *et al.* (1962) using rumen contents taken from recently fed (<5 hr) reindeer at slaughter. Heat production of the egesta amounted to 5% of resting metabolism which was 1.7 kcal · kg^{-1} · hr^{-1} or 128 kcal · kg$^{-3/4}$ · day^{-1}. The rate of production per kilogram of egesta was one-third to one-half the heat production of 1 kg of average body tissue. The importance of food type on the heat of fermentation in reindeer has not been investigated and thus, no conclusion can be drawn as to whether the values obtained by Hammel *et al.* (1962) are maximal. Provided that the sum of fermentative heat production and the other components of the specific dynamic effect substitute for regulative heat production, the effectiveness of the small amount of heat produced depends on the slope of the line relating rate of metabolism with ambient temperature (Scholander *et al.*, 1950). For a well-furred animal the slope is shallow (Irving, 1964b) and the effect could be important (Hammel *et al.*, 1962).

A stoichiometry between organic matter disappearance and the production of volatile fatty acids, methane, hydrogen, and heat has been found for commercial forages given to sheep and cattle (Walker, 1965; Hungate, 1966). Studies of ruminal fermentation patterns of arctic ruminants are required to determine if winter diets favor nonoxidative heat production. If it can be shown that the heat so produced is capable of at least substituting for the energy costs of melting ice and snow and raising forage dry matter and free water to deep body temperature, it may be possible to conclude if this is of adaptive significance.

Comparison of Caribou and Lemming Nutritional Strategies

Water Intake and Energy Metabolism

Unfortunately, studies on N, glucose and water metabolism in small arctic mammals are not as detailed as those for *Rangifer*. Holleman and Dieterich (1973) have determined water turnover in a number of rodents originating from many environments but reared under comparable laboratory conditions (Figure 6). Their work indicates that two arctic/subarctic species, *Microtus abbreviatus* and *M. oeconomus* have water turnover rates above the interspecies lines of both Adolph (1949) and Richmond *et al.* (1962). In contrast, results for the semiarid and desert species, *Chinchilla laniger, Acomys cahirinus,* and *Meriones unguiculatus* were below the interspecies line and was interpreted as evidence for evolution of a low rate of water turnover. This interpretation must be treated with caution for it does not take into account seasonal changes in dietary water content or intake. For example, when the reindeer data of Cameron and Luick (1972) are compared with the interspecies line of Richmond *et al.* (1962) (Figure 7), it is clear that water turnover rates determined in summer lie above and those for winter lie below the interspecies line. Preliminary comparisons of water metabolism in *Clethrionomys rutilis* suggests that the flux of field-caught specimens in winter is below the interspecies line, their laboratory reared counterparts lie slightly above it (Holleman, personal communication).

Although the lemming may ingest little snow, it must ingest free water contained in herbage and that in turn must be thawed and raised to deep body temperature. Knowledge is required of the temperatures of

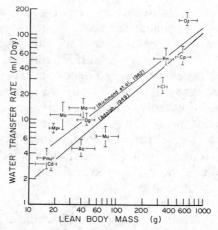

Figure 6 Relationship between water transfer rate and lean body mass in rodents (Holleman and Dieterich, 1973). Also shown are the interspecific lines of Adolph (1949) and Richmond *et al.* (1962). All animals were raised under laboratory conditions. *Dicrostonyx groenlandicus* (Dg) was obtained from Umnak Island (Alaska), other species are represented by *Microtus oeconomus macfarlani* (Mo), *M. pennsylvanicus* (Mp) and *M. abbreviatus* (Ma). These data suggest subarctic species have not evolved a low rate of water metabolism since the results for each species lay on or above the interspecies line.

plants consumed and of the subnivian environment (particularly the feeding runways and nests) to determine this energy cost to the animal. Morrison (1966) has made an intensive summary of the biometerological environment of the subnivian space compared with the surface. Clearly, a 10-cm depth of packed snow has the effect of minimizing daily temperature variation by reducing convective and conductive heat loss (Johnson, 1957; Morrison, 1966; Hart, 1971). In spite of this effective microclimate, conditions may not be suitable for reproduction and postnatal care without the construction of nests. A lactating lemming has an array of strategies available to it with respect to maintaining nest temperature. In a theoretical treatment of this concept, MacLean (1973) shows that nest temperatures are a function of heat loss plus heat production from the female and her offspring. A well-insulated nest cools slowly and warms quickly, while the converse is true for a poorly insulated nest. The warming curve depends on the time the female is in the nest and the cooling curve is tempered by heat produced by the offspring. Thus, the feeding strategy (many short feeding bouts compared with fewer, longer bouts) largely governs the temperature regime of the nest. It is clear that low food availability may affect survival of offspring

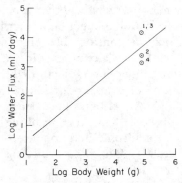

Figure 7 Seasonal changes in the water metabolism in reindeer in relation to interspecies line of Richmond *et al.* (1962). 1, Spring maximum for grazing reindeer; 2, winter minimum for grazing reindeer; 3 and 4, maximum and minimum values, respectively, for reindeer given high or low protein rations and held in winter photoperiod at −10° to −20°C (modified from Cameron, 1972).

by altering feeding behavior such that the length of feeding bouts may not allow sufficient time for heating the nest.

Thermoregulation and Heat Production

It is beyond the scope of this chapter to review in detail thermoregulation and metabolism of the small arctic mammals. Readers are referred to reviews by Morrison (1964, 1966), Irving (1964a,b, 1972) and Hart (1971). The work reviewed by these authors shows that changes in pelage insulation of small arctic mammals in response to cold acclimatization is less than for the large mammals. Hence, avoidance of long-term exposure to cold by making use of the subnivian microclimate, huddling, and nest building are behavioral adaptations. As judged by elevated resting and summit metabolism in cold acclimated compared with controls, or of winter acclimatized wild-caught compared with summer wild-caught rodents, *Microtus oeconomus* and *C. rutilis,* it can be argued that these species are prepared for and can withstand short-term bouts of cold exposure (Rosenmann and Feist, unpublished observation). These latter species are not necessarily comparable with *Lemmus* and *Dicrostonyx* for they are subarctic and there may be differences in their reproductive patterns in winter. Comparisons of cold acclimation of *Lemmus* and *Dicrostonyx* suggests the latter are more cold resistant as judged from their critical thermal minimum (Ferguson and Folk, 1970) and pituitary–adrenal responses (Andrews and Ryan, 1971).

The production of heat in cold acclimatized arctic and subarctic rodents is by shivering and nonshivering thermogenesis. The contribution of nonshivering thermogenesis, as judged by the increase in O_2 consumption in response to catecholamine injection at thermoneutrality, to maximum O_2 consumption may be considerable (Hart, 1971). In general, this is in marked contrast to the large mammals in which thermogenesis in response to catecholamine injection is small (Whittow, 1971). Thus, in ruminants the main source of heat production below the thermoneutral range is probably through shivering; and at least for sheep and cattle, heat production may not meet heat loss, resulting in gradual hypothermia (Webster, 1966). Relief from such conditions can be achieved by behavioral strategies such as lying and crowding to minimize surface heat losses (Hammel et al., 1962).

Except for a small replacement of the shivering component by physical activity at extremely low temperatures in small arctic rodents, the possibility of substitution for regulative heat production in rodents has been discounted (Hart, 1971). However, the possibility that some species may use the same muscles for exercise as for shivering cannot be discounted and raises the possibility of substitution. West and Norton (this volume) have discussed the role of exercise in replacing regulative heat production in birds. In the redpoll (Acanthis flammea) this becomes apparent between temperatures of −30° and −42°C (Pohl and West, 1973).

With respect to high metabolic capacities, small arctic mammals when acclimatized to cold, show similar adaptations as small arctic birds (West and Norton, this volume) but quite different from those of large mammals. For example, the thermal insulation of caribou increases markedly in winter resulting in critical temperatures probably lower than −52°C (Hart et al., 1961). Thus, a decline in resting metabolism (Segal, 1962) and the conservation of energy and nutrient reserves is not precluded by constant cold stress. From the review of West and Norton (this volume) a similar strategy is apparent for large birds, such as the snowy owl (Nyctea scandiaca), in which an increase in insulation is achieved through greater plumage density in winter.

The Dependence of Phagic Behavior on Total Energy Demand

The high rates of metabolism required for thermoregulation and reproduction in small mammals must be met by high rates of food intake (see for example Mayer, 1967). In the Barrow ecosystem, there is good evidence for a direct dependence of temporal changes in population size of Lemmus on the nutrient status of forage (Pitelka and Schultz, cited by Bunnell, 1973; Schultz, 1969). Specifically, hypotheses have been formulated based on a dependence of fecundity on above-threshold levels of N, P, and Ca in the vegetation (the "nutrient threshold" hypothesis) and a dependency of nutrient levels in herbage on the flow of nutrients through the various trophic levels in response to the pulsed removal of nutrients by periodic high lemming density (the "nutrient recovery" hypothesis; Schultz, 1964).

Laboratory studies on effects of diet on cold acclimation and acclimatization of small rodents have been reviewed by Hart (1971). Interactions or influences of diet have been noted based on restriction of food intake, the specific dynamic effect of the food, the water content, ratio of fat:carbohydrate:protein and the thyroxine content. Hart concludes that reports are conflicting and it is clear that more work is warranted.

Acknowledgments

I would like to thank participants in the IBP-U.S. Tundra Biome program, particularly G. O. Batzli, H. Melchior, B. R. Thomson, and T. Skogland, for the use of unpublished data. Collegues in the Institute of Arctic Biology, including R. D. Cameron, D. D. Feist, L. Irving, J. R. Luick, S. J. MacLean, P. R. Morrison, D. W. Norton, M. R. Rosenmann, and G. C. West, have my thanks for their comments and assistance in the preparation of this manuscript.

My research has been supported by the Office of Polar Programs and the International Biological Program of the National Science Founcation (NSF Grant GV-29342), the U.S. Atomic Energy Commission [AEC Contract (45-1)-2229-TA3] and the National Science Foundation (NSF Grant GB-29281).

Logistic support at Prudhoe Bay was made available through a grant to the Tundra Biome Center, University of Alaska, from the Prudhoe Bay Environmental Subcommittee.

References

Adolph, E. F. (1949). Quantitative relations in the physiological constitutions of mammals. *Science* **109**, 579–585.

Andrews, R. V., and Ryan, K. (1971). Seasonal changes in lemming pituitary-adrenal response to cold exposure. *Comp. Biochem. Physiol.* **40A**, 979–985.

Armstrong, D. G. (1965). Carbohydrate metabolism in ruminants and energy supply. *In* "Physiology of Digestion in the Ruminant," (R. W. Dougherty, ed.), pp. 272–288. Butterworths, Washington, D.C.

Arnold, G. W. (1970). Regulation of food intake in grazing ruminants. *In* "Physiology of Digestion and Metabolism in the Ruminants," (A. T. Phillipson, ed.), pp. 265–276. Oriel Press, Newcastle upon Tyne.

Baile, C. A., and Mayer, J. (1970). Hypothalamic centres: feedbacks and receptor sites in the short term control of feed intake. *In* "Physiology of Digestion and Metabolism in the Ruminant," (A. T. Phillipson, ed.), pp. 254–263. Oriel Press, Newcastle upon Tyne.

Ballard, F. J., Hanson, R. W., and Kronfeld, D. S. (1968). Gluconeogenesis and lipogenesis in tissue from ruminant and non-ruminant animals. *Fed. Proc.* **28,** 218–231.

Banfield, A. W. F. (1954). Preliminary investigation of the barren ground caribou. *Can. Wildl. Serv. Wildl. Manage. Bull.* Ser. 1, Nos. **10A, 10B,** 1–79, 1–112.

Batzli, G. O. (1973a). Population determination and nutrient flux through lemmings. *U.S. Tundra Biome Data Rep.* 73–19.

Batzli, G. O. (1973b). The role of small mammals in arctic ecosystems. Proc. Fourth IBP *Meet. Second. Product. Small Mammal Populations.* November 1973, Warsaw, Poland.

Baumgardt, B. R. (1970). Control of feed intake in the regulation of energy balance. *In* "Physiology of Digestion and Metabolism in the Ruminant," (A. T. Phillipson, ed.), pp. 235–253. Oriel Press, Newcastle upon Tyne.

Bergerud, A. T., and Nolan, M. J. (1970). Food habits of hand-reared caribou *Rangifer tarandus* L. in Newfoundland. *Oikos* **21,** 348–350.

Bergerud, A. T., and Russell, L. (1964). Evaluation of rumen food analysis for Newfoundland caribou. *J. Wildl. Manage.* **28,** 809–814.

Blaxter, K. L. (1962). "The Energy Metabolism of Ruminants." Thomas, Springfield Illinois.

Bliss, L. C., Courtin, G. M., Pattie, D. L., Riewe, R. R., Whitfield, B. W. A., and Widden, P. (1973). Arctic tundra ecosystems. *Annu. Rev. Ecol. Syst.* **4,** 359–399.

Bowen, S. (ed.) (1971). The structure and function of the tundra ecosystem. *Progr. Rep. Proposal Abstr.* **1.**

Bowen, S. (ed.). (1972). *Proc. 1972 Tundra Biome Symp.* Lake Wilderness Center, Univ. of Washington, 3–5 April 1972.

Bunnell, F. L. (1973). Computer simulation of nutrient and lemming cycles in an arctic tundra wet meadow ecosystem. *U.S. Tundra Biome Rep.* **73.**

Cameron, R. D. (1972). Water metabolism by reindeer *(Rangifer tarandus).* Ph.D. thesis, Univ. of Alaska, Fairbanks, Alaska.

Cameron, R. D., and Luick, J. R. (1972). Seasonal changes in total body water, extracellular fluid, and blood volume in grazing reindeer. *Can. J. Zool.* **50,** 107–116.

Cameron, R. D., White, R. G., and Luick, J. R. (1975). The accumulation of water in reindeer during winter. *Proc. 1st Int. Reindeer Caribou Symp.* 9–11 August 1972, Fairbanks Alaska (in press).

Chemical Engineering Handbook, 3rd Ed. (1950). McGraw Hill, New York.

Church, D. C., Smith, G. E., Fontenot, J. P., and Ralston, A. T. (1971). "Digestive Physiology and Nutrition of Ruminants," Vol. 2, pp. 737–762. D. C. Church, O.S.U. Book Stores, Corvallis, Oregon.

Cocimano, M. R., and Leng, R. A. (1967). Metabolism of urea in sheep. *Brit. J. Nutr.* **21,** 353.

Conrad, H. R., Pratt, A. D., and Hibbs, J. W. (1964). Nutritive evaluation of summer range forage with cattle. *J. Dairy Sci.* **47,** 54–62.

Courtright, A. M. (1959). Range management and the genus *Rangifer:* A review of selected literature. M.Sc. thesis, Univ. of Alaska, Fairbanks, Alaska.

Deardon, B. L., Pegau, R. E., and Hansen, R. M. (1975). Plant fragment discernibility in caribou rumens. *Proc. 1st Int. Reindeer Caribou Symp.* 9–11 August 1972, Fairbanks, Alaska (in press).

Dehority, B. A. (1975a). Characterization studies on rumen bacteria isolated from Alaska reindeer. *Proc. 1st Int. Reindeer Caribou Symp.* 9–11 August 1972, Fairbanks, Alaska (in press).

Dehority, B. A. (1975b). Rumen ciliate protozoa of Alaskan reindeer and caribou. *Proc. 1st Int. Reindeer Caribou Symp.* 9–11 August 1972, Fairbanks, Alaska (in press).

Fell, B. F., Campbell, R. M., and Boyne, R. (1964). Observations on the morphology and nitrogen content of the alimentary canal in breeding hill sheep. *Res. Vet. Sci.* **5,** 175.

Ferguson, J. H., and Folk, G. E., Jr. (1970). The critical thermal minimum of small rodents in hypothermia. *Cryobiology,* **7,** 44–46.

Fisher, K. C., Dawe, A. R., Lyman, C. P., Schönbaum, E., and South, F. E., Jr. (1967). Mammalian Hibernation III. *Proc. 3rd Int. Symp. Natur. Hibern.* 13–16 September 1965, Toronto. American Elsevier, New York.

Giesecke, D. (1970). Comparative microbiology of the alimentary tract. *In* "Physiology of Digestion and Metabolism in the Ruminant," (A. T. Phillipson, ed.), pp. 306–318. Oriel Press, Newcastle upon Tyne.

Griffin, D. R., Hammel, H. T., Johnson, H. M., and Rawson, K. S. (1951). The comparative physiology of temperature regulation and thermal insulation. *Arctic Aeromedi. Lab. Tech. Document. Rep. Contract* No. AF-33(038)-12764.

Hale, M. E. (1967). "The Biology of Lichens." Edward Arnold, London.

Hammel, H. T., Houpt, T. R., Andersen, K. L., and Skjenneberg, S. (1962). Thermal and metabolic measurements on a reindeer at rest and in exercise. *Arctic Aeromed. Lab. Tech. Document. Rep.* AAL-TDR-61-54.

Hanson, W. C., Whicker, F. W., and Lipscomb, J. F. (1975). Lichen forage ingestion rates of free-roaming caribou estimated with fallout cesium-137. *Proc. 1st Int. Reindeer Caribou Symp.* 9–11 August 1972, Fairbanks, Alaska (in press).

Hart, J. S. (1971). Rodents. *In* "Comparative Physiology of Thermoregulation," (G. C. Whittow, ed.), Vol. II, Chap. 1, pp. 1–149. Academic Press, New York.

Hart, J. S., Héroux, O., Cottle, W. H., and Mills, C. A. (1961). The influence of climate on metabolic and thermal responses of infant caribou. *Can. J. Zool.* **39,** 845–856.

Head, M. J. (1953). The effect of pregnancy and lactation in the ewe on the digestibility of the ration with a note on the partition of nitrogen in the foetus at full term. *J. Agri. Sci.* **43,** 214.

Hemming, J. E. (1971). The distribution and movement patterns of caribou in Alaska. *Alaska Dep. Fish Game Game Tech. Bull.* No. **1.**

Hoffman, R. A. (1964). Terrestrial animals in cold: hibernators. *In* "Handbook of Physiology," (D. B. Dill, E. F. Adolph and C. G. Wilber, eds.), Section 4: Adaptation to the Environment, pp. 379–403. Amer. Physiol. Soc., Washington, D.C.

Holleman, D. F., and Dieterich, R. A. (1973). Body water content and turnover in several species of rodents as evaluated by the tritiated water method. *J. Mammal.* **54**, 456–465.

Holling, C. S. (1966). The strategy of building models of complex ecological systems. *In* "Systems Analysis in Ecology," (K. E. F. Watt, ed.), Chap. 8, pp. 195–214. Academic Press, New York.

Houpt, T. R. (1959). Utilization of blood urea in ruminants. *Amer. J. Physiol.* **197**, 115–120.

Houpt, T. R. (1963). Urea utilization by rabbits fed a low-protein ration. *Amer. J. Physiol.* **205**, 1144–1150.

Houpt, T. R., and Houpt, K. A. (1971). Nitrogen conservation by ponies fed a low-protein ration. *Amer. J. Vet. Res.* **32**, 579–588.

Hungate, R. E. (1966). "The Rumen and Its Microbes." Academic Press, New York.

Irving, L. (1964a). Temperature regulation of large arctic land mammals. *Fed. Proc.* **23**, 1198–1201.

Irving, L. (1964b). Terrestrial animals in cold: birds and mammals. *In* "Handbook of Physiology" Section 4 (D. B. Bill, E. F. Adolph and C. G. Wilber, eds.), Adaptation to the Environment, pp. 361–377. Amer. Physiol. Soc., Washington, D.C.

Irving, L. (1972). "Arctic Life of Birds and Mammals Including Man." Springer-Verlag, New York.

Jacobson, E. and Skjenneberg, S. (1975). Some results from feeding experiments with reindeer. *Proc. 1st Int. Reindeer Caribou Symp.* 9–11 August 1972, Fairbanks, Alaska (in press).

Jakimchuk, R. D. (1975). Distribution and movements of the Porcupine caribou herd in the Yukon Territory. *Proc. 1st Int. Reindeer Caribou Symp.*, 9–11 August 1972, Fairbanks, Alaska (in press).

Johnson, H. McC. (1957). Winter microclimates of importance to Alaskan small mammals and birds. *Alaska Aeromed. Lab. Tech. Rep.* 57–2.

Jones, D. I. H. (1972). The chemistry of grass for animal production. *Outlook Agric.*, **7**, 32–38.

Kelsall, J. P. (1962). "The Caribou." Queen's Printer and Controller of Stationary, Ottawa, Canada.

Kennedy, G. C. (1967). Ontogeny of mechanisms controlling food and water intake. *In* "Handbook of Physiology," (C. F. Code, ed.), Sect. 6. pp. 337–351, ed. by Waverly Press, Inc., Baltimore, Maryland.

Kleiber, M. (1961). "The Fire of Life." Wiley, New York.

Klein, D. R. (1967). Interactions of *Rangifer tarandus* (reindeer and caribou) with its habitat in Alaska. *VII Int. Congr. Game Biol. Helsinki, 1967. Finnish Game Res.* **30**, 289–293.

Klein, D. R. (1968). The introduction, increase and crash of reindeer on St. Matthew Island. *J. Wildl. Manage.* **32,** 350 – 367.

Klein, D. R. (1970a). Food selection by North American deer and their response to over-utilization of preferred plant species. *In* "Animal Populations in Relation to their Food Resources," (A. Watson, ed.), *Brit. Ecol. Soc. Symp.,* No. **10,** pp. 25 – 46. Blackwell Scientific Publications, Oxford and Edinburgh.

Klein, D. R. (1970b). Tundra ranges north of the boreal forest. *J. Range Mange.* **23,** 8 – 14.

Leng, R. A. (1970). Glucose synthesis in ruminants. *Advan. Vet. Sci.* **14,** 209 – 260.

Lent, P. C. (1966). The caribou of north western Alaska. *In* "Environment of the Cape Thompson Region, Alaska," (N. J. Wilimovsky and J. N. Wolfe, ed.), pp. 481 – 517. USAEC Division of Tech. Inform. Ext., Oak Ridge, Tennessee.

Lent, P. C. (1973). Behavioral and ecological study of the Nunivak Island muskox population. *Alaska Coop. Wildl. Res. Unit Quart. Prog. Rep.* **24**(4), 7 – 9.

LeResche, R. E. (1975). The international herds: present knowledge of the Steese-Fortymile and Porcupine herds. *In Proc. 1st Int. Reindeer Caribou Symp.,* 9 – 11 August 1972, Fairbanks, Alaska. (in press).

Lindsay, D. B. (1970). Carbohydrate metabolism in ruminants. *In* "Physiology of Digestion and Metabolism in the Ruminant," (A. T. Phillipson, ed.), pp. 438 – 451. Oriel Press, Newcastle upon Tyne.

Longhurst, W. M., Oh, H. K., Jones, M. B., and Kepner, R. E. (1968). A basis for the palatability of deer forage plants. *Trans. N. Amer. Wildl. Nat. Resour. Conf.* **33,** 181 – 192.

Luick, J. R., White, R. G., and Reimers, E. (1971). Investigation of the adaptive significance of winter growth patterns in female reindeer calves. *Proc. 22nd Alaska Sci. Conf. AAAS.* Fairbanks, Alaska. p. 12.

Luick, J. R., Person, S. J., Cameron, R. D., and White, R. G. (1973). Seasonal variations in glucose metabolism of reindeer (*Rangifer tarandus* L.) estimated with [U-^{14}C]glucose and [3-^{3}H]glucose. *Brit. J. Nutr.* **29,** 245 – 259.

Lyman, C. P., and Dawe, A. R. (1960). Mammalian hibernation. *Proc. 1st Int. Symp. Natural Mam. Hibn.* 13 – 15 May 1959, Dedham, Mass. *Bull. Mus. Comp. Zool.,* Vol. **124.** Cambridge, Mass.

MacLean, S. F. (1973). The subnivian climate in the life of the brown lemming: a computer simulation. *In* "Climate of the Arctic." AAAS-AMS Conf., 15 – 17 August 1973, Fairbanks, Alaska (Abstr.).

Mayer, J. (1967). General characteristics of the regulation of food intake. *In* "Handbook of Physiology," (C. F. Code, ed.), Sect. 6. pp. 3 – 9. Waverly Press, Baltimore, Maryland.

McClymont, G. L. (1967). Selectivity and intake in the grazing ruminant. *In* "Handbook of Physiology," (C. F. Code, ed.), Sect. 6, pp. 129 – 137. Waverly Press, Baltimore Maryland.

McCown, B. H., and Tieszen, L. L. (1972). A comparative investigation of periodic trends in carbohydrate and lipid levels in arctic and alpine plants. *Proc. 1972 Tundra Biome Symp.,* (S. Bowen, ed.), pp. 40–45. 3–5 April 1972, Lake Wilderness Center, Univ. of Washington.

McDonald, I. W. (1952). The role of ammonia in ruminal digestion of protein. *Biochem. J.* **51,** 86.

McDonald, I. W. (1968). The nutrition of grazing ruminants. *Nutr. Abstr. Rev.* **38,** 381.

McEwan, E. H. (1968). Growth and development of the barren-ground caribou. II. Postnatal growth rates. *Can. J. Zool.,* **46,** 1023–1029.

McEwan, E. H. (1970). Energy metabolism of barren ground caribou *(Rangifer tarandus). Can. J. Zool.* **48,** 391–392.

McEwan, E. H., and Whitehead, P. E. (1970). Seasonal changes in the energy and nitrogen intake in reindeer and caribou. *Can. J. Zool.* **48,** 905–913.

Melchior, H. R. (1971). Abundance, feeding behavior and impact of the brown lemming on tundra vegetation. *In* "The Structure and Function of the Tundra Ecosystem," (S. Bowen, ed.), Vol. 1, pp. 92–96.

Melchior, H. R. (1972). Summer herbivory by the brown lemming at Barrow, Alaska. *Proc. 1972 Tundra Biome Symp.,* (S. Bowen, ed.), pp. 136–138. 3–5 April 1972, Lake Wilderness Center, Univ. of Washington.

Montgomery, M. J., and Baumgardt, B. R. (1965). Regulation of food intake in ruminants 2. Rations varying in energy concentration and physical form. *J. Dairy Sci.* **4,** 1623–1628.

Mooney, H. A. and Billings, W. D. (1960). The annual carbohydrate cycle of alpine plants as related to growth. *Amer. J. Bot.* **47,** 594–598.

Morrison, P. (1964). Adaptation of small mammals to the arctic. *Fed. Proc.* **23,** 1202–1206.

Morrison, P. R. (1966). Biometeorological problems in the ecology of animals in the arctic. *Int. J. Biometeorol.* **10,** 273–292.

Palmer, L. (1934). Raising Reindeer in Alaska. *U.S. Dep. Agr. Misc. Publ.* 207.

Pegau, R. E. (1968). Reindeer range appraisal in Alaska. M.Sc. thesis, Univ. of Alaska, Fairbanks, Alaska.

Pegau, R. E., Bos, G. N. and Neiland, K. A. (1973). Caribou report. *Proj. Progr. Rep. Alaska Dep. Fish Game.* **14,** 1–68.

Person, S. J., White, R. G., and Luick, J. R. (1975). *In vitro* digestibility of forages utilized by *Rangifer tarandus. Proc. 1st Int. Reindeer Caribou Symp,* 9–11 August 1972, Fairbanks, Alaska (in press).

Pitelka, F. A. (1957). Some aspects of population structure in the short-term cycle of the brown lemming. *Cold Springs Harbor Symp. on Quantitative Biol.* **22,** 237–251. Long Island Biol. Lab., New York.

Pitelka, F. A. (1972). Cycle pattern in lemming populations near Barrow Alaska. In *Proc. 1972 Tundra Biome Symp.,* (S. Bowen, ed.), pp. 132–135. 3–5 April 1972, Lake Wilderness Center, Univ. of Washington.

Pohl, H. and West, G. C. (1973). Daily and seasonal variation in metabolic response to cold during rest and forced exercise in the common redpoll. *Comp. Biochem. Physiol.* **45A,** 851–867.

Reilly P. E. B., and Ford, E. J. H. (1971). The effects of different dietary contents of protein on amino acid and glucose production and on the contribution of amino acids to gluconeogenesis in sheep. *Brit. J. Nutr.* **26**, 249–263.

Richmond, C. R., Langham, W. H., and Trujillo, T. T. (1962). Comparative metabolism of tritiated water by mammals. *J. Cell. Comp. Physiol.* **59**, 45–53.

Scholander, P. F., Hock, R., Walters, V., and Irving, L. (1950). Adaptation to cold arctic and tropical mammals and birds in relation to body temperature, insulation and basal metabolic rate. *Biol. Bull.* **99**, 259.

Schultz, A. M. (1964). The nutrient-recovery hypothesis for Arctic microtine cycles. *In* "Grazing in Terrestrial and Marine Environments," (D. J. Crisp, ed.), pp. 57–68. Symp. No. 4, *Brit. Ecol. Soc.* (ed. by) Blackwell, Oxford.

Schultz, A. M. (1969). A study of an ecosystem: the arctic tundra. *In* "The Ecosystem Concept in Natural Resource Management," Chap. V. pp. 77–93. Academic Press, New York.

Scotter, G. W. (1967). The winter diet of barren-ground caribou in northern Canada. *Can. Field Natur.* **81**, 33–39.

Segal, A. N. (1962). The periodicity of pasture and physiological functions of reindeer. *In* "Reindeer in the Karelian ASSR," *Akad. Nank Petrozavodsk* pp. 130–150. (Transl. Dep. Secretary of State Bur. Trans., Canada.)

Silver, H., Colovos, N. F., Holter, J. B., and Hayes, H. H. (1969). Fasting metabolism of white-tailed deer. *J. Wildl. Manage.* **33**, 490–498.

Skjenneberg, S., and Slagsvold, L. (1968). Rein Driften. Univ. forlaget, Oslo/Bergen/Tromsø.

Skjenneberg, S., Fjellheim, P., Gaare, E., and Lenvik, D., (1975). Reindeer with esophageal fistula in range studies. *Proc. 1st Int. Reindeer Caribou Symp.* 9–11 August 1972, Fairbanks, Alaska (in press).

Skogland, T. (1975a). Preliminary data on summer use by *Rangifer* of the arctic coastal plains vegetation at Prudhoe Bay, Alaska. Data Report, U.S. Tundra Biome Program (in preparation).

Skogland, T. (1975b). Wild reindeer range use and selectivity in southern Norway. *Proc. 1st Reindeer Caribou Symp.,* 9–11 August 1972, Fairbanks, Alaska (in press).

Skoog, R. D. (1968). Ecology of the caribou *(Rangifer tarandus granti)* in Alaska. Ph.D. thesis, Univ. of California, Berkeley, California.

South, F. E., Hannon, J. P., Willis, J. R., Pengelley, E. T., and Alpert, N. R. (1972). "Hibernation and Hypothermia, Perspectives and Challanges," 3–8 January 1971, Snowmass-At-Aspen, Colorado. Elsevier, New York.

Suomalainen, P. (1964). Mammalian Hibernation. II. *Proc. 2nd Int. Symp. on Natural Mam. Hibn.* 27–30 August 1962, Helsinki. *Am Acad. Sci. Fenn.* Series A, IV. Suomalainen Tiedeakatemia, Helsinki.

Tener, J. S. (1965). "Muskoxen in Canada." Queen's Printer, Ottawa, Canada.

Thompson, D. Q. (1955). The role of food and cover in population fluctuations of the brown lemming at Point Barrow, Alaska. Trans. 20th N. Amer. Wildl. Conf., pp. 166–176.

Thomson, B. R. (1971). Wild reindeer activity. *In* "Report from the Grazing

Project of the Norwegian IBP Committee." July–December 1970, Hardan-gervidda. Viltundersøkelser, Trondheim, Norway.

Thomson, B. R. (in preparation). Behavior and activity of caribou at Prudhoe Bay, Alaska. Data Report U.S. Tundra Biome Program.

Tilley, J. M. A. and Terry, R. A. (1963). A two-stage technique for the *in vitro* digestion of forage crops. *J. Brit. Grassl. Soc.* **18** 104–111.

Wales, R. A., Milligan, L. P., and McEwan, E. H. (1975). Urea recycling in cari-bou, cattle and sheep. *Proc. 1st Int. Reindeer Caribou Symp.* 9–11 August 1972, Fairbanks, Alaska (in press).

Walker, D. J. (1965). Energy metabolism and rumen microorganisms. *In* "Phys-iology of Digestion in the Ruminant," (R. W. Dougherty, ed.), pp. 296–310 Butterworth's, Washington, D.C.

Webster, A. J. F. (1966). The establishment of thermal equilibrium in sheep exposed to cold environments. *Res. Vet. Sci.* **7,** 454.

Westerling, B. (1975). Effect of changes in diet on the reindeer rumen mucosa. *Proc. 1st Int. Reindeer Caribou Symp.,* 9–11 August 1972, Fairbanks, Alas-ka (in press).

White, R. G., and Gau, A. M. (1975). Volatile fatty acid production in the ru-men and cecum of reindeer. *Proc. 1st Int. Reindeer Caribou Symp.,* 9–11 August 1972, Fairbanks, Alaska (in press).

Whittow, G. C. (ed.) (1971). Ungulates. *In* "Comparative Physiology of Ther-moregulation." Vol. II, Chap. 3, pp. 191–281. Academic Press, New York.

Wolff, J. E., and Bergman, E. N. (1972). Gluconeogenesis from plasma amino acids in fed sheep. *Amer. J. Physiol.* **223,** 455–460.

Wood, A. J., Cowan, I. McT., and Nordan, H. C. (1962). Periodicity of growth in ungulates as shown by deer of the genus *Odocoileus. Can. J. Zool.,* **40,** 593–603.

Zhigunov, P. S. (ed.) (1961). "Reindeer Husbandry," 2nd Edi. (Translation from Russian by M. Fleishmann.) Israel Program for Scientific Translations, Jeru-salem.

Ecological Adaptations of Tundra Invertebrates

Stephen F. MacLean, Jr.

Department of Biological Sciences
and
Institute of Arctic Biology
University of Alaska
Fairbanks, Alaska

Introduction

The existence of latitudinal gradients in species diversity is a basic observation of biogeography. The variety or diversity of most higher plant and animal taxa decreases as one nears the poles. Similar gradients in diversity are seen with increasing altitude, fewer species occur at higher elevations. The end points of these latitudinal and altitudinal gradients lie in the tundra communities of the high arctic, antarctic, and alpine regions of the world.

Much insight into the factors causing these gradients has come from broad comparisons of faunal or floral assemblages occurring at different latitudes or altitudes. Additional insight remains to be gleaned from careful examination of the physiological and ecological characteristics which adapt species for existence under the environmental conditions that prevail at particular places along major gradients. The tundra, as an end point, is ideally suited for such an analysis. This offers, of course, only one justification for the study of ecological and physiological characteristics of tundra organisms. Plant and animal life reaches the limits of its existence in extreme arctic, antarctic, and high alpine tundra. The species that occur under such circumstances probably demonstrate the limits of physiological and evolutionary adaptability under extreme conditions.

This chapter outlines the patterns of diversity found in the invertebrate component of the tundra communities of the world. The characteristics of tundra environments, and the physiological and ecological responses of invertebrates to these, are then discussed. Thus, it is hoped, the role of the environment in determining the diversity, function, and importance of invertebrates in the tundra ecosystem will be revealed. Additional information, particularly on quantitative aspects of tundra invertebrate populations and their role in ecosystem function, will be forthcoming soon when the results of studies conducted under the International Biological Program are published.

The distribution and physiological and ecological attributes of most groups of tundra invertebrates is very poorly known. As in other areas, the Insecta have received the most study, and the reviews of Downes (1962, 1964, 1965) and Oliver (1963, 1968) dealing with arctic insects are particularly useful. Research on the Antarctic subcontinent and subantarctic islands has emphasized systematics and biogeography (Gressitt, 1967 and 1970), although valuable ecological observations appear in the volumes edited by Gressitt (1967, 1970), and Gressitt and Strandtmann (1971). The most extensive survey of adaptations to alpine existence is that of Mani (1962, 1968) dealing with high-altitude insects.

Composition of Tundra Invertebrate Faunas

The invertebrate fauna of arctic tundra is depauperate in number of species and higher taxa (Table 1). Of the approximately 27 orders of Insecta (depending upon taxonomic scheme) found world wide, 24 occur in the British Isles and 18 have been collected in the vicinity of a single tropical forest site, the El Verde field station, Puerto Rico (Drewry, 1970). In contrast, 17 orders occur on Greenland (Henriksen, 1939), 12 near Point Barrow, Alaska (Hurd, 1958), 8 at Lake Hazen, Ellesmere Island, Canada, 6 on Bathurst, 7 on Devon Islands, Canada, and only 5 at Isachsen, Ellef Ringnes Island, Canada (McAlpine, 1964). The number of reported species shows a similar decline, from over 650 on Greenland to approximately 250 at Barrow and Lake Hazen and 37 at Isachsen. Figure 1 represents arctic areas of North America mentioned in text.

The reduction in species does not occur in all taxa equally. In the Annelida, Enchytraeidae are abundant and relatively diverse, while Lumbricidae are reduced or absent altogether. The Prostigmata make up

Table 1 Composition of the Insect Faunas of Selected Tundra Sites

Insect order	World[b] N	%	England[c] N	%	Greenland 60°–84° N[d] N	%	Barrow, Alaska, 71° 20′ N[e] N	%	Lake Hazen, 81° 49′ N[f] N	%	Devon Island, 75° 40′ N[g] N	%	Bathurst Island, 75° 43′ N[h] N	%	Isachsen, Ellef Ringnes Island, 78° 47′ N[i] N	%	Hardangervidda, Norway, 60° 36′ N[j] N	Antarctica[a,k] N
Collembola	2000	0.3	305	1.5	41	6.8	32	13.8	14	5.7	13	11.8	6	9.8	8	21.6	33	19
Ephemeroptera	2000	0.3	46	0.2	1	0.2	0	–	0	–	0	–	0	–	0	–	3	0
Odonata	4870	0.7	42	0.2	0	–	0	–	0	–	0	–	0	–	0	–	0	0
Orthoptera	22500	3.3	47	0.2	2	0.3	0	–	0	–	0	–	0	–	0	–	1	0
Mallophaga	2675	0.4	260	1.3	42	7.0	17	17.3	–	–	–	–	3	4.9	1	2.7	4	37
Anoplura	250	–	26	0.1	5	0.8	3	1.3	–	–	–	–	1	1.6	0	–	0	4
Thysanoptera	4500	0.5	183	0.9	5	0.8	2	0.9	3	1.2	0	–	0	–	0	–	2	0
Hemiptera	23000	3.4	499	2.5	5	0.8	1	0.4	0	–	0	–	0	–	0	–	3	0
Homoptera	32000	4.7	912	4.6	12	2.0	1	0.4	4	1.6	0	–	0	–	0	–	9	0
Neuroptera	4670	0.7	64	0.3	3	0.5	0	–	0	–	0	–	0	–	0	–	1	0
Coleoptera	290000	41.2	3707	18.8	44	7.3	12	5.2	4	1.6	4	3.6	0	–	0	–	74+	0
Trichoptera	4450	0.7	188	1.0	7	1.1	5	2.2	1	0.4	1	0.9	0	–	0	–	3	0
Lepidoptera	112000	16.3	2187	11.1	41	6.8	8	3.4	19	7.8	9	8.2	1	1.6	1	2.7	48	2
Diptera	86000	12.2	5199	26.4	275	45.8	120	51.7	142	58.2	47	42.7	47	77.0	26	70.3	84	0
Hymenoptera	105000	14.9	6191	31.4	87	14.5	30	12.9	57	23.4	36	32.7	3	4.9	1	2.7	35+	0
Total Orders	27		24 or 25		17		12		8+		6+		6		5		16	5
Total species	704,600		19,698		600		232		244		110		61		37		313+	67

[a]This list reflects the intense collecting of parasitic insects that has occurred, and thus is not wholly comparable to the others.

[b]Borror and DeLong, 1971.

[c]Data from various sources.

[d]Henriksen, 1939; Wolff, 1964.

[e]Hurd, 1958.

[f]Downes, 1964.

[g]J. K. Ryan, March, 1973 (unpublished).

[h]Danks and Byers, 1972.

[i]McAlpine, 1965a, b.

[j]Östbye (1969) and informal reports of the Norwegian IBP tundra program.

[k]Gressitt, 1963, 1967.

[l]It is likely that parasitic insects of the orders Mallophaga and Anoplura also occur here.

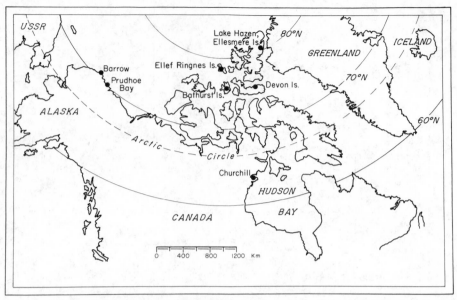

Figure 1 The arctic areas of North America, showing locations of sites mentioned in text.

an unusually high proportion of the mite (Acarina) population (Douce, 1973). Springtails (Collembola), and flies (Diptera) are particularly well represented in the arctic fauna. Collembola comprise about 0.3% of the insect species of the world, but 14% of the Barrow insect fauna, and 22% of the insect species at Isachsen. Abundance of these groups is similarly high, and they may be of major importance in arctic tundra ecosystems.

A conspicuous feature of arctic tundra is the predominance of Diptera. This order forms about 12% of the insects of the world, 26% of the insect fauna of Great Britain, 43% in Greenland, 44% on Devon Island, over 50% at Barrow, Alaska and Lake Hazen, Canada, over 60% on Spitzbergen, and over 70% on Ellef Ringnes and Bathurst islands.

The parasitic Hymenoptera, such as Ichneumonidae and Braconidae, are relatively well represented in arctic insect faunas. In contrast, the Coleoptera, which predominate world wide, are rather insignificant in the arctic, forming between zero and 6% of the insect species at each of the arctic sites I have mentioned. The sucking insects are also poorly represented; for example, there is but one hemipteran (Saldidae) and one homopteran (Cicidellidae) in the 230 insects reported for Barrow. Thus, it is clear that the arctic insect fauna is not a small but random sample of the earth's insects. Rather, the environment has acted as a differential filter favoring particular taxonomic groups.

The trophic structure of the arctic Invertebrata, similarly, differs from that of other parts of the world. Herbivores are striking in their scarcity. Plant grazing groups such as Orthoptera are absent altogether, and plant sucking insects are few in numbers of species and individuals. A large proportion of tundra invertebrates belong to the broad category "saprovores"—animals that ingest dead plant and animal remains. Many of these actually assimilate the bacteria, fungi, yeasts, etc., that are responsible for decay, while others digest and assimilate the dead organic substrate. This is a heterogeneous assemblage about which we know very little. Among the saprovores of arctic tundra are many nematodes, Enchytraeidae, Acarina, Collembola, and larvae of Diptera.

The trophic structure of the tundra invertebrate fauna is clearly related to taxonomic structure. The causal sequence (trophic structure derives from the fact that certain invertebrate taxa are favored, or *vice versa*) remains to be explored. It is interesting to note that these same trends in faunal composition are seen in the tundralike moor lands of Great Britain (Moor House; Table 1).

The geography of the antarctic region differs from the arctic, with important consequences. The north pole lies near the center of a polar sea, which greatly ameliorates the climate of surrounding land masses. The south polar region occupies a large continental land mass covered by an ice cap extending some 3000 m above sea level. The Antarctic peninsula extends to 63° S latitude, a latitude that is well within the boreal forest zone of the northern hemisphere; yet the terrestrial arthropod fauna of Antarctica consists of only 21 free-living insect species, 55 free-living mites, and 56 parasitic Acarina and Insecta (Gressitt, 1967). Only two free-living higher insects occur, both Diptera of the family Chironomidae. The Antarctic thus resembles the Arctic in that Acarina, Collembola, and Diptera are the persistent forms under the most severe climatic conditions.

Unlike the islands of the Canadian Arctic archipelago, the subantarctic islands are distant from the nearest land mass and surrounded by an unfrozen, turbulent sea. Endemism, rare in the arctic, is common in the invertebrates of the subantarctic islands, and accidents of biogeography play a significant role in shaping the fauna. The islands resemble the arctic in having few orders, with Acarina, Collembola, and Diptera among the most important. They differ from arctic regions in the greater abundance of Coleoptera.

The geography of alpine tundra is likewise important in shaping the invertebrate fauna. Alpine tundra generally exists as islands of habitat of various sizes, surrounded at lower elevations by forest, plains, and other ecosystem types. While certain species of alpine tundra invertebrates have obvious affinities with arctic forms, numerically the alpine fauna may be derived, in large part, from the fauna of surrounding ecosystems. Schmoller (1971) found that all species of Carabidae and Arachnida from Colorado alpine tundra also occurred below tree line. Edwards (1972) recorded 10 insect orders and at least 141 species in the wind-borne "fallout" on snowfields in alpine tundra above taiga forest in interior Alaska. In view of this large and diverse input, it is difficult to separate the true, successful alpine species from species which breed but maintain a population only with input of individuals from below tree line, and species occurring only as accidentals (Alexander, 1964). Locally extinct populations may be quickly replaced by new colonizers in alpine tundra, while extinctions in arctic tundra may be of more lasting importance to faunal diversity. Thus, considering alpine tundra as "islands" of habitat, the equilibrium species composition would shift in the direction of greater diversity due to the high rate of colonization (MacArthur and Wilson, 1967).

Areas with steep topography provide nonalpine habitats in close proximity to alpine tundra and, in addition, generate the air currents that transport arthropods. Thus, the gently rolling tundralike moorlands of the northern Pennines in Great Britain support 19 insect orders (Nelson, 1971) while 17 orders have been collected from the alpine tundra of the steeper Hardangervidda area in Norway by workers in the Norwegian IBP tundra program. This is a greater diversity than occurs at any of the arctic tundra sites. Within the alpine zone diversity decreases with elevation, as both distance from source areas and climatic severity increase.

Characteristics of Tundra Environments

We may list several characteristics of the tundra environment that are important for invertebrate animals and may require particular physiological adaptations:

1. Low winter temperature. Air temperatures of −40°C and below are encountered during the winter in the tundra zone. Similar and even colder temperatures occur in the northern boreal forest zone, or taiga; however, ground surface temperatures differ in the two zones. Precipitation is greater in the forest zone, creating an insulating snow layer of greater depth. Tundra areas tend to be areas of little precipitation and shallow snow. In the absence of protection afforded by trees, the snow in the tundra region is heavily influenced by wind. Some areas are blown free of snow altogether, leaving the ground surface exposed to ambient air temperatures. Where the snow remains it may develop a platelike or lamellar structure of high density and poor insulating property. Further, at least in the arctic and antarctic regions, tundra invertebrates are confined to a layer of seasonally thawing ground (the "active layer") lying above perennially frozen ground, or permafrost. Near Barrow, Alaska, the equilibrium temperature of permafrost is −10.6°C (Brewer, 1958). Thus, during winter the ground surface is surrounded by cold above and below, and quickly drops to low temperatures. Kelley and Weaver (1969) reported that the ground surface temperature near Barrow averages below −8°C for 8 months, and below −15°C for 4 months. MacLean *et al.* (1974) found a mean of less than −20°C at the ground surface in January, February, March, and the first half of April in a year of lighter than average snowfall. In March, 25 measurements made on 6 days averaged −26.2°C under an average of 28.6 cm of snow. No measurements were made on windswept areas devoid of snow. Temperature there must follow air temperature, and reach minima of −40° to −50°C.

2. *Short growing seasons.* The snow-free season may be 90 days or less, leaving only a short time for growth and reproduction. The frost-free season, the period between the last freezing temperature in spring and the first freezing temperature in fall, is of almost no meaning in a true polar or high altitude climate. At Barrow, Alaska, for example, the long-term average daily minimum temperature is below freezing for 324 days of the year, and freezing temperatures may occur even at the height of the summer season. It is important to note, however, that biologists frequently underestimate the length of the period of activity, particularly for soil dwelling organisms. Even after daily minimum and even mean temperatures fall below 0°C the soil may remain in an unfrozen state. Loss of energy from the soil is counteracted by latent heat of fusion released as water changes state to ice. As a result the soil column remains isothermal at or close to 0°C, although the surface layers may be frozen. This is the "zero curtain" phenomenon. Cold adapted organisms are able to remain active at 0°C, thus lengthening the period of activity by several weeks. After all water has changed to ice soil temperature drops rapidly to the winter values mentioned above, and all activity ceases.

3. *Low temperature during the growing season.* The long-term average daily mean air temperature at Barrow, and the temperatures recorded in two seasons, one warmer than average (1972) and one cooler than average (1973), are shown in Figure 2. The expected daily mean air temperature is below 5°C throughout the season. Temperature ex-

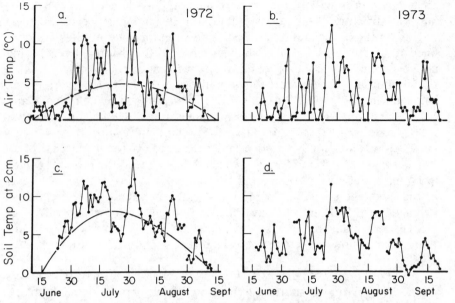

Figure 2 *a,* Daily mean air temperature recorded at U.S. Weather Bureau Station, Barrow, Alaska. Discontinuous curve, 1972; smooth curve, long-term average. *b,* Daily mean air temperature recorded at Barrow, Alaska, in 1973. *c,* Daily mean soil temperature recorded 2 cm below the surface of a low polygon rim at Barrow, Alaska. Discontinuous curve, 1972; smooth curve estimate of "normal" conditions, taking account of excursions in air temperature from the long-term mean (after MacLean 1973). d, Daily mean soil temperature recorded at −2 cm in 1973

ceeds 10°C on only the warmest days, and on many days temperature scarcely rises above 0°C. Thus, growth and reproduction must be accomplished at air temperatures that are below the minima for activity of many temperate species.

Two factors act to ameliorate the microclimate near the ground at latitudes above the Arctic (and Antarctic) circle. At latitudes above 67°N and S the possible amount of solar radiation (i.e., in the absence of cloud cover) increases with latitude (Danks and Oliver, 1972, quoting Gavrilova, 1966). Further, the diel range of sun altitude declines progressively with latitude, increasing the likelihood that the energy balance will remain positive throughout the day (Corbet, 1969). In the absence of near surface temperature inversions, the ground temperature will remain above the air temperature recorded at standard screen height, and diurnal temperature variations are small. As a result of this, edaphic factors influencing cloud cover are of greater importance than latitude in determining summer climate. Lake Hazen, at 81°49′ N, has a warmer climate (and greater invertebrate diversity) than does Bathurst Island (75°43′ N) or Ellef Ringnes Island (78°47′ N). In arctic Alaska the Point Barrow area (71°20′ N), at the convergence of the Beaufort and Chukchi seas, is exceptionally cool and foggy. Coastal localities in either direction (southwest or southeast) are significantly warmer, and exceptionally steep climatic gradients exist between coastal and inland tundra localities (Clebsch and Shanks, 1968). This is reflected in floral (Clebsch and Shanks, 1968) and faunal composition. For example, the number of recorded species of crane flies (Diptera, Tipulidae) increases from 4 at Barrow to 14 at Prudhoe Bay (70°16′ N). The number of recorded butterfly species is 5 at Barrow, 12 at Prudhoe Bay, and 23 at Kavik Camp, 90 km inland from Prudhoe Bay (Philip, personal communication).

The temperature regime of alpine tundra is quite different. During the day, with reduced atmospheric filtering, the radiation load may be quite high, resulting in very high temperatures, especially on the ground surface. In the evening, reradiation may be equally high and temperatures may fall precipitously. Thus, the daily temperature range is much greater than in the Arctic and becomes a factor in physiological adaptation to the environment (Remmert and Wunderling, 1969). Ballard (1972), investigating soil temperatures in subalpine British Columbia, found that at the time of the annual radiation maximum (21–22 June), the diurnal range in soil temperature 1 cm below bare ground was 35°C, and 5 cm below bare ground it was 20°C. At a depth of 5 cm below an herbaceous meadow, the diurnal range was nearly 17°C, and ground surface temperatures in the meadow probably exceeded 49°C. In contrast, on 21–22 June the diurnal temperature range 5 cm under arctic tundra at Barrow varied between 0.7° and 3.3°C (12 measurements). Even at the peak of the season, when maximum temperature gradients are developed, the diurnal temperature variation at 5 cm rarely exceeded 6°C. Thus, alpine organisms must be able to tolerate much wider variations in environmental temperature than arctic or antarctic tundra organisms.

4. Low primary productivity.   All of these factors, plus others discussed by Tieszen and Wieland, Courtin and Mayo, and McGown (this volume) result in low annual primary production, hence a relatively small amount of energy available to animal species. This may be important in determining length of food chains, invertebrate abundance and diversity, and the relative importance of various trophic types.

5. Weakness of photoperiodic cues.   In arctic and antarctic areas, the sun is continuously above the horizon for part of the growing season. Diurnal and seasonal information comes in the form of changes in light intensity, quality, and angle of incidence rather than major changes involving alternation of light and dark periods. Under overcast conditions these cues may be masked altogether. This may raise problems in the daily and seasonal timing of physiological processes and activities.

Adaptation to Tundra Environments

For convenience, adaptation to the special problems of existence in the tundra is treated under several categories. Actually, these form a suite of interrelated adaptations expressed in various degrees and combinations by the various groups of invertebrate animals.

1. Microhabitat selection. When the annual heat budget is small, small deviations from average conditions may have great ecological and physiological importance. The annual aboveground heat budget of Barrow, Alaska (Figure 2a) expressed as C° days above freezing, is 238 C° days. If, by microhabitat selection, an animal were able to achieve an average 1°C increase over the 90 days of the growing season, the heat budget would increase by 90C° days, or 32%.

Figure 2c and d shows the daily mean temperature recorded in 1972 and 1973 at a depth of 2 cm below the surface of a low polygon rim, a slightly elevated feature in the array of patterned ground that results from frost action in wet arctic and alpine sites (Hussey and Michelson, 1966). The smooth curve of Figure 2c is drawn to represent "average" conditions, taking into account excursions of air temperature from the long-term mean (Figure 2a). The total heat budget calculated from this curve is 440C° days above freezing, an increase of 55% over air temperature. The effect is greatest where solar radiation is high and less where cloud cover and fog limit ambient radiation. Invertebrates clearly derive a significant thermal advantage in existing in the soil rather than the air. This could be one factor contributing to the dominance of soil-dwelling saprovores over surface-active herbivores in arctic tundra.

Where possible, animals may move during the day or season to optimize the heat budget. Haufe (1957) found that the larvae of mosquitoes aggregate in the surface waters of the warmest parts of pools, and move clockwise around the pool during the day as the warmest point changes due to the changing position of the sun. Corbet (1966) observed that females of *Aedes nigripes* at Lake Hazen oviposit around midday and only when directly insolated. Thus, their eggs are placed on the south-facing banks of ponds and experience warmer temperatures as a result. The eggs of *Aedes impiger* are deposited in cracks on south-facing banks, and derive a similar advantage.

The dense cushions of mosses and such characteristic tundra plants as *Saxifraga oppositifolia* and *Dryas integrifolia* may capture radiation and warm well above ambient temperature, providing a favorable heat budget for invertebrate development and activity (Courtin and Mayo, this volume). Kevan (1972) observed heliotropism — orientation toward the sun — in the flowers of several arctic plant species. This concentrates radiation on the reproductive structures, resulting in temperatures of up to 10°C above ambient (Kevan, 1973). Many arctic insects bask in flowers, and heliotropism may be a mechanism for attracting pollinators (Hocking and Sharplin, 1965).

Kevan and Shorthouse (1970) investigated basking as a mechanism of behavioral thermoregulation in arctic butterflies. By selection of substrate and orientation toward the sun, butterflies were able to elevate their body temperature 10°C or more above ambient. The dark color (melanism) and hairy body that characterize many arctic insects contribute to the capture and retention of the energy of radiation. *Belgica antarctica,* the southernmost occurring higher insect species, is likewise melanic and is frequently seen basking (Peckham, 1971).

High altitude melanism is a common feature of alpine insects (Mani, 1968). This is often attributed to the need for protection from ultra-violet radiation; however, the existence of parallel increases in the frequency of pigmented species with latitude and altitude (e.g., Rapoport 1969 for Collembola) suggests that absorption of radiation and increase in body temperature is the most important selective basis of melanism.

2. Life cycles. In speaking of temperate invertebrates the length of the life cycle is expressed as number of generations per season. In considering tundra invertebrates we find ourselves increasingly asking, How many years per generation? The known incidence of extended life cycles in tundra invertebrates is summarized in Table 2. The life cycles of few tundra invertebrates have been investigated; however, it seems certain that, when more data are available, this will prove to be a very common means of dealing with the short growing season and limited heat budget of the tundra.

Flexibility is another feature of the life cycle of arctic species. (Downes, 1965; Oliver, 1968; MacLean, 1973). During unfavorable years pupation may not occur, with individuals remaining as larvae for 1 or more additional years. This adaptation of extended and flexible life cycles is analogous to the perennial growth form of arctic plants. The future of the population is not dependent upon the success in any one year, as would be the case for annual species. The population perseveres even if unfavorable conditions lead to the failure of reproduction in any one year.

Table 2 Cases of Prolonged Life Cycles in High Latitude and High Altitude Invertebrates.

Species	Order:Family	Location	Duration	Reference
Pardosa glacialis	Araneae:Lycosidae	Lake Hazen, NWT Canada	6–7 years	Leech (1966)
Tarentula exasperans			6–7 years	
Pardosa concinna	Araneae:Lycosidae	Alpine tundra, Colorado	2 years	Schmoller (1970)
Pardosa tristis			2 years	
Haplodrassus signifer	Araneae:Gnaphosidae	Alpine tundra, Colorado	2? years	Schmoller (1970)
Gnaphosa muscorum			2? years	
Gnaphosa mima			2? years	
Drassodes sp. nov.			2? years	
Pulvinaria ellesmerensis	Homoptera: Coccoidea	Lake Hazen	As many as 5 years	Richards (1964)
Pterostichus brevicornis	Coleoptera: Carabidae	Taiga, Interior Alaska	14–36 months	Kaufmann (1971)
Pterostichus spp.	Coleoptera: Carabidae	Barrow, Alaska	2 or more years	MacLean, unpubl.

Species	Taxonomy	Location	Duration	Reference
Upis ceramboides	Coleoptera: Tenebrionidae	Taiga, Interior Alaska	16–25 months	Kaufmann (1969)
Gynaephora (=Byrdia) groenlandica	Lepidoptera: Lymantriidae	Lake Hazen	2 or more years / "Perhaps as many as 5" years"	Oliver et al. (1964) / Downes (1965)
G. rossi				
Olethreutes inquietana	Lepidoptera: Tortricidae	Lake Hazen	"at least 2 years"	MacKay and Downes (1969)
Olethreutes mengelana			2 years; exceptionally, 1 year	
Tipula carinifrons	Diptera:Tipulidae	Siberia	2 years	Chernov and Savchenko (1965)
Tipula carinifrons	Diptera:Tipulidae	Barrow, Alaska	4 or more years	MacLean and Clement, in prep.
Tipula arctica	Diptera:Tipulidae	Greenland	2 years	Nielsen (1910)
Tipula excisa	Diptera:Tipulidae	Norway	2 years	Hofsvang (1973)
Pedicia hannai	Diptera:Tipulidae	Barrow, Alaska	4 or 5 years	MacLean, 1973
Culicoides spp.	Diptera; Ceratopogonidae	Churchill, Manitoba	2 years	Downes (1962)
Procladius sp.	Diptera; Chironomidae	Lake Hazen, NWT	3 or more years	Oliver (1968)
Diamesa valkanovi	Diptera: Chironomidae	Finse, Norway	2 years; exceptionally, 1 year	Saether (1968)
Diamesa davisi				
Chironomus hyperboreus	Diptera: Chironomidae	Saskatchewan, Canada	2 years	Rempel (1936)

The existence of life cycles of more than 1 year leads to overlapping generations and the coexistence of several year-classes in a single population. Thus, the high density and biomass of certain tundra insect species may be a direct result of low annual productivity and the resulting prolonged life cycle (MacLean, 1973). Care must be taken in interpreting density and biomass values for tundra invertebrates.

While pupation may be prevented and the life cycle prolonged in unfavorable years, the reverse—accelerated pupation in favorable years—apparently does not occur (MacLean and Pitelka, 1971). Danks and Oliver (1972) argue that an obligate diapause prior to pupation is included in the life cycles of arctic insects as a mechanism preventing unseasonal emergence, for instance, late in the season in an unusually warm year. It should be noted that an extended life cycle is not necessarily a flexible one. A species may be rigidly bound in a life cycle that involves several years, and the coexistence of larvae in several stages of development (Dahl, 1970) is not, in itself, evidence of flexibility.

The length of the life cycle of arctic insects derives almost entirely from the larval period. The adult existence is usually brief, and is often devoted entirely to reproduction. Females of three abundant crane flies occurring near Barrow, Alaska emerge from pupation with fully developed ova, copulate within hours, and lay their complement of eggs within a day or so of emergence. In arctic blackflies (Simuliidae) development of the eggs begins during pupation, and in at least two species the eggs are mature at the time of emergence (Downes, 1965). Reduction of adult life span reaches an extreme in the Norwegian species *Prosimulium ursinum*. This species is parthenogenetic. Most individuals fail to emerge from the pupa; the eggs are shed into the stream when the abdominal wall ruptures (Carlsson, 1962). Thus, there is essentially no adult stage.

Oliver (1968) observed that follicular development occurred in the pupae in chironomids at Lake Hazen, but maturity was not reached until $2\frac{1}{2}-4$ days after emergence. Even in these species, however, the adults did not feed and egg maturation was completed using nutrient material accumulated during the larval stage. Surprisingly, some species can mature a second egg batch after the first has been laid (Oliver, 1968), a characteristic not seen in the arctic Tipulidae.

Ryan (personal communication) found that female moths of the genus *Byrdia* at Devon Island, Northwest Territory, Canada, have matured most of their complement of eggs in the pupal stage. Mating proceeds immediately, so that the first cluster of fertilized eggs is deposited on the cocoon itself.

Females of the antarctic midge *Belgica antarctica* apparently mature their eggs in the pupal stage, and eggs are generally deposited in a single mass of 30–50 eggs within a day or two of the emergence of the female (Strong, 1967). Females were observed to live for a week or so after oviposition, but no more than one egg mass was observed for a single female.

By completing most of the life cycle in the larval stage, usually protected by the soil, tundra invertebrate species limit the length of time that the critical reproductive phase is exposed to the uncertainties of the severe climate, and to surface-dwelling predators as well.

With the reduced adult life span, a morphological reduction of adult insects is often found. Wing reduction (brachyptery or aptery) is frequently found. Two of the three abundant crane flies near Barrow, *Tipula carinifrons* and *Pedicia hannai,* have brachypterous females. In *P. hannai* reduction involves leg length, eyes, antennae, and mouth parts as well (Tjeder, 1963). Byers (1969) argued that cold temperature, which limits the power of flight, is primarily responsible for the evolution of wing reduction; however, the tendency toward retention of wings by males indicates that there must be opposing selective pressures involved. Winter crane flies (*Chionea* spp.) gain a 4% advantage in egg production by replacing the flight muscles with eggs in the thorax (Byers, 1969), an advantage that would not accrue to males. Females of many species are so laden with mature eggs at emergence that, even if fully winged, flight would be difficult at best. With the reduced mobility that accompanies winglessness in females, the responsibility for mate location falls entirely upon the males, and wings may be retained for that purpose. Still, at the prevalent environmental temperatures encountered in midseason near Barrow, males of *T. carinifrons* and *P. hannai* are capable of feeble fluttering movement over the tundra surface at best, and do not engage in free flight. When brought into the laboratory and warmed to room temperature they are able to fly. On the Pribilof Islands, males of *P. hannai,* as well as females, are brachypterous (Tjeder, 1963).

In contrast to vertebrate homeotherms (Bergmann's rule), there is a tendency toward smaller body size in tundra representatives of a number of invertebrate taxa. Mani (1962) cited evidence for alpine insects. Hemmingsen and Jensen (1957) found that mean body length of *Tipula arctica* in Greenland decreases about 4.5% per 10° increase in latitude. This decrease is, presumably, the result of shorter growing seasons and lower temperatures, which reduce growth rate at higher latitudes. Thus, life cycle length and adult body size are both evolutionary responses to length and temperature of the growing season. Since potential fecundity is related to body size, decreased body size means reduced fecundity.

Alternatively, a species might maintain body size by increasing the life cycle length; this, however, increases the period of vulnerability to mortality prior to reproduction. The actual life cycle and morphological characteristics of any tundra species probably represent a compromise between considerations of fecundity and probability of survival in maximizing individual reproductive success.

Arctic mosquitoes offer a conspicuous contrast to the trend of prolonged life cycles, short adult life span, and morphological reduction of adults seen in many other tundra Diptera. All species, apparently, have annual life cycles. Eggs laid in summer hatch at melt-off the following spring. Larval development occurs rapidly, leading to pupation and emergence of adults. Corbet and Danks (1973) investigated life cycle characteristics and phenology of the two high arctic mosquitoes, *Aedes nigripes* and *A. impiger,* at Lake Hazen, Ellesmere Island, Northwest Territory. They found that adult activity persisted for over a month after emergence has ceased. Both sexes took flower nectar as an energy source. During this prolonged activity period females were able to complete three or possibly even four gonadotrophic cycles.

The annual life cycle leaves arctic mosquitoes particularly vulnerable to the vagaries of the arctic climate. Cold weather at Lake Hazen during the summer of 1964 led to a severe reduction in egg laying, and hence emergence of adults in 1965 (Corbet and Danks, 1973). Two successive cold seasons could easily lead to extinction of the population. This is far less likely when several generations of larvae (future generations of adults) coexist in the relatively protected environment of the soil at any one time.

Autogeny—completion of ovarian development and egg laying without the benefit of a blood meal in biting flies—can be considered adaptive reduction of the life cycle. Corbet (1967) observed that both *Aedes impiger* and *A. nigripes* at Lake Hazen could lay reduced complements of eggs if deprived of a blood meal. This facultative autogeny gives individuals the advantage of high fecundity if a blood meal can be obtained, while allowing some amount of reproduction (and continuation of the population) even if poor weather or a shortage of suitable hosts should prevent the taking of a blood meal. *Aedes communis* is apparently always autogenous at Fort Churchill, Manitoba, although further south it appears to be a normal biting species (Hocking, 1960). Eight of the nine black fly species in arctic Canada are autogenous, as are the tundra species of *Culicoides* (Diptera: Ceratopogonidae) (Downes, 1965). Thus, if harrassment by biting flies becomes an annoyance in arctic tundra, one need only think of what it might have been but for autogeny!

One of the two antarctic midges, *Belgica antarctica,* is wingless, while the other, *Parochlus steinenii,* is winged. These species are believed to have life cycles of about 1 year, but with considerable flexibility, depending upon local circumstances and variation in seasons (Wirth and Gressitt, 1967; Peckham, 1971).

The life cycles of tundra microarthropods — mites and Collembola — remain to be investigated. Janetschek (1967) found the antarctic springtail *Gomphiocephalus hodgsoni* overwintering in all stages, with the possible exception of eggs. He concluded, on the basis of a statistical analysis of population size distribution, that the time needed to reach sexual maturity (minimum generation time) was 38.5 days at Cape Crozier, allowing two generations per season, and 49.2 days at Mount England, where one generation was completed per year. The full life cycle, however, extended over two seasons at Cape Crozier and three seasons at Mt. England. Peterson (1971) reported that this species may complete two generations in "good" summers, and only one generation in others. He found individuals overwintering in all stages, including the egg.

The life history of *Aeropedellus clavatus*, a high altitude grasshopper occurring in the Colorado Rockies, was investigated by Alexander and Hilliard (1964). They found an obligate diapause, apparently involving more than one season, in the egg stage; however, postembryonic development and the life cycle are completed in a single season. The total period from hatching to adult is approximately 6 weeks. This is accomplished, in part, by a reduction in the life cycle from five juvenile instars, typical of most Acrididae, to only four. This is seen in other boreal Acrididae. Apparently this group adapts to tundra conditions by reduction rather than prolongation of the life cycle. The scarcity or absence of grasshoppers from tundra may indicate the limitation of this mode of adaption.

Extended life cycles have been observed in at least two subarctic beetles (Kaufmann, 1969, 1971); however, in these species the life cycle involves extension of adult life. Arctic carabid beetles overwinter in both larval and adult stages near Barrow, indicating a life cycle involving 2 or more years. The vast majority of arctic insects overwinter as larvae or prepupae, and perhaps the tendency to overwinter as adults limits the success of Coleoptera under arctic conditions.

3. Resistance to winter cold.   In general, cold-climate insects may pass the winter in either of two manners: they may supercool, and thus avoid the formation of ice crystals, or they may freeze solid but, by various mechanisms, avoid tissue damage due to freezing. The actual physiological mechanisms are far from understood. The subject has recently been reviewed by Asahina (1969), Salt (1969), and Cloudsley-Thompson (1970), and will not be treated in detail here.

Several temperatures are of importance to poikilotherm under cold conditions. The chill-coma temperature is the minimum temperature at which activity is possible; the freezing point is the warmest temperature at which tissues will freeze; and the supercooling point is the minimum temperature that can be reached without freezing. Sømme and Östbye (1969) found that the chill-coma temperature is less than the freezing point in some winter-active insects; thus, they are capable of muscular and metabolic activity in a supercooled state.

Both supercooling and freeze-tolerance are facilitated by high concentrations of glycerol and other polyhydric alcohols in the hemolymph (Miller, 1969; Baust and Miller, 1970). Glycerol is synthesized in fall, possibly by anaerobic catalysis of glycogen; it remains in high concentration over the winter, and disappears in spring. However, some species are able to survive freezing even in the absence of glycerol, and other species with high glycerol content have a relatively high supercooling point (Sømme, 1964, 1965). Other mechanisms are clearly involved. Scholander et al. (1953) showed that dehydration was an important contributor to freeze tolerance in arctic Chironomidae. Presumably, by reducing the volume of intracellular water, the formation of damaging ice crystals is prevented. Concentration of tissue solutes due to dehydration is not sufficient to explain the decrease in supercooling point seen in winter acclimated larvae (Salt, 1969).

In areas where the temperature of the overwintering habitat does not fall far below 0°C metabolism may continue throughout the winter. Conradi-Larsen and Sømme (1973a,b) showed that overwinter survival of beetles enclosed in ice in Norway depended both on cold-hardiness and on their ability to tolerate oxygen deficiency. They recorded 100% survival after 127 days in an oxygen-free atmosphere at 0°C. During anoxia the beetles developed an oxygen debt and high concentrations of lactate and alanine accumulated in the hemolymph.

In arctic tundra freezing of the active layer proceeds upward from the permafrost table and downward from the surface. Unfrozen tundra may persist for a considerable period, trapped between frozen ground above and below. Decomposition may continue at and even below 0°C, exhausting the soil oxygen supply and leading to general anaerobiosis. Thus, tolerance of oxygen deficiency may be a general feature of overwintering tundra invertebrates, particularly since many lowland tundra soils are saturated with water by late summer and are generally low in oxygen.

The glycerol content falls and freeze tolerance disappears within 36 hr of thawing and exposure to temperatures above 0°C (Baust and Miller, 1970). Remmert and Wisniewski (1970) noted low resistance to cold in mites and Collembola collected during the summer on Spitzbergen. The avoidance of freezing temperatures during the summer is thus of importance to tundra invertebrates. In the relatively warm 1972 summer season at Barrow (Figure 2) the daily minimum air temperature was 0°C or below on 29 days in June, 16 days in July, 9 days in August, and continuously following 7 September. Soil temperature at −2 cm, however, remained continuously above 0°C following thawing. This offers another important reason for the preponderance of soil-dwelling over surface-active invertebrates in arctic climates.

Resistance to cold in alpine invertebrates has not been investigated. Where temperatures may fall well below freezing each night due to reradiation to a clear sky we might expect to find retention of supercooling or freezing-resistance mechanisms during the summer season. Schmoller (1971) has observed that the alpine spider and beetle fauna may be divided into day-active and night-active species which experience very different micro-climates. These differences may be reflected in adaptations relating to cold tolerance and metabolism.

4. Metabolic adaptations. The degree of metabolic adaptation to tundra conditions remains in dispute. Scholander *et al.* (1953) found only slight physiological adaptation in the metabolic rate (displacement of the metabolic rate/temperature curve toward cold temperatures) of terrestrial poikilotherms near Barrow, Alaska. They concluded that the most important adaptive mechanism was microhabitat selection. Aquatic invertebrates, in contrast, showed considerable but incomplete metabolic adaptation, relative to temperature and tropical forms. McAlpine (1965a) noted that most adult insects were collected walking rather than flying on Ellef Ringnes Island, Northwest Territory, and Downes (1962) observed that bumblebees can forage and pollinate flowers in this way. In 1971 we collected large numbers of the moth *Barrovia fasciata* on sticky boards placed on the ground surface at Barrow; K. W. Philip (personal communication), collecting by conventional means at the same time, obtained none. Their distribution around the outside of each board indicated that the moths had walked onto the surface. These observations suggest that an evolutionary adjustment of behavior has occurred in response to reduced metabolic capacity.

Still, the existence of chill-coma temperatures below the tissue freezing point indicates that some adjustment of physiological capacity in response to low temperature must have occurred. We have found that arctic tundra crane fly larvae and adults, Saldidae, and Enchytraeidae respire actively at +0.5°C Tilbrook and Block (1972) found cold adaptation, particularly in the immature stages, in the antarctic collembole *Cryptopygus antarcticus*, since these had a higher metabolic rate than temperate Collembola at comparable temperatures.

Metabolic rate or respiration, as measured by oxygen consumption or CO_2 production at a particular temperature, is only part of the question of metabolic adaptation. Equally important are the changes in metabolic rate with changing temperature, and the relationship of metabolic rate to the total bioenergetic budget. The relationship of metabolic rate to temperature is usually expressed by a Q_{10} value—the proportional change in metabolic rate that occurs with a 10° change in temperature. Values around 2.5–3 are most commonly reported. The Q_{10} value is constant only if the metabolic rate:temperature relationship is exponential over the entire range of measurement (Howard, 1971). Measurement of metabolic rate must be made at least three, and preferably more, temperatures spanning the normal range of activity of the species in question.

Many species tend toward a linear increase in metabolic rate with temperature. In this case the Q_{10} value increases as metabolic rate approaches zero, and Q_{10} is of value only over the particular range of measurement. Species with such a pattern show a metabolic rate that is lower than expected (from the exponential model) at high and low temperatures (Figure 3). The latter may be particularly important for tundra invertebrates.

We have found a constant Q_{10} (exponential relationship between metabolic rate and temperature) in both male and female adult *Tipula carinifrons* near Barrow (MacLean and Clement, in preparation); however, Q_{10} increased at lower temperatures, indicating deviation from the exponential model, in adult male *Pedicia hannai* and in adult *Chiloxantus stellatus* (Hemiptera:Saldidae) (Testa and MacLean, in preparation).

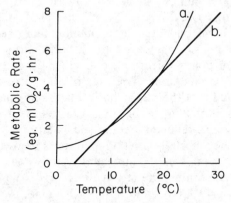

Figure 3 Possible relationships between metabolic rate and temperature: a, the exponential model—Q_{10}, is constant; b, the linear model—Q_{10}, increases at low temperatures, decreases at high temperatures.

Larvae of both crane fly species show increasing Q_{10} values at low temperatures.

Hofsvang (1972) calculated linear regression lines for oxygen consumption and temperature for all stages of *Tipula excisa;* however, the goodness of fit was largely a result of the small number of data points involved. Calculations made from his data show that the relationship is more nearly exponential for adults, and falls off rapidly for early instar larvae.

Tilbrook and Block's (1972) data for the antarctic collembole *Cryptopygus antarcticus* show this tendency in the extreme. For the smallest size class (mean = 3.0 μg) the ratio of increase in metabolic rate is greater between 2° and 6°C than between 6° and 10°C. Metabolic rate changes 11.47-fold over the entire 8° temperature range. For animals in the second size class (10.2 μg) the ratio of metabolic increase is independent of temperature, as predicted by the exponential model. For the three larger size classes Q_{10} is less between 2° and 6°C than between 6° and 10°C, indicating a steeper than exponential rise in metabolic rate with temperature. However, for the largest size class (92.8 μg) the metabolic increase is only 1.79-fold over the 2° – 10°C range. Thus, in these insects the smallest animals show a large metabolic decline at low temperatures, while the largest animals show very little metabolic decline at low temperatures. Later data (Block and Tilbrook, 1975) collected from animals taken directly from the field showed that respiration rate of the smallest size class rose sharply as temperature was increased from 0° to 5°C, then fell slightly between 5° and 10°C. Animals of intermediate size gave a linear response to increasing temperature, while respiration rate of the largest animals fit the exponential model. The overall response from 0° to 10°C was greatest for the largest size classes, in contradiction of the data reported earlier for animals maintained in laboratory culture (Tilbrook and Block, 1972).

Thus, while the data are sparse, there appears to be a pattern of changing metabolic response to temperature as development proceeds. The significance of this can only be interpreted in relation to other parameters of the bioenergetic budget. The total amount of energy ingested is equal to the energy egested as feces, *(F)* plus the energy of assimilation *(A):*

$$I = F + A$$

the assimilated energy is partitioned into energy of metabolism or respiration, *(R)* and production *(P):*

$$A = R + P$$

Thus:

$$I = F + R + P$$

Temperature and body size may affect each of these parameters. If low temperature has a severe depressing effect on the ability of an individual to ingest or assimilate energy, for example, then depression of the metabolic rate would be adaptive. Adaptation to tundra conditions involves the ability to maintain a positive energy balance (positive P, or R less than A) at low temperatures, rather than simply maintaining a high metabolic rate.

We might imagine three distinct patterns in the metabolic response of an invertebrate animal to temperature (Figure 4). (I) The rate of assimilation may be greater than the rate of respiration at all temperatures. Such an organism could grow and complete the life cycle under both temperate and cooler arctic or alpine conditions. (II) The rate of assimilation increases more rapidly with increasing temperature than does respiration rate. Thus, the amount of energy available for growth increases with temperature. Such an organism may be unable to complete the life cycle at low temperatures because of an unfavorable energy balance. (III) The rate of respiration increases more rapidly with temperature than does assimilation. Such a pattern might occur in an obligate arctic or alpine organism that is able to maintain a positive energy balance only at low temperatures.

A particularly useful metabolic parameter is the ratio of energy of growth or production to respiration (P/R). MacLean (1973) found that the P/R ratio of the arctic crane fly *Pedicia hannai* is near 1 in the early larval stages, but falls to a very low value in the fourth and final instar. Thus, the accumulation of energy in growth becomes increasingly difficult. This may contribute to the long larval life of this species, rather

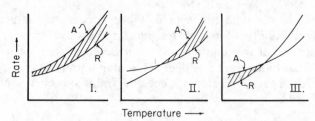

Figure 4 Some possible variations in the response of assimilated energy *(A)* and energy lost as respiration *(R)* to temperature. The hatched area *(A* greater than *R)* indicates energy available for production. These curves show only the part of the temperature range ordinarily encountered by the organism in the field. Productive energy must approach zero at very high and very low temperatures.

than low temperature *per se*. At 0.5° and 5°C, metabolic rate is appreciable; however, no larval growth could be detected after 2 months in the laboratory at 5°C. In keeping with this, larval growth in the field is poor early and late in the season, when soil temperature is less than 5°C. Thus, *Pedicia hannai* appears to show the type II (Figure 4) metabolic pattern. If this is so, this species owes its existence in the arctic to the warmer days of midsummer and the occasional clear, warm days on which soil temperature rises above normal. The species would be an opportunist, tolerating arctic conditions but depending upon more temperate conditions for growth. Dalenius (1965) and Peckham (1971) observed that maximum microhabitat temperatures have the greatest effect on the maturation of antarctic microarthropods.

Hofsvang (1973) found that the P/R ratio of *Tipula excisa* in arctic-alpine Norway was 1.97 during the summer season, but 0.82 over the life cycle as a whole. The difference was in part explained by the fact that respiration continues during the winter although growth ceases.

In contrast, according to O. A. Saether (quoted in Hågvar and Østbye 1973), many larvae of the chironomid subfamily Orthocladiinae seem to grow only at temperatures below 5°C, and may be at rest during the summer when water temperature rises above 5°C. Thus, they seem to follow the type III (Figure 4) pattern with, perhaps, an obligate quiescence during the summer to minimize the period of negative energy balance. This represents an interesting and important mode of physiological adaptation to tundra conditions, and we should hope that additional data will soon be forthcoming.

Tilbrook and Block (1972), as discussed above, found the greatest metabolic depression with cold temperature in Collembola of the smallest size class. If the ability to secure and process food (i.e., assimilation) declined equally with temperature in all size classes, the smaller individuals would be at a distinct advantage at low temperature relative to the P/R ratio. They would be able to maintain a favorable individual energy balance (positive P) at lower temperatures and thus would tend toward the type I, or even type III (Figure 4) metabolic pattern. The relationship of the various parameters of the bioenergetic budget to temperature clearly requires investigation in temperate as well as tundra organisms if we are to understand physiological adaptation to the environment.

The integrated output of the bioenergetic budget under natural conditions is seen as growth rate. Haufe and Burgess (1956) determined the growth response of mosquito larvae to temperature near Ft. Churchill, Manitoba, by comparing development periods in pools of different temperature. The three species with geographic ranges extending into the tundra *(Aedes nigripes, A. impiger,* and *A. communis)* are the first mosquitoes to emerge each season at Churchill; hence, they complete development with the smallest heat sum. The lowest threshold for development (34°F = 1.2°C) occurs in *A. impiger*. The thermal constant (days × degrees above the threshold) required to complete development in this species is comparable to subarctic species; however, the low threshold allows larvae of *A. impiger* to quickly complete development following spring melt-off, even under arctic conditions. The other truly high arctic mosquito, *A. nigripes*, requires a heat sum of about 20% greater than that required by *A. impiger* (Corbet and Danks, 1973). *Aedes nigripes* is the only mosquito occurring at Barrow and on Spitzbergen, indicating that geographic range of arctic mosquitoes is not determined by metabolic (or bioenergetic) adaptation alone.

Haufe and Burgess (1956) also reported a difference in thermal constant between males and females of a given species. This allows males to emerge several days before females. At lower temperatures, however, the effect upon development time of this difference in thermal constant is magnified and the difference in emergence dates of males and females is increased. The absence of subarctic species from some tundra localities may be due as much to dissynchrony in emergence of the sexes as to absolute failure of larval development.

5. *Timing mechanisms.*   Two distinct activity rhythms are of significance to tundra invertebrates: seasonal and diurnal or diel. These have been studied best in relation to the emergence and swarming activities of adult insects, especially Diptera. Research on rhythms in other functions and invertebrate groups might prove quite rewarding.

Snow melt in tundra locations usually occurs shortly before the summer solstice, when photoperiodic cues are at a minimum. In many species, at least of Diptera, development proceeds rapidly following snow melt and the thawing of tundra ponds, so that the bulk of adult insect activity occurs early in the season before a distinct pattern of alternating light and dark periods develops. Emergence of adults of a species can be strikingly synchronous. MacLean and Pitelka (1971) found that the period of time encompassing the middle 67% of the emergence of three species of crane flies near Barrow varied from 3.8 to 11.6 days. The latter occurred in an unusually cold season when the emergence was protracted. Hadley (1969) observed a comparable degree of synchrony in a small moorland crane fly, *Molophilus ater*, in Great Britain. Danks and Oliver (1972) observed the emergence of a given species of aquatic chironomids at Lake Hazen and found that emergence of a given species was highly synchronized within a pond, but varied between ponds based upon depth and exposure. Similar results for mosquitoes were reported by Corbet and Danks (1973). Haufe and Burgess (1956), as discussed above, used the variation in emergence patterns of mosquitoes in different ponds at Ft. Churchill to calculate temperature threshold and thermal constant required for development.

Between-season and between-habitat variations in the timing of emergence are clearly related to temperature. In the cold 1969 and 1973 seasons at Barrow, emergence was delayed and protracted in duration (MacLean and Pitelka, 1971; MacLean and Clement, in progress). At Lake Hazen, Danks and Oliver (1972) observed that (1) the time of first emergence from the same pond in different years was related to pre-emergence water temperature; (2) emergence was later and more synchronous from deeper, colder water; and (3) emergence occurred later in deeper, colder ponds. They concluded that emerging individuals were at the same developmental stage (fully grown, final instar larvae) at the beginning of each season, and pupated without further feeding immediately following the thaw. Thus, timing of emergence is determined by metabolic temperature summation, and synchrony results from the similarity in thermal regime which the pupae experience. No external cues, such as photoperiod, are necessary. Downes (1965) suggested that synchronization in the absence of external cues is most easily achieved in species that pupate at or soon after the melt-off. This may in part explain the observation that many arctic insects emerge early in the season, before the thermal peak of the season.

At Barrow crane fly pupae are not found until shortly before emergence begins; however, the emergence patterns fit the hypothesis of Danks and Oliver. It appears that the mechanism initiating pupation is easily triggered. Final instar larvae of *Tipula carinifrons* removed from the tundra in August 1973, after nightly freezing of the tundra surface had begun, initiated pupation when kept under warmer conditions (10°C following brief exposure to room temperature during weighing) for a period of time (L. E. Clement, research in progress). It appears that a particular cohort of fourth instar larvae destined to complete the life cycle at the next emergence period (and this does not include all of the larvae in the fourth instar at a time; MacLean, 1973) is set for pupation by freezing conditions. Pupation is then triggered by the next occurrence of warm soil conditions. This is not likely to occur in fall because of the shallow sun angle and diminishing photopériod.

Downes (1965) suggested that dormancy in arctic insects may be a direct response to prevailing temperature, rather than a diapause controlled by more remote stimuli. This would favor rapid resumption of growth when favorable conditions return in spring. It is apparent, however, that the external cue—freezing temperatures—is of great importance in timing the life cycle. Danks and Oliver (1972) refer to this as a "diapause" although, at least in crane flies, the obligate cessation of activity usually associated with diapause is lacking. Hofsvang (1973) found that larvae of *Tipula excisa* collected from Norwegian alpine tundra in winter became active after a few seconds warming in the palm of the hand. If this is truly a diapause, (a) it involves only temperature as both initiating and terminating stimulus, without the necessary intervention of photoperiod (the short days of fall and winter); and (b) it is easily broken. Such a mechanism is unlikely to occur in alpine tundra species; there, warm days may alternate with freezing nights throughout the summer season, and we may expect that preparation for pupation and emergence is set by some other environmental change.

There is a natural attempt to attribute synchronous emergence to the compression of events in the short arctic summer. Other factors may be equally or more important. The short functional adult life span makes prompt location of a mate particularly important. Mate location may be made more difficult by wing reduction in one or both sexes and the absence of mating swarms, and by low temperature which may decrease mobility. These factors make emergence into a high density population of particular selective advantage, thus selecting for intraspecific synchrony. MacLean and Pitelka (1971) point out that intense predation upon adult insects by birds (West and Norton, this volume) would select against insects emerging into a low density population. This would select for both intra- and interspecific synchrony of emergence as a predator swamping mechanism. Interspecific synchrony in emergence is certainly a conspicuous feature, at least among Diptera, in arctic tundra.

The diel periodicity of emergence seems to result from a direct response to environmental temperature (Corbet, 1966; Danks and Oliver, 1972). Air temperature is likely to be fluctuating around the lower threshold for mating activities, and changes in light intensity may not accurately indicate conditions above the ground or water. Further, diel changes in light intensity at high latitudes are relatively small. Syrjämäki (1968) found the mean ratio between night and day light intensities during July on Spitzbergen (78° N) to be 1:4. Such variations may be masked by changes in cloud cover.

Danks and Oliver (1972) found that the threshold for pupal ecdysis for chironomids at Lake Hazen (approximately 7°C) was higher than the threshold for pupation (4° or 5°C) or larval development (approximately 1°C). This promotes both seasonal and diel synchrony of emergence, and assures that the adults do not emerge into an environment in which they cannot fly. Such a mechanism leads us to expect the largest emergence on the first warm day following a sequence of cool (less that 7° for chironomids at Lake Hazen) days. Our observations of crane fly emergence at Barrow support this hypothesis.

In some cases, particularly on warm days, Danks and Oliver (1972) recorded a bimodal pattern of emergence. The first peak occurred as the rising temperature passed the threshold for ecdysis. The second, later peak was attributed to accelerated pupal development at the maximum daily temperature.

For insects that have already emerged, some synchronization of activity via photoperiodism may occur. Thus, Corbet (1966) interpreted small morning and afternoon peaks in mosquito activity at Lake Hazen as vestiges of dawn and dusk maxima that characterize mosquito activity further south. Syrjämäki (1968) believed that photoperiodism may play a part in the midday maximum in activity of the chironomid *Smittia extrema* on Spitsbergen. *Trichocera borealis* (Diptera: Trichoceridae) showed no diel periodicity in swarming activity. Papi and Syrjämäki (1963) showed that the diel fluctuations in light intensity at 69° N are sufficient to set the sun orientation rhythm in a wolf spider, *Lycosa fluviatilis* (Araneae: Lycosidae). The meaningful question, as Danks and Oliver (1972) pointed out, is not whether organisms can detect the slight summer diel light intensity changes at high latitudes, but whether light is a useful measure of what is important for their existence.

Acknowledgments

Original research reported herein and the preparation of the manuscript were supported by the National Science Foundation under Grant GV29342 to the University of Alaska. It was performed under joint NSF sponsorship of the International Biological Program and Office of Polar Programs, and was conducted under the auspices of the U.S. Tundra Biome Program. Participation in the Amherst, Massachusetts, meeting of the Ecological Society of America and A.I.B.S. was supported by a travel grant from the A.I.B.S.

References

Alexander, G. (1964). Occurrence of grasshoppers as accidentials in the Rocky Mountains of northern Colorado. *Ecology* **45**, 77–86.

Alexander, G., and Hilliard, J. R. (1964). Life history of *Aeropedellus clavatus* (Orthoptera: Acrididae) in the alpine tundra of Colorado. *Ann. Entomol. Soc. Amer.* **57**, 310–317.

Asahina, E. (1969). Frost resistance in insects. *Advan. Insect. Physiol.* **6**, 1–42.

Ballard, T. M. (1972). Subalpine soil temperature regimes in southwestern British Columbia. *Arctic Alpine Res.* **4**, 139–146.

Baust, J. G., and Miller, L. K. (1970). Variations in glycerol content and its influence on cold hardiness in the Alaskan carabid beetle, *Pterostichus brevicornis*. *J. Insect Physiol.* **16**, 979–990.

Block, W., and Tilbrook, P. J. (1975). Respiration studies on the antarctic collembolan *Cryptopygus* antarcticus at Signy Island, South Orkney Islands. *Oikos,* **26** (in press).

Borror, D. J., and DeLong, D. M. (1971). "An Introduction to the Study of Insects," 3rd Ed. Holt, Rinehart, and Winston, New York.

Brewer, M. C. (1958). Some results of geothermal investigations of permafrost in northern Alaska. *Trans. Amer. Geophys. Union* **39**, 19–26.

Byers, G. W. (1969). Evolution of wing reduction in Crane Flies (Diptera: Tipulidae). *Evolution* **23**, 346–354.

Carlsson, G. (1962). Studies on Scandinavian black flies. *Opusc. Entomal. Suppl.* 21.

Chernov, Y. I., and Savchenko, E. N. (1965). Ecology and preimaginal development phases of the arctic *Tipula (Pterolachisus) carinifrons* Holm. (Diptera: Tipulidae). *Zool. Zh.* **44**(5), 777–779.

Clebsch, E. E. C., and Shanks, R. E. (1968). Summer climatic gradients and vegetation near Barrow, Alaska. *Arctic* **21**(3), 161–171.

Cloudsley-Thompson, J. L. (1970). Terrestrial invertebrates. *In* "Comparative Physiology of Thermoregulation," (C. G. Whittow, ed.), vol. I pp. 15–77, Academic Press, New York.

Conradi-Larsen, E., and Sømme, L. (1973a). Anaerobiosis in the over-wintering beetle *Pelophila borealis*. *Nature (London)* **245**, 388–390.

Conradi-Larsen, E., and Sømme, L. (1973b). The overwintering of *Peolophila borealis* Payk. II. Aerobic and anaerobic metabolism. *Norsk Ent. Tidsskr.* **20**, 325–332.

Corbet, P. S. (1966). Diel patterns of mosquito activity in a high arctic locality, Hazen Camp, Ellesmere Island, N.W.T. *Can. Entomol.* **98**, 1238–1252.

Corbet, P. S. (1967). Facultative autogeny in arctic mosquitoes. *Nature (London)* **215**, 662–663.

Corbet, P. S. (1969). Terrestrial microclimate: amelioration at high latitudes. *Science* **166**, 865–866.

Corbet, P. S., and Danks, H. V. (1973). Seasonal emergence and activity of mosquitoes (Diptera: Culicidae) in a high-arctic locality. *Can. Entomol.* **105**, 837–872.

Dahl, C. (1970). Distribution, phenology, and adaptation to arctic environment in Trichoceridae (Diptera). Oikos, **21**, 185–202.

Dalenius, D. (1965). The acarology of the Antarctic regions. *In* "Biogeography and Ecology in Antarctica," (J. van Mieghem and P. van Oye, eds.), *Monogr. Biol.* **15**, 414–430.

Danks, H. V., and Byers, J. R. (1972). Insects and arachnids of Bathurst Island, Canadian arctic archipelago. *Can. Entomol.* **104**(1), 81–88.

Danks, H. V., and Corbet, P. S. (1973). Sex-ratios at emergence of 2 species of high-arctic *Aedes* (Diptera: Culcidae). *Can. Entomol.* **105**(4), 647–651.

Danks, H. V., and Oliver, D. R. (1972). Diel periodicities of emergence of some high arctic Chironomidae (Diptera). *Can. Entomol.* **105**(6), 903–916.

Douce, G. K. (1973). The population dynamics and community analysis of the Acarina of the arctic coastal tundra. Unpubl. M.S. Thesis, Univ. of Georgia, Athens.

Downes, J. A. (1962). What is an arctic insect? *Can. Entomol.* **94**, 143–162.

Downes, J. A. (1964). Arctic insects and their environment. *Can Entomol.* **96**, 279–307.

Downes, J. A. (1965). Adaptation of insects in the Arctic. *Annu. Rev. Entomol.* **10**, 257–274.

Drewry, G. (1970). A list of insects from El Verde, Puerto Rico. *In* "A Tropical Rain Forest: A Study of Irradiation and Ecology at El Verde, Puerto Rico," (H. T. Odum and R. F. Pigeon, eds.), *U. S. A. T. Energy Comm.* pp. E-129–E-150.

Edwards, J. S. (1972). Arthropod fallout on Alaskan snow. *J. Arctic Alpine Res.* **4**(2), 167–176.

Gavrilova, M. K. (1966). Radiation climate of the arctic. Israel Program Sci. Translat., Jerusalem.

Gressitt, J. L. (ed.) (1963). Insects of Antarctica and subantarctic islands. *In* "Pacific Basin Biogeography," pp. 435–442. Bishop Museum Press, Honolulu.

Gressitt, J. L. (ed.) (1967). Entomology of Antarctica. *Amer. Geophys. Union, Antarctic Res. Ser.* No. 10.

Gressitt, J. L. (ed.) (1970). Subantarctic entomology, particularly of South Georgia and Heard Island. *Pac. Inst. Monogr.* **23**.

Gressitt, J. L., and Strandtmann, R. (eds.) (1971). Advances in Antarctic and far southern entomology. *Pac. Inst. Monogr.* **25**.

Hadley, M. (1969). The adult biology of the crane-fly *Molophilus ater Meigen*. *J. Anim. Ecol.* **38**, 765–790.

Hågvar, S., and Østbye, E. (1973). Notes on some winter-active chironomidae. *Norsk Ent. Tidsskr.* **20**, 253–257.

Haufe, W. O. (1957). Physical environment and behavior of immature stages of *Aedes communis* (Diptera: Culicidae) in subarctic Canada. *Can. Entomol.* **89**, 120–139.

Haufe, W. O., and Burgess, L. (1956). Development of *Aedes* (Diptera: Culicidae) at Fort Churchill, Manitoba, and prediction of dates of emergence. *Ecology* **37**, 500–519.

Hemmingsen, A., and Jensen, B. (1957). The occurrence of *Tipula (Vestiplex) arctica* Curtis in Greenland and its decreasing body length with increasing latitude. *Medd. Grønland.* **159**(1), 1–20.

Henriksen, K. L. (1939). A revised index of the insects of Grønland. *Medd. Grønland.* **119**(10), 112 pp.

Hocking, B. (1960). Northern biting flies. *Annu. Rev. Entomol.* **5**, 135–152.

Hocking, B., and Sharplin, C. D. (1965). Flower basking by arctic insects. *Nature London* **206**, 215.

Hofsvang, T. (1972). *Tipula excisa* Schum. (Diptera: Tipulidae) life cycle and population dynamics. *Norsk. Ent. Tidsskr.* **19**, 43–48.

Hofsvang, T. (1973). Energy low in *Tipula excisa* Schum. (Diptera: Tipulidae) in a high mountain area, Finse, South Norway. *Norw. J. Zool.* **21**, 7–16.

Howard, P. J. A. (1971). Relationship between activity of organisms and temperature and the computation of the annual respiration of microorganisms decomposing leaf litter. IV Colloquium Pedobiologiae, Dijon. Paris: *Inst. Nat. Recherche Agr.*, pp. 198–205.

Hurd, P. D., Jr. (1958). Analysis of soil invertebrate samples from Barrow, Alaska. *Arctic Inst. of No. Amer. Final Rep.*, 24 pp.

Hussey, K. M., and Michelson, R. W. (1966). Tundra relief features near Point Barrow, Alaska. *Arctic* **19**, 162–184.

Janetschek, H. (1967). Growth and maturity of the springtail, *Gomphiocephalus hodgsoni* Carpenter, from South Victoria Land and Ross Island. *In* "Entomology of Antarctica," (J. L. Gressitt, ed.), pp. 295–305. Amer. Geophys. Union, Antarctic Res. Ser. 10.

Kaufmann, T. (1969). Life history of *Upis ceramboides* at Fairbanks, Alaska. *Ann. Entomol. Soc. Amer.* **62**(4), 922–923.

Kaufmann, T. (1971). Hibernation in the arctic beetle, *Pterostichus brevicornis*, in Alaska. *J. Kansas Entomol. Soc.* **44**, 81–92.

Kelley, J. J., Jr., and Weaver, D. F. (1969). Physical processes at the surface of the arctic tundra. *Arctic* **22**(4), 425–437.

Kevan, P. G. (1972). Heliotropism in some arctic flowers. *Can. Field Natur.* **86**, 41–44.

Kevan, P. G. (1973). Flowers, insects, and pollination ecology in the Canadian high arctic. *Polar Rec.* **16**, 667–674.

Kevan, P. G., and Shorthouse, J. D. (1970). Behavioral thermoregulation by high arctic butterflies. *Arctic* **23**(4), 268–279.

Leech, R. E. (1966). The spiders (Araneida) of Hazen Camp 81°49′ N, 71°18′ W. *Quest. Entomol.* **2**, 153–212.

MacArthur, R. H., and Wilson, E. O. (1967). "The Theory of Island Biogeography." Princeton Univ. Press, Princeton, New Jersey.

MacKay, M. R., and Downes, J. A. (1969). Arctic Olethreutinae (Lepidoptera: Tortricidae). *Can. Ent.* **101**, 1048–1053.

MacLean, S. F., Jr. (1973). Life cycle and growth energetics of the arctic crane fly *Pedicia hannai antenatta*. *Oikos* **24**(3), 436–443.

MacLean, S. F. Jr., and Pitelka, F. A. (1971). Seasonal patterns of abundance of tundra arthropods near Barrow. *Arctic* **24**(1), 19–40.

MacLean, S. F., Jr., Fitzgerald, B. M., and Pitelka, F. A. (1974). Population cycles in arctic lemmings: winter reproduction and predation by weasels. *Arctic Alpine Res.* **6**, 1–12.

Mani, M. S. (1962). "Introduction to High Altitude Entomology." Methuen, London.

Mani, M. S. (1968). "Ecology and Biogeography of High Altitude Insects." Dr. W. Jank N.V., The Hague.

McAlpine, J. F. (1964). Arthropods of the bleakest Barren Lands: Composition and distribution of the arthropod fauna of the northwestern Queen Elizabeth Islands. *Can. Entomol.* **96**, 127–129.

McAlpine, J. F. (1965a). Insects and related terrestrial invertebrates of Ellef Ringnes Island. *Arctic* **18**, 73–103.

McAlpine, J. F. (1965b). Observations on anthophilous Diptera at Lake Hazen, Ellesmere Island. *Can. Field Natur.* **79**, 247–252.

Miller, L. K. (1969). Freezing tolerance in an adult insect. *Science* **166**, 105–106.

Nelson, J. M. (1971). The invertebrates of an area of Pennine moorland within the Moor House Nature Reserve in Northern England. *Trans. Soc. Brit. Entomol.* **19**, 173–235.

Nielsen, J. C. (1910). A catalogue of the insects of North-East Greenland, with descriptions of some larvae. Part II of I. *Medd. Grønland.* **43**, 55–68.

Oliver, D. R. (1963). Entomological studies in the Lake Hazen area, Ellesmere Island, including lists of species of Arachnida, Collembola, and Insecta. *Arctic* **16**, 175–180.

Oliver, D. R. (1968). Adaptations of arctic Chironomidae. *Ann. Zool. Fenn.* **5**(1), 111–118.

Oliver, D. R., Corbet, P. S., and Downes, J. A. (1964). Studies on arctic insects: the Lake Hazen project. *Can Entomol.* **96**, 138–139.

Østbye, E. (1969). Records of Coleoptera from the Finse area. *Norsk Entomol. Tidsskr.* **16**, 41–43.

Papi, F., and Syrjämäki, J. (1963). The sun-orientation rhythm of wolf spiders at different latitudes. *Arch. Ital. Biol.* **101**, 59–77.

Peckham, V. (1971). Notes on the chironomid midge *Belgica antarctica* Jacobs at Anvers Island in the maritime antarctic. *Pac. Ins. Monogr.* **25**, 145–166.

Peterson, A. J. (1971). Population studies on the Antarctic collembolan *Gomphiocephalus hodgsoni* Carpenter. *Pac. Ins. Monogr.* **25**, 75–98.

Rapoport, E. H. (1969). Gloger's rule and the pigmentation of Collembola. *Evolution* **23**, 622–626.

Remmert, H., and Wisniewski, W. (1970). Low resistance to cold of polar animals in summer. *Oecologia,* **4**, 111–112.

Remmert, H., and Wunderling, K. (1969). Temperature differences between arctic and alpine meadows and their ecological significance. *Oecologia* **4**, 408–210.

Rempel, J. G. (1936). The life history and morphology of *Chironomus hyperboreus. J. Biol. Bd. Can.* **2**, 209–221.

Richards, W. R. (1964). The scale insects of the Canadian Arctic (Homoptera: Coccoidea). *Can. Entomol.* **96**, 1457–1462.

Saether, O. A. (1968). Chironomids of the Finse area, Norway, with special reference to their distribution in a glacier brook. *Arch. Hydrobiol.* **64**, 426–483.

Salt, R. W. (1969). The survival of insects at low temperatures. *In* "Dormancy and Survival," *Symp. Soc. Exp. Biol.* **23**, 331–350

Schmoller, R. (1970). Life histories of alpine tundra Arachnida in Colorado. *Amer. Midl. Natur.* **83**, 119–133.

Schmoller, R. R. (1971). Habitats and zoogeography of alpine tundra Arachnida and Carabidae (Coleoptera) in Colorado. *Southwest. Natur.* **15**(3), 319–329.

Scholander, P. F., Flagg, W., Walters, V., and Irving, L. (1953). Climatic adaptation in arctic and tropical poikilotherms. *Physiol. Zool.* **26**, 67–92.

Sømme, L. (1964). Effects of glycerol on cold hardiness of insects. *Can. J. Zool.* **42**, 87–101.

Sømme, L. (1965). Further observations on glycerol and cold-hardiness in insects. *Can. J. Zool.* **43**, 765–770.

Sømme, L., and Østbye, E. (1969). Cold-hardiness in some winter active insects. *Nor. Entomol. Tidsskr.* **16**, 45–48.

Springett, J. A. (1970). The distribution and life histories of some moorland Enchytraeidae (Oligochaeta). *J. Anim. Ecol.* **39**, 725–737.

Strong, J. (1967). Ecology of terrestrial arthropods at Palmer Station, Antarctic Peninsula. *In* "Entomology of Antarctica," (J. L. Gressitt, ed.), pp. 357–371. Amer. Geophys. Union Antarctic Res. Ser. 10.

Syrjämäki, J. (1968). Diel patterns of swarming and other activities of two arctic Dipterans (Chironomidae and Trichoceridae) on Spitzbergen. *Oikos* **19**, 250–258.

Tilbrook, P. J., and Block, W. (1972). Oxygen uptake in an Antarctic collembole *Cryptopygus antarcticus*. *Oikos* **23**, 313–317.

Tjeder, B. (1963). Three subapterous craneflies from Alaska. *Opusc. Entomol.* **28**, 229–241.

Wirth, W. W., and Gressitt, J. L. (1967). Diptera: Chironomidae (Midges). *In* Entomology of Antarctica, (J. L. Gressitt, ed.), pp. 197–203. Amer. Geophys. Union Antarctic Res. Ser. 10.

Wolff, N. L. (1964). The Lepidoptera of Greenland. *Medd. Grønland.* **159**(11), 1–74.

Metabolic Adaptations of Tundra Birds

George C. West and David W. Norton

Institute of Arctic Biology
University of Alaska
Fairbanks, Alaska

Introduction

The study of metabolic adaptations may proceed through various complementary forms of inquiry. Metabolic processes may be examined from either the anabolic or the catabolic side of the equation, at the organismic or the suborganismic level, and on a quantitative (rates of energy flow) or a qualitative basis (dietary selection or depot energy substrates). We have outlined a series of dichotomies within which we will attempt to summarize what is and what is not known of the metabolic attributes of birds that spend all or part of their life cycle on high latitude tundra (Table 1). Two contrasts are brought out in the ensuing discussion: the strategic distinction between permanent residents and summer visitors to arctic and alpine tundra, and the differences in thermoregulatory strategy exercised by large- versus small-bodied birds.

Much of the metabolic information available on arctic birds is based on respiratory metabolism measurements at different ambient temperatures. In reference to Table 1, therefore, modern inquiry which began in the late 1940s, centered on whole-bird metabolic rates in the context of thermal balance and only more recently have other aspects been considered or measured. From the earliest investigations (Scholander *et al.*,

Table 1 Outline of Known or Suspected Types of Metabolic Response

---

A. Quantitative aspects of metabolism
   1. Organismic (whole-animal) energetics
      a. Thermal balance: regulation of body temperature
      b. Mobility and productive processes
   2. Suborganismic energetics
      a. Rates of organ and cellular metabolism for maintenance
      b. Rates of organ and cellular metabolism for locomotion and in productive
         activity
B. Qualitative aspects of metabolism
   1. Organismic (whole-animal) aspects
      a. Dietary substrates and selectivity
      b. Depot storage products
   2. Suborganismic aspects
      a. Digestion and assimilation
      b. Intermediary metabolic enzymes and substrates

1950a,b,c; Irving and Krog, 1954, 1955; Irving *et al.,* 1955) to the more recent (West, 1968, 1972a,b; Gessaman, 1972; Norton, 1973; Pohl and West, 1973), this focus of inquiry indicates that we tropical homeotherms have been quite properly impressed with the energetic problems facing birds in cold-dominated environments and with the ability of birds to solve these problems. Tundra residence therefore forces birds to generate adaptive solutions to the total range of metabolic aspects as outlined in Table 1. A review of the various problems and solutions as we know them follows the two main strategies of bird species toward tundra occupancy. These options may be described by the phrase, "take it or leave it."

The Two Strategies

The "Take It" Strategy

Those species that remain as permanent residents in the arctic tundra are few in number. The snowy owl *(Nyctea scandiaca),* raven *(Corvus corax),* the willow ptarmigan *(Lagopus lagopus),* and occasional redpolls *(Acanthis hornemanni* and *A. flammea)* are the most conspicuous. Farther south in the taiga forests, where temperatures reach lower extremes, other species reside which must endure similar climatic hardships as on the tundra. In discussing energetic adaptations of tundra permanent residents, examples can therefore be drawn from taiga species.

We see five categories of environmental problems that must be solved by permanent residents of tundra in winter: (1) the duration of the winter season; (2) short or no hours of daylight; (3) factors promoting heat loss, including low temperatures, high wind velocity, radiative, conductive, and evaporative heat loss; (4) relative uniformity of the habitat; and (5) a food supply limited in variety.

Duration of Winter.   On the arctic tundra of northern Alaska, the Canadian Archipelago, in northern Scandinavia and the Soviet Union, the sun does not rise above the horizon in winter for a varying length of time from a few days at the Arctic Circle to 3 months in the arctic islands. The duration of the cold and snow covered portion of the year extends from October to April at the Arctic Circle and from the end of August until late June in the arctic islands. Permanent residents are thus faced with 8 – 10 months of what to us would seem energetically to be extremely costly for survival of populations of homeotherms.

The long duration of winter creates an increased annual energy demand because of the lower environmental temperatures. The long winter also means a much shortened growing season in which to produce vegetative matter required by arctic herbivores. Insectivorous birds cannot remain in the Arctic in winter and permanent residency of predatory birds is dependent on cyclic populations of small mammals and on ptarmigan.

Day Length.   Despite the length of the winter and the sunless days, there is a long period of twilight, enough apparently for daylight-dependent birds to find food. There are indications that arctic birds increase their activity time in the low intensity illumination of arctic winter as compared to summer (Pohl, 1972), and it appears that this ability may be unique to arctic and subarctic members of the same species that also reside at lower latitudes (Pohl, personal communication).

We know that despite the low light intensities of long arctic winter days, birds maintain a substantial activity period. At Fairbanks, Alaska (65° N latitude), redpolls have been observed to be active for about 10 hr in midwinter when the day length was only a little over 3 hr (Pohl, in preparation) and willow ptarmigan are active for about 5.5 hr (Figure 1; West, 1968). Personal observation at 69° N latitude in January indicates that ptarmigan are feeding, flying, and calling when it is hardly light enough for man to see. Despite some recent studies in the Scandinavian arctic (Aschoff *et al.,* 1970) little is known about the activity patterns of arctic tundra birds in the wild, in part because of the problems of acquiring information on free living birds in the field.

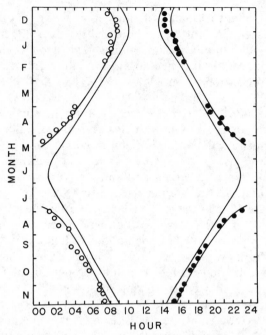

Figure 1   Onset (o) and end (●) of activity of caged willow ptarmigan
maintained under natural conditions of light and temperature at Fairbanks, Alaska. The outer lines indicate beginning and end of civil
twilight; the inner lines indicate sunrise and sunset at the cage site.
Data points during May, June, and July are lacking since the birds
were continuously active over the 24-hr period (modified from West,
1968).

Heat Loss.   Tundra birds in winter become physiologically acclimatized to the cold temperatures through insulative and metabolic means.
Large birds such as the snowy owl and willow ptarmigan have greater
plumage densities which decrease their heat loss in winter. The snowy
owl has the lowest heat loss coefficient (thermal conductance) recorded
for birds (Gessaman, 1972), a value three to four times lower than that
of the well-insulated willow ptarmigan (West, 1972a).

The increased insulation in large birds (>300 g) allows them to extend their lower critical temperature to near 0°C, and to maintain homeothermy at low temperatures with an energy output at −40°C of 1.7 to
2.3 times the resting rate at thermal neutrality (Table 2). The emperor
goose *(Anser canagica)* population is resident in Alaska and adjacent
Siberian waters. Water temperatures on the northern breeding grounds
do not differ greatly from those of the more southern wintering areas al-

Table 2 Resting Metabolic Rate at Thermal Neutrality (SMR), Lower Critical Temperature (T_c), and the Increase in Resting Rate Over SMR at $-40°C$ of Arctic and Alpine Permanent Resident Species of Birds

Species	Season	Body weight (g)	SMR (cm^3 $O_2 \cdot g^{-1} \cdot hr^{-1}$)	T_c (°C)	RMR at $-40°C$ $\times$ SMR	Reference
Anser canagica	Summer	2800	0.63	-2	1.93	Morehouse and West (in preparation)
Nyctea scandiaca	Winter	1800	0.40	2.5	2.28	Gessaman (1972)
Corvus corax	Winter	850	1.78	-5	1.68	Veghte and Herreid (1965)
Lagopus lagopus	Winter	590	1.06	-6.3	1.74	West (1972a)
Lagopus lagopus	Summer	536	1.30	7.7	2.52	West (1972a)
Lagopus mutus	Winter	450	1.40	4.5	1.91	West (1972a)
Lagopus leucurus	Summer	326	1.30	6.5	2.41	Johnson (1968)
Perisoreus canadensis	Winter	70	2.18	5.0	2.17	Veghte (1964)
Acanthis flammea	Winter	14	6.13	7.0	2.69	Pohl and West (1973)
Acanthis flammea	Summer	14	4.02	23.5	3.84	West (1972b)

305

though air temperatures in winter may be somewhat colder. From our preliminary study, it appears that these large waterfowl possess excellent insulation, so that in summer their lower critical temperature remains below 0°C (Table 2).

The resting metabolic rate at thermal neutrality of these larger birds is low in winter corresponding to the 0.72 power of body weight (Lasiewski and Dawson, 1967), while the resting metabolic rate of the small redpoll is some 30% higher in winter than would be predicted on the basis of weight (West, 1972b). Therefore, an increase in metabolism of 2.7 times the thermal neutral rate means a relatively greater energy cost for the small redpoll than for the larger owl or ptarmigan (Table 2). The winter resting metabolic rate of willow ptarmigan at −40°C is 40% lower than in the summer at a comparable temperature and the metabolic rate required to sustain a winter willow ptarmigan at −40°C would only sustain the same bird at −10°C in the summer because of insulative differences (West, 1972a).

Studies are currently underway to determine the resting metabolic rate of subarctic ravens (Schwann, in preparation). Veghte and Herreid (1965) estimated the metabolic rate of ravens from radiometric determinations of feather insulation and indicated an increase in metabolic rate at −40°C of 1.86 times the thermal neutral rate (Table 2).

Small birds cannot increase their insulation to the same degree as can large birds. Pohl (in preparation) weighed the feathers of common redpolls and found that the plumage of winter caught birds was 20% heavier than that of summer birds. Nevertheless, we have shown that despite this plumage increase, the winter metabolic rate is higher than the summer rate at comparable temperatures below thermal neutrality (Pohl and West, 1973). In winter, small birds have a high resting rate at thermal neutrality which can be explained by the fact that in winter, the birds are never exposed to thermal neutral temperatures, and when so exposed, they are not capable of lowering their metabolic rate to the expected value in the 1- or 2-hr duration of a metabolism test (Table 2; West, 1972b). If the measured rate in winter equalled the predicted rate (or summer rate) then at −40°C, the increase in metabolism would have to be 3.8 times the resting rate, much higher than the increase required of larger birds.

What small birds lack in increased insulation, however, they make up for in metabolic capability. Winter acclimatized redpolls tested at −50°C during both day and night maintained normal body temperatures for the duration of tests which lasted over 3 hours. Summer acclimatized birds had lower metabolic rates at −50°C associated with slightly lower body temperatures, but it was concluded that adults can maintain sustained high metabolic rates at all seasons (Pohl and West, 1973). Furthermore, juvenile redpolls still in their first plumage were capable of higher metabolic rates per gram-hour than the adults but for a shorter period of time.

This ability to evolve heat at low temperatures is apparently due to shivering in resting birds (West, 1965). The question arises of how much additional energy the birds must expend when they move about in search of food. This activity consists mostly of hopping along branches or the snow surface searching for birch seeds. In tests where redpolls were forced to exercise by hopping in a rotating drum, we found that the increased heat production due to exercise was additive in constant increments to that required for maintenance of homeothermy from near 0° to −30°C during winter (Pohl and West, 1973). However, at lower temperatures, substitution occurred with no increase in metabolic rate until, at the lowest temperature used for exercising birds in the fall (−42°C), the redpolls were no longer able to maintain homeothermy for more than a few minutes (Figure 2). In winter, one test at −44°C indicated an increased ability to produce heat while exercising and in summer, a similar test showed a marked decrease in ability.

Flying from branch to branch probably does not increase the metabolic rate greatly above that required for hopping or moving along branches in search of seeds. Longer flights to other trees in winter are more costly. Calculating from the equation of Hart and Berger (1972) for an estimate of the cost of flight, the rate would be a little over nine times the resting rate at thermal neutrality, i.e., the redpoll must add almost 9.5 $cm^3O_2 \cdot min^{-1}$ to its 3.9 $cm^3O_2 \cdot min^{-1}$ at −40°C to fly. These figures, however, are subject to some error since to our knowledge, no testing of flight metabolism has been made at low ambient temperatures and we assume that flight, like hopping activity, is additive to that of thermoregulation. Locomotion, and especially flight, moreover, deny the active bird of optimal conformation of the surface insulation for impeding heat loss (cf. Hart and Héroux, 1955).

That these small homeotherms are capable of extremely high metabolic rates has been demonstrated by tests using a helium–oxygen atmosphere by Rosenmann and Morrison (1974) which indicates the redpolls can increase their resting metabolic rate 5.5 times the minimum rate measured during day time (Pohl and West, 1973). There is no question then, that despite their small size, the 12- to 15-g redpolls have the metabolic capacity to exist in the Arctic provided they can find enough food in the time available for feeding.

In the arctic tundra, low temperatures are often accompanied by winds. By increasing convective heat loss, wind causes an increase in metabolism at a rate approximately equivalent to the square root of the

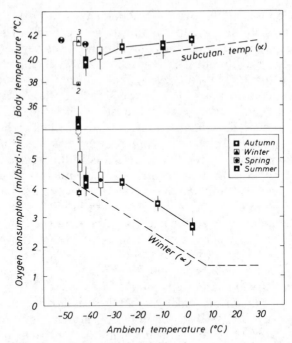

Figure 2   Oxygen consumption and body temperature as a function of ambient temperature during forced exercise in common redpolls measured at different seasons. Data points are means; bars are ±2 S.E.; vertical lines are ±1 S.D. The two dashed lines are from data on resting redpolls measured at daytime (α) during winter. The circles (●) in the upper diagram are mean body temperatures of redpolls after resting in the dark for 1 hr at the test temperature (from Pohl and West, 1973).

air speed (Figure 3; Gessaman, 1972). A snowy owl sitting on the tundra at −40°C on a still day, requires 0.91 cm³O₂·g⁻¹·hr⁻¹ to maintain homeothermy, but if the wind comes up to about 7.5 m·sec⁻¹, this rate is increased 2.4 times. No studies have been made on the effect of wind velocity on small birds, but one can suppose that the increase would be greater since the surface area available for convective heat loss is relatively larger and the insulation relatively poorer than in larger birds.

Habitat Uniformity.   Despite a high degree of microrelief in the tundra which has a great effect in summer on plant growth, occurrence of small mammals, and even nesting of tundra birds, the situation in winter is radically altered by blowing snow which fills many of the depressions

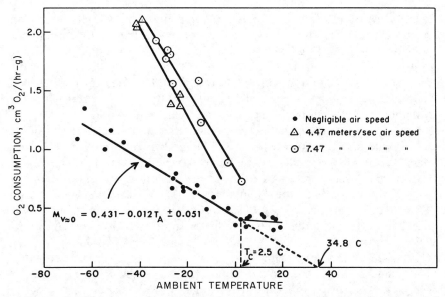

Figure 3 Relation of oxygen consumption to ambient temperature of four female snowy owls at negligible air speed and of three owls at air speeds of 4.47 and 7.47 m · sec⁻¹ (from Gessaman, 1972).

and tends to smooth out irregularities in the tundra surface. Where willow *(Salix)* or alder *(Alnus)* brush grows above the snow line, or along river and stream cuts, some relief from blowing snow can be found. Some tundra birds, however, such as ptarmigan (Irving, 1960) and redpolls create their own relief by burrowing in the snow, thereby apparently conserving energy through the added insulation of the snow (Sulkava, 1969).

Desert birds can increase heat loss through their feet at high ambient temperatures by conduction to cooler substrates (e.g., water), but it is doubtful if heat loss through the feet of arctic birds is an important avenue of heat loss in the cold. The actual surface contact of feet to the substrate is greatly minimized in arctic birds either through foot feathering (ptarmigan) or the rough surface of the corneal scales on toe pads. When ambient temperatures are above freezing, foot temperatures may be only a degree or two higher, but when substrate temperatures fall below freezing, blood flow is increased to maintain sensitive tissues above freezing while surface corneal scales may drop below freezing. The vascular system and its control for heat regulation in the feet of arctic birds, especially the web-footed species, have not been described.

Food Supply. Because of the relative uniformity of habitat, plant species diversity is low and only a few species of plants are available as food for wintering birds in arctic tundra. To be available, plants must grow above the surface of the snow since birds, unlike caribou *(Rangifer)* rarely remove snow from the ground surface for finding food. There are several species of willow, alder, and birch *(Betula)* which are available to browsing birds such as ptarmigan. Studies on the arctic willow ptarmigan indicate that 94% of their diet in winter consists of the catkin buds and terminal twigs of willow and of that, 80% may be of a single species *(S. alaxensis).* The variety of willow and the inclusion of other species, e.g., birch, increases in the diet southward into the tundra-taiga ecotone south of the Brooks Range in Alaska (West and Meng, 1966). Rock ptarmigan *(Lagopus mutus)* in winter prefer birch (86%) over willow (6%) in the alpine tundra of interior Alaska while interior willow ptarmigan maintain a preference for willow (89%) (Weeden, 1969). White-tailed ptarmigan *(Lagopus leucurus)* in Alaska depend on alder while further south in the alpine tundra of the Rocky Mountains where there is no competition from other ptarmigan species, they eat willow in winter (Weeden, 1967; Braun and May, 1972). The rather neat partitioning of the three main dietary items among the three species of ptarmigan in Alaska (willow for willow ptarmigan, birch for rock ptarmigan, and alder for white-tailed ptarmigan) is a result of habitat preference and interspecific competition (Weeden, 1969; Moss, 1973).

In other regions of circumpolar arctic tundra, food preference of ptarmigan shifts according to availability (Seiskari, 1957; Peters, 1958; Gelting, 1937; and others). The energy content of these diets is relatively uniform, with birch being more energy rich than willow (West and Meng, 1966). Ability to utilize the energy available in the browse, however, is rather low, approaching 45% (West, 1968; Moss, 1973), which is similar to the digestive efficiency of grazing small arctic mammals (Melchior, 1972) and tundra ruminants (White, this volume).

Redpolls consume primarily birch seeds in winter, and although many individuals migrate south into the taiga, populations are present in the brush-covered areas of tundra throughout the winter where birch is available. No field studies have been made, however, of redpolls on the tundra in winter.

As mentioned above, permanent residency of the large predatory birds depends on populations of a food supply. Snowy owls, for example, depend on microtine rodents, which exhibit cyclic fluctuations in numbers (Pitelka, 1972). Caged snowy owls required four to seven 60-g lemmings per day in northern Alaska which clearly indicates the dependence of these owls on high population densities of lemmings

(Gessaman, 1972). Gyrfalcons *(Falco rusticolus)* depend in part on populations of ptarmigan which cycle in interior Alaska alpine tundra (Weeden and Theberge, 1972). Observations of numbers of ptarmigan in the Arctic have been so sporadic that we can not say if their populations vary significantly over the years.

Vegetative browse in winter contains from 40–55% water (Irving *et al.,* 1964) which exists in the form of ice. When ice or snow is consumed, whether in the tissues of plants or alone for drinking water, it must be heated from ambient temperature to body temperature, as much as 80°C when the environmental temperature is at −40°C. In addition, a caloric input of approximately 80 cal·g⁻¹ must be made to melt the ice. Therefore, the intake of 1 g of water at −40°C costs a bird 160 calories. Willow ptarmigan consume 150–200 g of fresh willow buds per day that contain about 50% of their weight as ice. The metabolic cost of melting the ice and raising the temperature of the water approximates 25–30 kcal·day⁻¹, or about 18% of the total estimated daily energy expenditure (West, 1968).

With the extremely low humidities in the Arctic, especially in winter, evaporation of water from the respiratory tract must be considerable, requiring a substantial replacement of water by melting of ice. But no work has been done to determine actual rates of evaporative water loss in arctic birds.

The "Leave It" Strategy

Birds absent from tundra ecosystems for all but the few weeks annually required to complete their breeding cycles might seem to be exempt from this discussion. In contrast to permanent residents, they do not experience the extreme low temperatures, high potential heat loss, nor, in the case of arctic tundra, the restricted day length of midwinter. They do, however, confront a series of environmental problems that are partly similar to those faced by winter birds, partly the opposite extreme conditions, and partly unrelated problems arising from the "leave it" strategy. We list seven such problems, as follows:

A. Direct factors
1. The shortness of the breeding season
2. Factors promoting heat loss, including low temperatures, wind, radiative and evaporative heat loss
3. Long or continuous daylight hours
4. Lack of vertical habitat structure (song perches, topographic relief)

>   5. Long-distance migrations between wintering and breeding
>   ranges
> B. Indirect factors
>   6. Vagaries of weather
>   7. Patchiness of suitable habitat through space and time

Of course, not all of these factors apply to all tundra situations, nor
to all species equally in a given area. Furthermore, where several do
occur simultaneously, it is presently impossible to distinguish, let alone
rank, their importance to avian metabolic processes.

Length of Breeding Season. The first five factors above all seem to
be reasonably directly related to the rates at which birds must be capable of metabolizing energy. Shortness of breeding season limits the
normal opportunity for birds to space a sequence of energetically expensive activities and processes. Holmes (1966a,b; 1971) has explored the
degree of overlap of molting and breeding in two populations of dunlins
(Calidris alpina). The extent of overlap is greater in the breeding population at Barrow (71° N latitude) than in that of Kolomak River, Alaska
(61° N latitude), as would be predicted on the basis of length of season
at those places. Other *Calidris* sandpipers at Barrow begin body molt
and extensive fat deposition simultaneously, as soon as they are freed
from the dependence of chicks. They almost certainly cannot complete
this molt before starting on southward migration, and the process is presumably arrested during migration (MacLean, 1969). These sandpipers
are obligate insectivores, and must await snow-melt before they can
occupy tundra. A delayed snowmelt can be reflected in their dates of initiating breeding (Figure 4). The time required to establish territory, pair,
lay eggs, and complete incubation averages approximately 25 days
among four species (Norton, 1973). MacLean and Pitelka (1971) demonstrated that the brief, sharp peak in seasonal emergence of adult insects, upon which the sandpiper chicks depend (Holmes, 1966c), occurs
about 1 month after snow-melt. Shortness of season, therefore, is to be
understood as the urgency surrounding initiation of breeding. This con-
straint raises the required rate of energy procurement and mobilization
by adults engaged simultaneously in several metabolically expensive activities such as courtship and egg formation (Norton, 1973).

Species whose feeding strategies permit them some use of tundra
resources before snow-melt include snow buntings *(Plectrophenax nivalis)* and snowy owls. Male snow buntings, in particular, exercise the op-
tion of early territory establishment (Norton, personal observation) and
spend as much as 5 months annually in high arctic localities (Pattie,

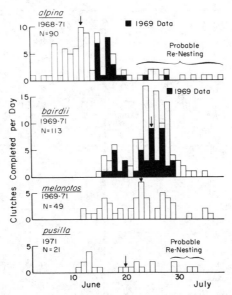

Figure 4 Clutch completion dates in four species of *Calidris* sandpipers at Barrow, Alaska. Median clutch completion dates are indicated by arrows. The 1969 completion dates are indicated for *C. alpina* and *C. bairdii* to compare the phenological effect of that year's delayed snow-melt on the two species (from Norton, 1973).

1972), but must do so at the expense of having to compensate metabolically for added heat loss because of wind and low temperatures, particularly during the arctic winter month of May.

Heat Loss. Heat loss may or may not be a problem to a particular tundra-breeding species. Undoubtedly, some adults experience warmer ambient temperatures on alpine and arctic breeding grounds than they do elsewhere during the rest of the year. On the other hand, the extensive coastal tundra regions of arctic and subarctic Canada and Alaska almost never afford ambient temperatures corresponding to the thermoneutral zones of temperate latitude birds (approximately 25°–35°C) (cf. Irving, 1972). We might expect, therefore, to find metabolically economical countermeasures in adults of species breeding in these areas. As in winter acclimatized permanent residents, increased insulation would reduce the steepness of the thermostatic heat requirement, and lower the critical temperature to appropriate levels reflective of ambient conditions. The calidridine sandpipers at Barrow, however, do not show any thermoneutral zone in resting metabolic rates, and therefore, must be

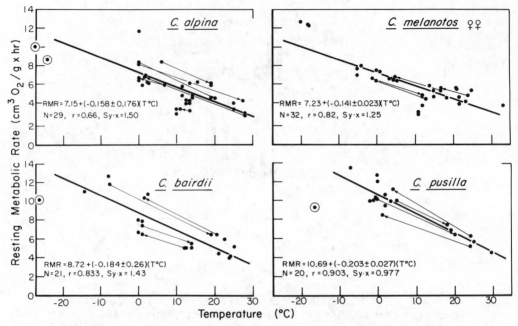

Figure 5 Oxygen consumption (RMR) as a function of temperature in adults of *Calidris* sandpipers at Barrow. Overall regression curves are shown as thick lines; arrows connect selected individuals' performances in successive runs at either higher or lower chamber temperatures; circled points indicate birds which failed to maintain body temperatures, values for which were not included in computation of least squares regression (from Norton, 1973).

expending energy continuously in thermoregulation (Figure 5). Respirometry studies on Devon Island Snow Buntings by D. L. Pattie, and on Barrow Lapland longspurs *(Calcarius lapponicus)* by T. W. Custer, may reveal whether these two passerine species follow the pattern of maintenance of low critical temperatures in summer shown by redpolls and species of greater body mass in winter (see above), or the pattern exhibited by summer sandpipers.

Heat loss is a more immediately critical problem for eggs and young than it is for adults. With few exceptions, nests on open arctic tundra are not remarkable for their insulative properties (cf. Irving and Krog, 1956). Effective extension of homeothermy to eggs therefore requires a high level of nest attendance by the incubating adult(s), lest the eggs cool rapidly to ambient temperatures. This requirement is generally met by the incubation schedules of calidridine sandpipers (Norton, 1972), but occasional long interruptions have been observed. These interruptions prompted a preliminary examination of freezing resistance in fresh eggs, and embryonic survival of low temperature exposure (Norton, personal observation). Unincubated eggs of *Calidris* species and of red phalaropes *(Phalaropus fulicarius)* could be supercooled to $-11°$ to $-14°C$ before sudden temperature increase at the shell surface indicated freezing, and the evolution of the heat of fusion. Survival and continued development by some embryos exposed to $-5°C$ for 12 hr, as well as hatchability and viability in the wild of chicks exposed as embryos for longer periods to temperatures near $0°C$, suggest that cryoprotective substances or mechanisms should be investigated, as they may relate to metabolic adaptations in arctic shorebirds.

Perhaps the most striking metabolic adaptation among breeding birds of the tundra is the recently discovered case of thermolability of calidridine sandpiper chicks (Norton, 1973). These chicks weigh less than 10 g at hatching and become independent of the nest and of adults (except for periods of brooding) within hours of hatching. Their small size, possession of only a thin downy plumage, and requirement for freedom to forage actively essentially rules out insulative specializations; their heat loss coefficients (reciprocal of insulation indices) average 2.4 times that of similar-sized adult redpolls (West, 1972b; Norton, 1973). Instead, free-living chicks consistently reduce the gradient between core and ambient temperatures by allowing body temperatures to drop to $30°-35°C$ while remaining functional, alert, and active. The energy not expended in counteracting heat loss across a gradient $10°C$ wider can be estimated by reference to Newton's law of cooling (Figure 6).

This hypothermia differs from all other cases so far described among birds. First, it is characteristic of active birds. Previous studies (Irving, 1955; Steen, 1958; Haftorn, 1972) related to measurements on resting or confined adults, generally at night. Secondly, in contrast to torpor (cf. Irving, 1964), chick hypothermia coincides with the period of rapid growth and maximum rates of biosynthesis. Indeed, hand-reared dunlin and Baird's sandpiper *(C. bairdii)* chicks grew better when caged at Barrow ambient temperatures than they did at room temperatures (Figure 7). Third, other studies of exothermy or thermolability in growing young birds have generally determined that endothermy develops gradually before fledging or independence from the nest is attained (cf. Bartholomew and Dawson, 1952; Maher, 1964; Bernstein, 1973; Theberge and West, 1973) but these sandpiper chicks showed no clear trend toward higher body temperatures during feeding as fledging approached at

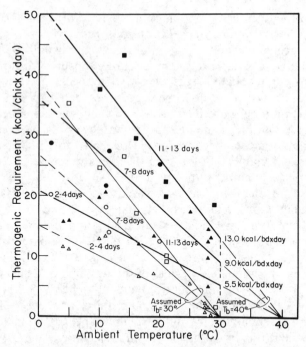

Figure 6 Estimated savings in metabolized energy derived by hypothermia by *Calidris bairdii* chicks of three different ages. Measured
heat loss coefficients were used, by correcting only the denominator
in the formulation $(cm^3\ C_2 \cdot g^{-1} \cdot hr^{-1})/(T_b - T_a)$ (from Norton, 1973).

15–20 days of age. The entire thermal strategy clearly invites closer
examination of both behavioral and neurophysiological ramifications,
and of the temperature-related function in digestive and other enzyme
systems.

Rock ptarmigan chicks are brooded extensively in inclement
weather, presumably because development of homeothermy does not
come until 5 days after hatching (Theberge and West, 1973; Anvik,
1969). The average amount of time available for foraging by the small
chicks which weigh from 18 to 30 g over the first 6 days of life averaged
96 min·24 hr⁻¹ on the alpine tundra of interior Alaska. This small
amount of time (6.7% of the day), however, provided sufficient foraging
time to secure enough energy to allow maintenance and growth of the
chicks (Theberge and West, 1973).

Day Length. Long or continuous daylight hours permit, or perhaps
force, birds on the tundra to remain active and alert, hence metabolically

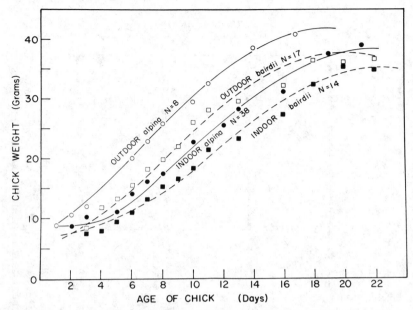

Figure 7 Comparison of mean daily weights as a function of age in indoor versus outdoor captive populations of *C. alpina* and *C. bairdii* chicks (from Norton, 1973).

active, to a greater degree than is the case elsewhere. To be sure, diel rhythms are not lost in most species (Cullen, 1954; Armstrong, 1954; Aschoff *et al.*, 1970; Norton, 1972) but there is a definite seasonal change in the activity pattern of willow ptarmigan in summer (West, 1968). The normal bimodal pattern is lost and activity remains continuous throughout the 24 hr (Figure 8). Light intensity and usually ambient temperatures continue to vary with a 24-hr periodicity. Nevertheless, birds unprepared to capitalize on favorable feeding conditions at unconventional hours would appear to be at a selective disadvantage. The predators upon eggs and young of small tundra birds near Barrow do not seem noticeably less active at midnight than at other hours, and therefore probably exact a consistent level of vigilance. T. W. Custer's ongoing study of Lapland Longspur time–activity budgets throughout the 24-hr period should provide information relevant to these speculations. There is a definite need for more research on circadian rhythms of arctic birds which so far have only been little studied.

Habitat Uniformity. A characteristic of small birds breeding in open country is the degree to which territorial advertisement is performed

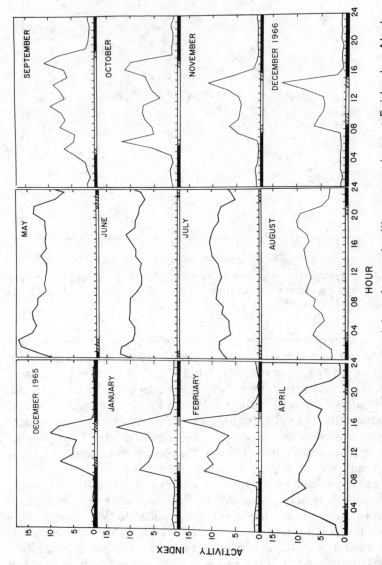

Figure 8 Annual pattern of gross activity of caged willow ptarmigan at Fairbanks, Alaska. Activity index is defined as the average number of 3-min intervals per hour in which a bird is active. The dark base line indicates night; the cross-hatched line, civil twilight; and the open line, daylight (from West, 1968).

during extended flight (cf. Pitelka *et al.,* 1973). Insofar as the lack of vertical dimension of tundra habitats increases the proportion of time that birds spend flying, it results in a metabolic investment, as indicated by oxygen consumption rates at least 8 – 14 times higher in flying, than in resting birds (Tucker, 1968; Hart and Berger, 1972; Berger and Hart, 1972).

Migration. We can view the remoteness of tundra breeding grounds from the wintering range of many species in the same manner. Long migrations before and after their annual sojourn on the tundra guarantees, in a sense, that those species are indeed capable of sustained mobilization of energy at high rates.

Thus far, we have been discussing five environmental factors associated with tundra systems that seem directly to require control by summer birds over rates of energy metabolism. Energy-conservative adaptations (e.g., insulative) among adults in the size range, 20 – 150 g, are not apparent in the best-known species, calidridine sandpipers, nor for summer breeding redpolls (Pohl and West, 1973). The capacity for sustained high metabolic rates may prove to be a distinguishing feature of all such birds, as more species are studied. The one exception to this pattern of prodigal energy expenditure is that of thermolability in chicks.

Weather and Habitat Pattern. In response to vagaries of weather and patchiness of suitable tundra habitats, tundra birds seem to have generated adaptive solutions in · behavioral, social, and morphological characteristics that parallel those seen in waterfowl (McKinney, 1973). These solutions tend to increase the flexibility of many species' approach to an unpredictable environment, and involve metabolic systems secondarily. Once again, calidridine sandpipers, which breed nearly exclusively on arctic and subarctic-alpine tundra exemplify this assertion. Pitelka *et al.* (1974) have analyzed the social systems (mating systems, spacing mechanisms, dimorphisms in morphology and behavior, etc.) of the 24 species in the subfamily Calidridinae as "adaptive resource exploitation strategies." An opportunistic approach to breeding characterizes 9 of the 24 species. These nine all have non-monogamous mating systems; all but one have no known site attachment (philopatry, nest site tenacity); and their pairbonds are fleeting or nonexistent. Thus, unbound by "tradition," they are freed to avoid unfavorable breeding sites and capitalize on favorable conditions elsewhere in any given year. In each of these species, typically only one adult incubates a given clutch. An obvious result of such division of labor is the theoretical doubling of that individual's energetic investment in incubation (see Figure 9). The single-sex incubation systems of the arctic-breeding phalaropes *(Phalaropus fulicarius* and *Lobipes lobatus)* suggest that specialization of the sexes may have occurred independently in different groups of tundra species. Furthermore, single-sex incubation in other groups at high latitudes (passerines, waterfowl) suggests that arctic incubation is feasible even for single adults that have little time to spend foraging. For example, female pectoral sandpipers *(C. melanotos)* incubate for all but 3.6 hr daily, but manage to forage effectively enough to avoid weight loss during the incubation period (Figure 10), although these females show greater excursions in body weight during incubation than do incubating adults of other species.

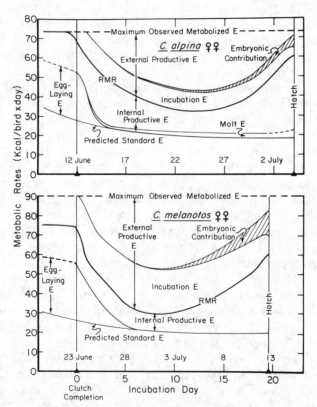

Figure 9 Comparison between estimated partial energy budget of female *Calidris* sandpipers representing two-sex incubation *(C. alpina)* and single-sex incubation *(C. melanotos)* (from Norton, 1973).

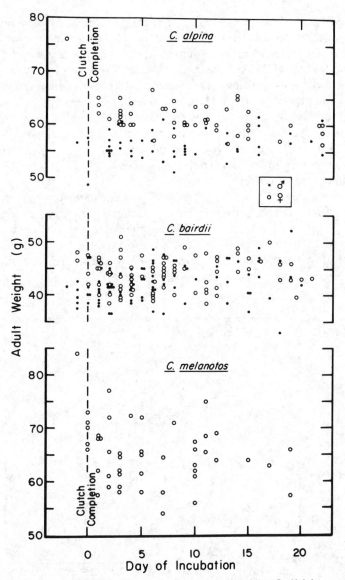

Figure 10 Body weight excursions in incubating *Calidris* sandpipers of three species over the duration of the incubation period (from Norton, 1973).

Breeding Season Adaptations of Both Strategies

Breeding tundra birds satisfy the energetic demands of maintenance and production on a variety of diets. The diets of some species of small birds are accurately known, such as those of tree sparrows *(Spizella arborea)* (West, 1973; Figure 11), Lapland longspurs (T. W. Custer, in preparation), snow buntings (D. L. Pattie, 1972; in preparation), and the *Calidris* species at Barrow (Holmes, 1966c). Animal protein supports tundra breeding by these species to a striking degree, often representing a complete reversal of food preferences during the breeding season, as in tree sparrows (Figure 11). Rock ptarmigan adults in Alaskan alpine situations are herbivorous, but Theberge and West (1973) determined that chick diets comprised 26% by weight of invertebrates between hatching and 6 days of age. This level of animal protein ingestion may represent mistakes in food recognition by inexperienced birds, but the energetic advantages of invertebrate food (higher caloric value, greater digestibility) suggest that the growth of young is optimally supported with some proportion of animal food, even in nominally herbivorous species, such as ptarmigan, and perhaps redpolls. There are only vague indications

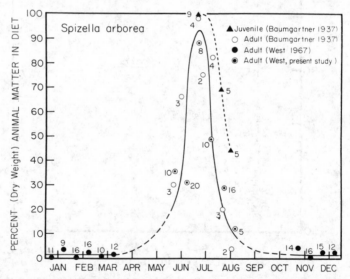

Figure 11 Monthly changes in the proportion of animal matter in the diet of tree sparrows. Summer data from birds collected near Churchill, Manitoba; winter data from central Illinois. Numbers beside data points indicate the number of stomachs analyzed (from West, 1973).

that the assumed exclusive herbivory of redpolls is relaxed during feeding of nestlings (Baldwin, 1968; Clement, 1968).

Presently, we know just enough about intermediary metabolic problems of tundra birds during the breeding season to whet the physiologist's appetite. MacLean (1969) studied the occurrence of fat in *Calidris* species at Barrow, and proposed that fat is generally more important as a metabolic substrate for species with opportunistic breeding strategies. Much could be learned about cycles of lipolysis and lipogenesis that occur in regular association with events of the annual cycle and the breeding cycle in particular. We have seen that the depot fats of redpolls accumulated during spring migration are rich (80%) in linoleic acid while during summer, the pattern is one of more even distribution of the principal fatty acids (West and Meng, 1968). We are just beginning to learn the external and internal controls of the deposition of specific fatty acid patterns in arctic birds. We can only guess at the significance of Norton's (1973) observations that free-living and outdoor-reared *Calidris* chicks developed only low levels of extractable body fat, whereas birds hand-reared at room temperatures on the same diet, and otherwise similar conditions, had much higher fat levels. Respiratory metabolism of breeding birds should at least include determination of respiratory quotients in the future to hint at the metabolic substrates being used.

Another observation related to nutrition and intermediary metabolism, concerns the importance of calcium to egg-laying birds. MacLean (1974) found that egg-producing female *Calidris* sandpipers at Barrow commonly ingest lemming *(Lemmus trimucronatus)* teeth and bone fragments. In response to his colleagues' skepticism that this occurrence represented effective calcium ingestion and mobilization, MacLean has measured the calcium content of whole fresh eggs, the concentrations of calcium in representative dietary items (excluding teeth), and the calcium contents of whole female carcasses. The results make it apparent that all the calcium in the female's body, even if mobilizable, would not supply the eggs with the quantities observed. Tundra arthropod larvae typical of sandpiper diets at the stage of egg-laying would also have to be eaten in great quantities to satisfy the calcium demand. Calcium must therefore come largely from the diet over a short period, and by process of elimination, we conclude that lemming teeth and bones are part of the equation. After all, these sandpipers lay clutches of four eggs in 4 days that together weigh as much as, or more than, the adult female.

Egg production by these sandpipers would be a metabolic exercise of considerable magnitude in even a warm environment. For instance, following King's (1973) procedure, the energy invested in production of a single egg by a female dunlin can be estimated at 2.46 times the female's basal metabolic rate. The dunlin's nearest rivals in King's (1973, his Table 4) list of 14 species are the cinnamon teal *(Anas cyanoptera)* and lesser scaup *(Aythya affinis)* in which the respective ratios are 2.39 and 2.11 times basal rates.

This review shows that at least some birds that utilize tundra resources to support breeding show little reticence in dissipating the energy they secure. It is worth pondering whether such metabolic extravagance is related to low avifaunal diversity, an abundance of food during the biologically active season, or to some other qualitative and quantitative peculiarities of tundra ecosystems.

Species that have spent the entire winter in the tundra may enjoy some advantages over species that migrate long distances. Their early presence implies best selection of suitable nesting ground and food supplies at break up. It is questionable, however, if there is any competition for tundra resources between resident and migrant species. Ptarmigan and redpolls are species populations that contain migratory and nonmigratory elements. The situation with redpolls is entirely unknown except that in some years, there are extensive migrations of both hoary and common redpolls through interior Alaska in spring (West *et al.*, 1968) and in fall when large flocks form (personal observation). In other years, the change in population density is scarcely noticeable. The northward extent of wintering and therefore of presence of individuals on the breeding grounds in spring may be dependent on food supply (the birch seed crop) or on overall population density. The migration routes and the extent of latitudinal movement of Alaskan redpoll populations are thus far unknown.

Willow ptarmigan of arctic Alaska have a definite migratory pattern which leaves the adult males on the breeding grounds north of the Brooks Range in winter, the juvenile males in the passes of the Brooks Range, and the females south of the range (Irving *et al.*, 1967). This distribution pattern may result in slightly different energy demands and definitely results in different diets of the four age – sex groups of the population (West and Meng, 1966). The old adult males which remain in the vicinity, or at least closest to the breeding grounds in winter, have the first choice of breeding territories as snow melts off in May and June. Juvenile males are present at 20% of the population in winter but substantial numbers of this group or of females do not arrive until June. Rock ptarmigan in the alpine-tundra of interior Alaska show a similar pattern (Weeden, 1964) but on an altitudinal instead of a latitudinal basis.

In the taiga, and perhaps in the tundra, certain predatory birds nest early in the season; this is perhaps an adaptive feature to capitalize on the supply of eggs and young of later nesting migrants which are then used to feed their own young. Ravens, great horned *(Bubo virginianus)* and other owls, and the gray jay are noteworthy examples.

In summary, our present understanding of metabolism in high latitude tundra-residing birds falls short of reasonable coverage of the topics outlined in Table 1. Several ongoing studies promise soon to bring us closer to combining thermal balance, activity budgets, and productive energy output, in documenting whole bird energetics for longspurs (T. W. Custer, in preparation) and shorebirds (Safriel, in preparation; Norton, in preparation). Further research is needed into diet selection, digestive, assimilative, and productive efficiencies. In particular, we should like to know how important metabolic substitution from the heat increments of feeding and of muscular activity is to birds in cold environments. When information from such studies becomes available, it may become clearer whether "tundra birds" constitute a natural grouping, functionally distinguishable from other groups by their bioenergetic and metabolic adaptations. Regardless of whether we eventually find it profitable to treat tundra birds as a natural assemblage, we expect that they will continue to be subjects for physiological inquiry, with increasing emphasis at the suborganismic level, where we have tried to outline some of the problems indicated by research to date.

Acknowledgments

The following grants and contracts aided in the support of the research contained in this review: GM-10402 from the National Institutes of Health; T-EC 00031 Training Grant from the National Institutes of Health; GV-29342 (Tundra Biome Program) from the National Science Foundation, Office of Polar Programs and International Biological Program. The data obtained by David Norton on *Calidris* at Barrow was made possible through cooperation with the Naval Arctic Research Laboratory, Office of Naval Research, and the Institute of Arctic Biology, University of Alaska.

References

Anvik, J. O. (1969). The development and maintenance of homeothermy in the rock ptarmigan *(Lagopus mutus)*. Unpublished B. Sc. thesis, Univ. of Brit. Columbia.

Armstrong, E. A. (1954). The behaviour of birds in continuous daylight. *Ibis* **96,** 1–30.

Aschoff, J., Gwinner, E., Kureck, A., and Müller, K. (1970). Diel rhythms of chaffinches *Fringilla coelebs* L., tree shrews *Tupaia glis* L. and hamsters *Mesocricetus auratus* L. as a function of season at the Arctic Circle. Oikos (Suppl.) **13,** 91–100.

Baldwin, P. H. (1968). Hoary Redpoll. *In* "Life Histories of North American

Cardinals, Grosbeaks, Buntings, Towhees, Finches, Sparrows, and Allies," (O. L. Austin, Jr., ed.). *U.S. Nat. Mus. Bull.* **237** (Pt. 1), 404.

Bartholomew, G. A., and Dawson, W. R. (1952). Body temperatures in nestling Western Gulls. *Condor* **54**, 58–60.

Berger, M., and Hart, J. S. (1972). Die Atmung beim Kolibri *Amazilia fimbriata* während des Schwirrfluges bei verschiedenen Umgebungstemperaturen. *J. Comp. Physiol.* **81**, 363–380.

Bernstein, M. H. (1973). Development of thermoregulation in Painted Quail, *Excalfactoria chinensis. Comp. Biochem. Physiol.* **44A**, 355–366.

Braun, C. F., and May, T. A. (1972). Colorado alpine tundra avifaunal investigations, 1966–71. *Proc. 1972 Tundra Biome Symp.* U.S. Tundra Biome, Univ. of Alaska, Fairbanks, pp. 165–168.

Clement, R. C. (1968). Common Redpoll. *In* "Life Histories of North American Cardinals, Grosbeaks, Buntings, Towhees, Finches, Sparrows, and Allies," (O. L. Austin, Jr., ed.). *U.S. Nat. Mus. Bull.* **237** (Pt. 1), 414.

Cullen, J. M. (1954). The diurnal rhythm of birds in the arctic summer. *Ibis* **96**, 31–46.

Gelting, P. (1937). Studies on the food of East Greenland ptarmigan. *Medd. Grønland* **116**, 1–96.

Gessaman, J. A. (1972). Bioenergetics of the snowy owl *(Nyctea scandiaca). Arctic Alpine Res.* **4**, 223–238.

Haftorn, S. (1972). Hypothermia of arctic tits in winter. *Ornis Scand.* **3**, 153–166.

Hart, J. S., and Berger, M. (1972). Energetics, water economy and temperature regulation during flight. *Proc. XVth Int. Ornithol. Congr.,* pp. 189–199.

Hart, J. S., and Héroux, O. (1955). Exercise and temperature regulation in lemmings and rabbits. *Can. J. Biochem. Physiol.* **33**, 428–435.

Holmes, R. T. (1966a). Breeding ecology and annual cycle adaptations of the red-backed sandpiper *(Calidris alpina)* in northern Alaska. *Condor* **68**, 3–46.

Holmes, R. T. (1966b). Molt cycle of the red-backed sandpiper *(Calidris alpina)* in western North America. *Auk* **83**, 517–533.

Holmes, R. T. (1966c). Feeding ecology of the red-backed sandpiper *(Calidris alpina)* in arctic Alaska. *Ecology* **47**, 32–45.

Holmes, R. T. (1971). Latitudinal differences in the breeding and molt schedules of Alaskan red-backed sandpipers *(Calidris alpina). Condor* **73**, 93–99.

Irving, L. (1955). Nocturnal decline in the temperature of birds in cold weather. *Condor* **57**, 362–365.

Irving, L. (1960). Birds of Anaktuvuk Pass, Kobuk and Old Crow. *U. S. Nat. Mus. Bull* **217**, 1–450.

Irving, L. (1964). Terrestrial animals in cold: birds and mammals. *In* "Adaptation to the Environment, Handbook of Physiology," (D. B. Dill, ed.) Sect. IV, pp. 361–77. Amer. Physiol. Soc., Washington, D.C.

Irving, L. (1972). "Arctic Life of Birds and Mammals including Man." Zoophysiology and Ecology 2, pp. 1–192. Springer-Verlag, New York.

Irving, L., and Krog, J. (1954). Body temperatures of arctic and subarctic birds and mammals. *J. Appl. Physiol.* **6,** 667–680.

Irving, L., and Krog, J. (1955). Temperature of skin in the arctic as a regulator of heat. *J. Appl. Physiol.* **7,** 355–364.

Irving, L., and Krog, J. (1956). Temperatures during the development of birds in arctic nests. *Physiol. Zool.* **29:** 195–205.

Irving, L., Krog, J., and Monson, M. (1955). The metabolism of some Alaskan animals in winter and summer. *Physiol. Zool.* **28,** 173–185.

Irving, L., West, G. C., and Krog J. (1964). Changes in water content of arctic plants during winter. *Proc. 15th Alaska Sci. Conf.,* 37.

Irving, L., West, G. C. Peyton, L. J., and Paneak, S. (1967). Migration of willow ptarmigan in arctic Alaska. *Arctic* **20,** 77–85.

Johnson, R. E. (1968). Temperature regulation in the white-tailed ptarmigan *(Lagopus leucurus). Comp. Biochem. Physiol.* **24,** 1003–1014.

King, J. R. (1973). Energetics of reproduction in birds. In "Breeding Biology of Birds," (D. S. Farner, ed.), pp. 78–107. Nat. Acad. Sci., Washington, D.C.

Lasiewski, R. C., and Dawson, W. R. (1967). A re-examination of the relation between standard metabolic rate and body weight in birds. *Condor* **69,** 13–23.

MacLean, S. F., Jr. (1969). Ecological determinants of species diversity in arctic sandpipers near Barrow, Alaska. Unpubl. Ph.D. thesis, Univ. of California, Berkeley, California.

MacLean, S. F., Jr. (1974). Calcium in the reproduction of arctic sandpipers: supply and demand. *Ibis* **116,** 552–557.

MacLean, S. F., Jr. and Pitelka, F. A. (1971). Seasonal patterns of abundance of tundra arthropods near Barrow, Alaska. *Arctic,* **24,** 19–40.

Maher, W. J. (1964). Growth rate and development of endothermy in the snow bunting *(Plectrophenax nivalis)* and lapland longspur *(Calcarius lapponicus)* at Barrow, Alaska. *Ecology* **45,** 520–528.

McKinney, F. (1973). Ecoethological aspects of reproduction. *In* "Breeding Biology of Birds," (D. S. Farner, ed.), pp. 8–21. Nat. Acad. Sci., Washington, D.C.

Melchior, H. R. (1972). Summer herbivory by the brown lemming at Barrow, Alaska. *Proc. 1972 Tundra Biome Symp.* U.S. Tundra Biome, Univ. of Alaska, Fairbanks, pp. 136–138.

Moss, R. (1973). The digestion and intake of winter foods by wild ptarmigan in Alaska. *Condor* **75,** 293–300.

Norton, D. W. (1972). Incubation schedules of four species of calidridine sandpipers at Barrow, Alaska. *Condor* **74,** 164–176.

Norton, D. W. (1973). Ecological energetics of calidridine sandpipers breeding in northern Alaska. Unpublished Ph.D. thesis, Univ. of Alaska, Fairbanks, Alaska.

Pattie, D. L. (1972). Preliminary bioenergetic and population level studies in high arctic birds. *In* "Devon Island I.B.P. Project, High Arctic Ecosystems." (L. C. Bliss, ed.). pp. 281–292. Univ. of Alberta, Edmonton.

Peters, S. S. (1958). Food habits of the Newfoundland willow ptarmigan. *J. Wildl. Manage.* **22,** 384–394.

Pitelka, F. A. (1972). Cyclic pattern in lemming populations near Barrow, Alaska. *Proc. Tundra Biome Symp. 1972* U. S. Tundra Biome, Univ. of Alaska, Fairbanks, 132–135.

Pitelka, F. A., Holmes, R. T. and MacLean, S. F., Jr. (1974). Ecology and evolution of social organization in arctic sandpipers. *Amer. Zool.* **14**, 185–204.

Pohl, H. (1972). Seasonal changes in light sensitivity in *Carduelis flammea*. *Naturwissenschaften* **59**, 518–519.

Pohl, H., and West, G. C. (1973). Daily and seasonal variation in metabolic response to cold during rest and forced exercise in the common redpoll. *Comp. Biochem. Physiol.* **45A**, 851–867.

Rosenmann, M., and Morrison, P. (1974). Maximum oxygen consumption and heat loss facilitation in small homeotherms by $He-O_2$. *Amer. J. Physiol.* **226**, 490–495.

Scholander, P. F., Walters, V., Hock, R., and Irving, L., (1950a). Body insulation of some arctic and tropical mammals and birds. *Biol. Bull.* **99**, 225–236.

Scholander, P. F., Hock, R., Walters, V., Johnson, F. and Irving, L. (1950b). Heat regulation in some arctic and tropical mammals and brids. *Biol. Bull.* **99**, 237–258.

Scholander, P. F., Hock, R., Walters, V., and Irving, L. (1950c). Adaptation to cold in arctic and tropical mammals and birds in relation to body temperature, insulation and basal metabolic rate. *Biol. Bull.* **99**, 259–629.

Seiskari, P. (1957). [On the winter feeding of the willow patrmigan.] *Suom. Riista* **11**, 43–47.

Steen, J. (1958). Climatic adaptation in some small northern birds. *Ecology* **39**, 625–629.

Sulkava, S. (1969). On small birds spending the night in the snow. *Aquito. Ser. Zool.* **7**, 33–37.

Theberge, J. B., and West, G. C. (1973). Significance of brooding to the energy demands of Alaskan rock ptarmigan chicks. *Arctic* **26**, 138–148.

Tucker, V. A. (1968). Respiratory exchange and evaporative water loss in the flying budgerigar. *J. Exp. Biol.* **48**, 68–87.

Veghte, J. H. (1964). Thermal and metabolic responses of the gray jay to cold stress. *Physiol. Zool.* **37**, 316–328.

Veghte, J. H., and Herreid, C. F. (1965). Radiometric determination of feather insulation and metabolism of arctic birds. *Physiol. Zool.* **38**, 267–275.

Weeden, R. B. (1964). Spatial separation of sexes of rock ptarmigan in winter. *Auk* **81**, 534–541.

Weeden, R. B. (1967). Seasonal and geographic variation in the foods of adult white-tailed ptarmigan. *Condor* **69**, 303–309.

Weeden, R. B. (1969). Foods of rock and willow ptarmigan in central Alaska with comments on interspecific competition. *Auk* **86**, 271–281.

Weeden, R. B., and Theberge, J. B. (1972). The dynamics of a fluctuating rock ptarmigan population in Alaska. *Proc. XV Int. Ornithol. Congr.* E. J. Brill, Leiden., pp. 90–106.

West, G. C. (1965) Shivering and heat production in wild birds. *Physiol. Zool.* **37**, 111–120.

West, G. C. (1968). Bioenergetics of captive willow ptarmigan under natural conditions. *Ecology* **49,** 1035–1045.

West, G. C. (1972a). Seasonal differences in resting metabolic rate of Alaskan ptarmigan. *Comp. Biochem. Physiol.* **42A,** 867–876.

West, G. C. (1972b). Effect of acclimation and acclimatization on the resting metabolic rate of the common redpoll. *Comp. Biochem. Physiol.* **43A,** 293–310.

West, G. C. (1973). Foods eaten by tree sparrows in relation to availability during summer in northern Manitoba. *Arctic* **26,** 7–21.

West, G. C., and Meng, M. S. (1966). Nutrition of willow ptarmigan in northern Alaska. *Auk* **83,** 603–615.

West, G. C., and Meng, M. S. (1968). Effect of diet and captivity on the fatty acid composition of redpoll *(Acanthis flammea)* depot fats. *Comp. Biochem. Physiol.* **25,** 535–540.

West, G. C., Peyton, L. J. and Savage, S. (1968). Changing composition of a redpoll flock during spring migration. *Bird-Banding* **39,** 51–55.

Part IV
Adaptations of Aquatic Organisms

Morphophysiological Adaptations in Unicellular Algae

Constantine Sorokin

Department of Botany
University of Maryland
College Park, Maryland

The relationships between factor, form, and function, though far from being simple in unicellular organisms, are, however, simplified compared to multicellular systems by the absence of the intricate interactions between organs, tissues, and individual cells characteristic of multicellular organisms. Unicellular algae, grown in well-defined and easily controllable aquatic environment, seem to be particularly suitable for studies of morphophysiological adaptations at the cellular level.

Adaptations in the Course of Cell Development

To compete and survive, an organism must be well adapted to its needs and environment at all stages of its development. At the cellular level, the significance and even existence of the physiological changes during growth division cycle, for lack of appropriate techniques, remained for a long time uncertain (Brachet, 1950).

The advance in physiological and biochemical investigations of the cell developmental cycle came with the introduction of the synchronization technique which was first developed for unicellular algae (Sorokin and Myers, 1954; Tamiya *et al.*, 1953) and later developed for other microorganisms. A discontinuous synthesis during the cell developmental cycle has been well established for DNA (Howard and Pelc, 1953), a number of enzymes, and for some other proteins (Mitchison, 1971). Fluctuations in the rates of metabolic processes such as photosynthesis (Sorokin, 1963a, 1965; Tamiya *et al.,* 1953), respiration (Sorokin and Myers, 1957; Talbert and Sorokin, 1971), enzyme activities (Schmidt, 1969), and growth (Sorokin, 1963b, 1964) also were generally ascertained for algal cells.

Compared to the progress in physiological and biochemical investigations, studies of the morphological structures related to the cell developmental cycle were until recently entirely confined to the mitotic transformations and movements of chromosomes. The larger part of the cell cycle—the interphase—has been assumed to be completely void of any detectable morphological events. Mitchison actually emphasized that "the most striking fact about the structure of the cell during the rest of the cycle is how little it changes at the level both of the light microscope and of the electron microscope" (Mitchison, 1971).

Shape of the Chloroplast and Photosynthetic Activity

Recently, conspicuous morphological changes in the shape of the chloroplast were demonstrated in the course of cell development of a green rod-shaped alga isolated in our laboratory from several freshwater habitats (Sorokin *et al.,* 1972). The reported observations were performed on cultures grown in light in liquid inorganic medium (Sorokin *et al.,* 1972). Autotrophically grown cells were usually $1.8-2.5$ μm in width and, under conditions of slow growth (high population density and/or low light intensity), $2-6$ μm in length. Each cell had a single parietal girdlelike chloroplast. In the absence of pyrenoids, the organism could be considered as a *Stichococcus*-type alga (Figure 1a) of the order Ulotrichales. Allowed to grow at higher rate, the cell remained nearly the same in width but increased in length, reaching up to $10-12$ μm (Figure 1b). Rapid extension of the cell was not followed by an equally extensive building of the body of the chloroplast. As the synthetic processes involved in the building of the chloroplast fell behind, the chloroplast, by extension, attenuation, and twisting, took the shape of an extended helix (Figure 1c and d).

In regard to relative rates of cell extension and chloroplast synthesis, and resulting changes in the extension and attenuation of the chloroplast, the growth-division cycle consisted of two phases: one of fast cell extension and lagging chloroplast synthesis, and another of slower or absent cell extension and relatively fast chloroplast synthesis. The phase of slow cell extension and relatively fast chloroplast synthesis began during

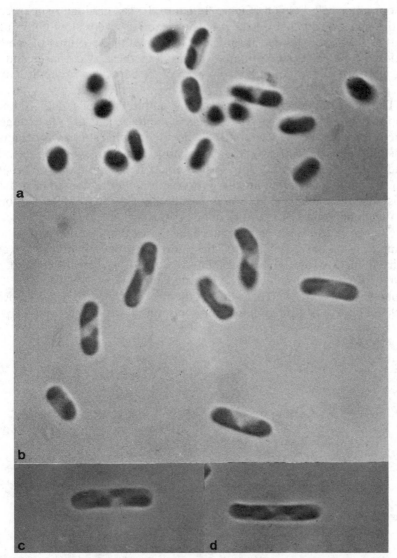

Figure 1 Development of helical chloroplasts in the *Stichococcus-*type alga. × 2000. a, Cells grown in a dense culture at low light intensity. Cell length from 2 to 6 μm. b, Cells grown under conditions more favorable for growth. Several cells have helical chloroplasts, each chloroplast with one turn of a helix. c and d, Chloroplasts have two complete turns of a helix.

or soon after cell division (Figure 2g,h,a,b). It was gradually superceded by the phase of intensive cell extension and relatively slow chloroplast synthesis which extended throughout the remaining portions of the cell cycle (Figure 2c–f). The relative duration of these two phases and the degree to which they differed from each other depended on environmental conditions.

The appearance in the same clonal culture of cells with different shapes of the chloroplast from highly compressed to greatly extended helical form would be, without cell developmental studies, uncomprehensible. These forms would be probably considered as representing genetically different organisms arising either from mutations or brought into the culture as contaminants. Observations in the course of growth-division cycle, however, indicated that the different morphological forms are developmental stages of the same organism.

Change in the form of the chloroplast goes parallel and is thus well adapted to the basic function of the chloroplast, photosynthesis. A generalized picture of the changes in the rate of photosynthesis in the course of cell development is presented in Figure 3 (Sorokin, 1957). Photosynthesis rate increases during the first part of the growth-division cycle and reaches a maximum after about one-third of the cycle is over.

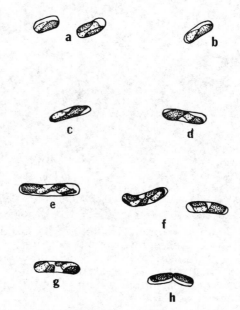

Figure 2 Schematic presentation of the development of a helical chloroplast during growth-division cell cycle.

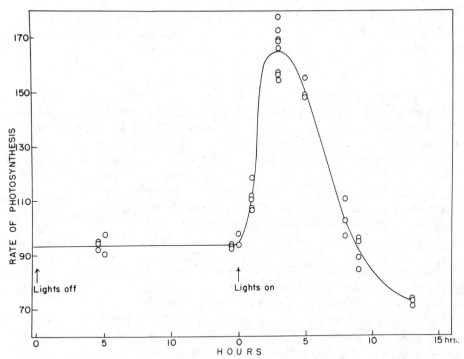

Figure 3 Rates of apparent photosynthesis in mm³O₂ · mm⁻³ packed cells · hour⁻¹ for cells of successive developmental stages of *Chlorella*.

This coincides with the period of relatively extensive building of the body of the chloroplast (Figure 2). Then the photosynthetic activity declines toward the end of the cycle and this coincides with the attenuation of the chloroplast caused by the lag in the building of the body of the chloroplast.

Changes in the chloroplast form and in the rate of photosynthetic function are also well adapted to external conditions. Under conditions of slow growth, the amplitudes of changes in the shape of the chloroplast and in the rate of photosynthetic activity during the cell cycle decrease and at a very slow growth rate the cycling disappears. There is no need to work fast and the development can proceed at an even and sluggish rate. The pronounced cycles in photosynthetic activity and in the changes in chloroplast synthesis are noticed only under external conditions conducive to fast growth. The cell growth puts a strain on the growth and extension of the chloroplast. As chloroplast growth falls behind, photosynthetic activity declines and the growth rate decreases.

Then, during cell division, the reverse takes place. The chloroplast synthesis and photosynthetic activity gradually increase to make the cycle possible.

Mitochondria and Respiration Activity

Another demonstration of morphological alterations in subcellular structures during the cell developmental cycle was recently produced for mitochondria. Electron microscope studies of the synchronously grown cells of *Chlamydomonas reinhardi* indicated that "giant mitochondria of various shapes were temporarily formed, probably by fusion of smaller mitochondria, in the algal cells at an intermediate stage of the growth phase of the cell cycle" (Osafune *et al.*, 1972). Later during the cell cycle, the giant mitochondria divided into smaller forms. The formation of giant mitochondria during the cell cycle was also observed in *Chlorella* and *Euglena* (Osafune *et al.*, 1972). Concomitant with the formation of giant mitochondria in *Chlamydomonas*, there was a decline in respiration rate. Respiration activity was restored to a higher level later during the cell cycle, the restoration being connected with the division of giant mitochondria into smaller forms (Osafune *et al.*, 1972).

Observations on the increase in respiration activity toward the end of the cell cycle need, however, verification in view of the difficulties involved in reaching consensus on the typical course of respiration activity during the cell developmental cycle. Beginning with the earlier observations on the respiration activity in single cells (Stefanelli, 1937; Zeuthen, 1946) and including the subsequent studies on synchronized cells (Cornutt and Schmidt, 1964; Nihei *et al.*, 1954; Reid *et al.*, 1963; Sasa, 1961; Soeder and Reid, 1967; Sorokin and Myers, 1957), the typical course of respiration activity during the cell cycle eluded general description. Not only observations by different investigators varied in detail, but agreement was lacking even on the basic and seemingly simple question as to whether respiration activity generally increases, declines, or remains constant during the cell cycle.

The diversity of opinions on the course of changes in respiration activity in the process of cell development was recently (Talbert and Sorokin, 1971) evaluated with regard to differences in the techniques of synchronization, in methods of culturing synchronized cells, and in the conditions during measurements of respiration rates. To exclude the effects of these accessory factors, observations were made on *Chlorella* cells separated into age groups by selective (centrifugation) synchronization and thus having identical prehistories. These observations were compared with measurements of respiration rates on cells synchronized by induced (light:dark cycles) synchronization. To avoid limitations imposed on the respiration rate by the possible scarcity of respiratory substrate, glucose was supplied in both series of observations as the exogenous source of carbon. Both techniques produced concordant results indicating that respiration activity of cells generally declines during the growth phase of the cell developmental cycle.

The above conclusion differs from the Osafune *et al.* (1972) observations on the restoration of respiration activity to a higher level during the later portion of the cell developmental cycle. The data of Osafune *et al.* can be possibly attributed to some peculiar environmental factors or to specific physiological condition of cells (preculture). In this connection, observations on synchronized cells of *Euglena gracilis* grown on different media (Calvayrac, 1970) are of considerable interest. The formation of giant chondriome was observed in cells grown in medium containing lactate and coincided with increased respiration activity. Respiration rates in the glutamate and malate media were lower and mitochondria were of normal size. Obviously, more observations are necessary on the morphology of mitochondria during the cell developmental cycle. To relate the form of the mitochondria to their function, not only the respiration activity, but also other yet unknown functions (Osafune *et al.*, 1972) must be taken into consideration.

Cell Wall Formation and Cell Growth

Interchange of the growth and division phases is, of course, the most dramatic demonstration of the periodicity of morphophysiological events during the cell developmental cycle. The division phase culminates in the formation of the new cell wall followed in unicellular organisms by the separation of daughter cells.

In the rod-shaped alga depicted in Figure 1, cell division begins with the division of the chloroplast (Figure 4a), followed by the division of the protoplast (Figure 4b). The transverse partition is then formed by the deposition of the wall material at the cell plate (Figure 5a). No visible cell material is deposited over the rest of the cell surface.

Before the separation of two daughter cells, the transverse partition splits into two (Figure 5b). The disjunction of the daughter cells in the rod-shaped algae occurs by softening of the parent cell wall in the region where the transverse partition becomes attached to the parent cell wall. The selective lysis of the narrow strip of the parent cell wall only where the transverse partition is attached to the parent cell wall is characteristic of the separation of rod-shaped unicellular algae.

The interchange of the formation of transverse partition and of the elongation of the rest of the cell wall is characteristic of many types of plant cells. The elongation may occur by apposition and/or intussuscep-

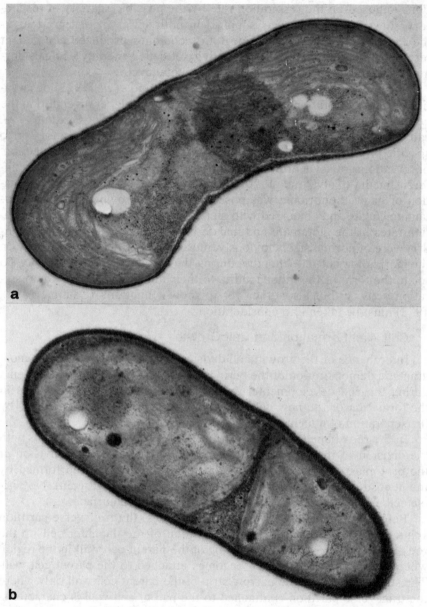

Figure 4 Cell division in the rod-shaped *Stichococcus*-type alga. a, A cell in the initial division stage. The chloroplast divided into two. × 20,000. b, The cell in a later division stage. The protoplasts of the daughter cells separate and the transverse partition is being built between them. × 21,000.

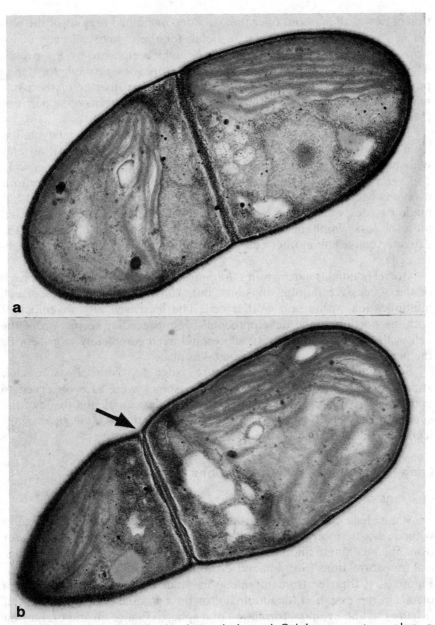

Figure 5 Cell division in the rod-shaped *Stichococcus*-type alga. a, The cell in the advanced division stage. The transverse partition is formed but is not yet split into two. × 25,000. b, Two daughter cells before disjunction. The transverse partition is split into two. The region of the parent cell wall where the transverse partition is attached to it (arrow) is weakened and soon will be completely dissolved. × 24,000.

tion of new wall material over the extended or limited regions of the parent cell wall. It was described in detail for the cylindrical cells of fission yeast *Schizosaccharomyces pombe,* which elongate by tip growth. The addition of new cell material at the tip goes through the larger portion of the cell cycle but stops during the last quarter of the cycle when the new cell wall material is being added to the transverse partition (Mitchison, 1957).

Periodicity of growth activity during the cell developmental cycle has been also demonstrated for *Chlorella* (Sorokin, 1963b, 1964), an alga with pattern of multiplication different from that of *Stichococcus.* In *Chlorella* (Sorokin and Corbett, 1975), a number of successive mitotic divisions occur within the mother cell wall. The process of cell wall formation is delayed until a later phase when cell walls are constructed more or less simultaneously around the entire surface of each of the daughter cells. The mother cell wall then bursts and releases the daughter cells.

Correspondingly, growth in *Chlorella* cells is not in phase with each of the successive mitotic divisions, but with the entire process of cell multiplication within one mother cell. The increased growth coincides with the portion of the developmental cycle preceding formation of the cell walls. The growth activity abates and even completely stops during the period when cell wall formation takes place.

Several other subcellular structures such as chloroplasts, nuclei, endoplasmic reticula, flagella, and dictyosomes were also observed to undergo morphological alterations during the developmental cycle of the synchronized cells (Osafune *et al.*, 1972) though the physiological significance of these changes is unknown.

Long-Lasting Reversible Adaptations

Transformation of Rod-Shaped Cells into Spherical Cells

Some algae can be grown either autotrophically or heterotrophically without drastic morphological alterations while others adapt to transfer from one medium to another by noticeable morphological and physiological transformations (Sorokin and Nishino, 1973). In the alga depicted in Figure 1, a transfer from inorganic medium into some organic media results in repression of longitudinal growth, a gradual swelling of the cell (Figure 6a) and eventual formation of a sphere (Figure 6b and c). During the transition stage, the ends of the originally rod-shaped cell can be seen protruding from the sphere (Figure 6b). Eventually, if not withdrawn into the body of the sphere during swelling of the cell, the protrusions disappear (Figure 6c) in the process of the first division of the

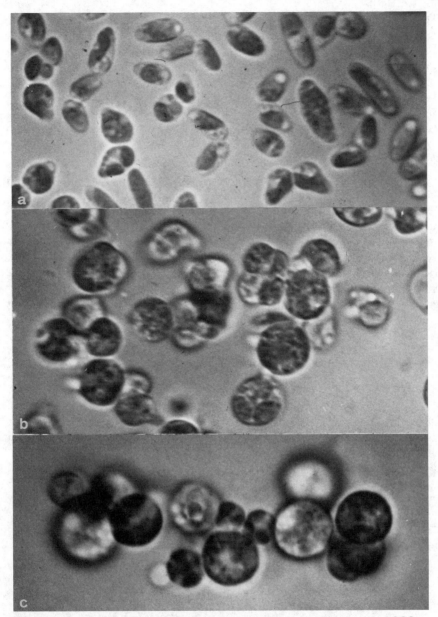

Figure 6 Transformation of rod-shaped cells into spheres. × 2000.
a, Autotrophically grown cells, such as depicted in Figure 1, after 1
day in tryptic soy broth. b, Cells after 4 days in tryptic soy broth. c,
Cells from a culture maintained by regular transfers for 10 months in
tryptic soy broth.

spherical cell. The details of transformation of the rod-shaped cells into spherical cells are shown schematically in Figure 7. The progress in the process of transformation and the percentage of the transformed cells are affected by the physiological conditions of the original cells and the environmental factors during transformation and vary among the different strains of the organism. Of all organic media tested, the most effective in the transformation of rod-shaped cells into spheres proved to be tryptic soy broth in the concentration of $10-20$ g $\cdot$ liter^{-1} of distilled water.

The conversion of the rod-shaped cells into spheres usually takes from several days up to $1-2$ weeks. Then, by regular transfers into fresh tryptic soy broth medium, the culture of spherical cells can be maintained without degeneration for several months. In one experiment a culture of spherical cells was maintained without degeneration for 10 months (Figure 6c). Fluctuations in the length of the period during which a culture of spherical cells can be maintained without degeneration may indicate that this period can be extended, though so far we were unable to maintain cultures as spheres indefinitely.

The obtained spherical cells superficially resemble spherical struc-

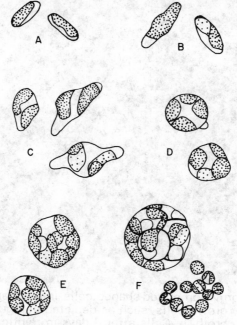

Figure 7 Schematic presentation of the transformation of rod-shaped cells into spheres.

tures produced from rod-shaped bacterial, fungal, and algal cells by the action of lysozyme, penicillin, or other agents causing either degradation of the already built cell wall or disruption of the synthesis of the new cell walls. A complete or partial removal of the cell wall is characteristic of these structures which depending on the degree of the removal of the cell wall have been called protoplasts or spheroplasts (Frey-Wyssling, 1967; Spizizen, 1962; Tulasne et al., 1960; Weibull, 1958).

The formation of spherical cells depicted in Figure 6 does not involve general degradation of the cell wall, though the pattern of formation of the cell wall in spherical cells is remarkably changed compared to that in the original rod-shaped cells. Cell division in the rod-shaped cells culminates in the formation of the transverse partition (Figure 5a). This portion of the wall of daughter cells is the only new section built in the process of cell division, the rest of the wall is that of the mother cell.

In the transformed spherical cells, the division, as in the rod-shaped cells, begins with the division of the chloroplast (Figure 8a) followed by the division of the nucleus and formation of the cell wall (Figure 8b). However, after each nuclear division, the cell wall is formed around the entire surface of each of the daughter cells (Figures 8b and 9a and b). Thus, a series of successive cell divisions of one original cell produces a series of successive generations of daughter cells each subsequent generation of cells within the cell wall of the preceding generation of cells. The formation of the cell wall does not involve an immediate lysis of the cell wall of the preceding generation of cells and thus each succeeding generation of daughter cells can be expected to be enclosed, in addition to their own cell wall, also by the walls of preceding generations of cells (Figure 9b).

Biologically, only the cell walls of the last generation of daughter cells and the wall of the original mother cell, until it releases the enclosed within it daughter cells, are necessary; all intermediate cell walls become superfluous. Some of these intermediate walls are eventually lysed before the liberation of the last generation of daughter cells from the mother cell wall but the lysis is not complete so that some daughter cells upon their release from the mother cell are in two's or four's covered and held together by the walls of the preceding generation of cells.

Reversion of Spheres into Rods and Properties of the Regenerated Rod-Shaped Cells

Eventually, reversion of the spherical cells into the rod-shaped cells takes place even if the culture is maintained by regular transfers to a fresh tryptic soy broth. The process is the reverse of the conversion of

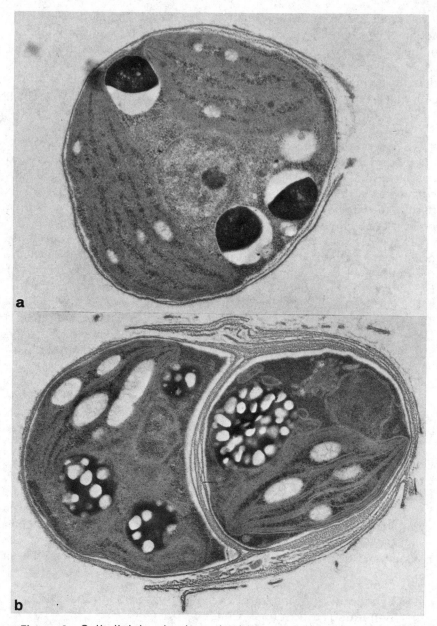

Figure 8 Cell division in the spherical cells transformed from the rod-shaped cells. a, A cell in the initial division stage. Chloroplast divided into two. × 25,000. b, The cell divided into two daughter cells. Notice the abundant formation of cell wall material. × 25,000.

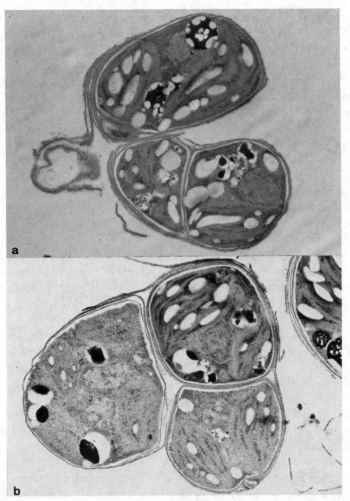

Figure 9 Cell division in the spherical cells transformed from the rod-shaped cells (continued). a, The next division within the spherical cell. Notice lysis of the wall of the preceding generation. × 12,000. b, Spherical cell in the same division stage as in (a). Lysis of the walls of the preceding generation less complete than in (a) and the continuous extension of these walls over the subsequent generation of cells is clearly visible. × 12,000.

rods into spheres. A cell gradually elongates with a concomitant decrease in width. The reversed rods can be maintained without further deterioration indefinitely by regular transfers into tryptic soy broth.

The process of reversion of spheres into rods can be expedited by transferring spherical cells from tryptic soy broth into inorganic medium and growing cultures autotrophically. The regenerated rods do not differ morphologically from the original rod-shaped cells. However, in their physiological characteristics, cultures of the rod-shaped cells obtained by reversion from the spherical cells remain markedly different for a prolonged time from the cultures of the rod cells which in their history did not experience the conversion into spheres. If, after a period of autotrophic growth, the regenerated rod cells are again inoculated into tryptic soy broth, their capacity to form spheres is noticeably lower than that of the rods which had no prehistory of conversion into spheres.

The original and regenerated rod-shaped cells differ also in their capacity for autotrophic and heterotrophic growth. In Table 1, growth rates of rod cells are given for four categories of cells with different prehistories. The original cells were continuously maintained under autotrophic conditions and thus never experienced a conversion into spheres. The regenerated cells were obtained by transfer of transformed spherical cells grown in tryptic soy broth into inorganic medium. After the transfer, the regenerated rods were grown autotrophically for different lengths of time—11, 46 or 153 days—before being used for growth measurements.

As seen in Table 1, growth rates under autotrophic conditions were invariably higher for all categories of cells than under heterotrophic conditions. Under autotrophic conditions, the growth rate for the original cells which in their prehistory were never exposed to heterotrophic conditions, was consistently higher than for regenerated cells and within the regenerated cells their capacity for autotrophic growth increased with the increase in the length of the period during which they were exposed to autotrophic conditions before their autotrophic growth rate was measured.

The reverse change in the growth rate was observed for regenerated rod-shaped cells under heterotrophic conditions. The heterotrophic growth rate for the original cells was lower than for any of the categories

Table 1 Growth Rates of the Original and Regenerated Rod-shaped Cells

Kinds of cells	Autotrophic conditions	Heterotrophic conditions
Original rods	5.24	2.24
Regenerated rods after:		
153 days in inorganic medium	4.56	2.40
46 days in inorganic medium	3.63	2.76
11 days in inorganic medium	4.02	2.84

of the regenerated cells. Within the regenerated cells, the capacity for heterotrophic growth declined with the increase in the length of the period during which the cells were exposed to autotrophic conditions after being transferred from the tryptic soy broth. However, even after 153 days in inorganic medium, regenerated rods remained markedly distinct in their growth characteristics from those which had never experienced transformation into spheres.

Summary

Modifications in the chloroplast shape during cell developmental cycle of some rod-shaped algae as well as transformations of these algae into spherical forms will be considered in regard to their magnitude, the involvement of hereditary factors, and reproducibility. The magnitude of the affected change can be evaluated by comparison with differences in the similar characteristics between the existing taxonomic groups.

A change in the chloroplast shape from a plate-like girdle to a helical band described to occur during the cell cycle of our organism involves spanning differences between forms known to belong to different orders of algae. Helical, often called spiral, chloroplasts have been described in four genera of green algae: *Spirogyra, Sirogonium, Genicularia,* and *Spirotenia* — all belonging to the order Zygnematales (Smith, 1950) or Conjugales (Fritsch, 1965). Rod-shaped algae with girdlelike chloroplasts, in which the change to helical shape was observed, could be classified as belonging to the genus *Stichococcus* of the order Ulotrichales. By manipulating experimental conditions, such as temperature and light intensity, the growth rate of the organism and the change from one shape of the chloroplast to another could be readily affected.

Transformation of the rod-shaped cells into spheres which, in our observations, could be then propagated as such for many generations, involved a basic change in the method of cell multiplication. Difference in the method of cell multiplication similar to that affected by the transformation of rod-shaped cells into spheres was considered by Fritsch (1965) sufficient to separate members of the order Chlorococcales possessing the so-called vegetative cell division into distinct family of Chlorosphaeraceae apart from other families of the order characterized by "asexual reproduction."

In vegetative cell division exemplified in our case by the original rod-shaped cells, daughter protoplasts are separated from one another by transverse partition which is joined laterally to the cell wall of the parent cell. The parent cell wall is not discarded in the process of division but is passed over to and then constitutes the larger portion of the cell walls of daughter cells.

In asexual reproduction characteristic of our transformed spherical cells, daughter cells arise within the parent cell wall. In the process of cell division, a new cell wall is formed around the entire surface of each daughter cell. The release of daughter cells occurs by rupture of the parent cell wall, the remnants of which, after liberation of daughter cells, are seen floating in the medium.

In another treatment, Herndon (1958) considered the distinction between vegetative cell division and asexual reproduction taxonomically important enough to remove the family of Chlorosphaeraceae from the order of Chlorococcales and to elevate it to the rank of the distinct order Chlorosphaerales. In our work, this taxonomic gap was bridged within a few days by a change in the environmental conditions.

Though the dependence of the change in the shape of the chloroplast and in the shape of the cell on experimental conditions was clearly demonstrated in our observations, the role of hereditary constitution of the organism in the susceptibility to environmental factors also became obvious. Three species of *Stichococcus* (*S. bacillaris*, *S. mirabilis*, and *S. chodati*), two species of *Hormidium* (*H. flaccidum* and *H. sterile*) and one species of the filamentous alga, *Ulotrix subtilissima*, all obtained from the Indiana Culture Collection, were subjected to experimental conditions similar to those which affected morphophysiological transformations in our organism. The reaction was generally negative. Specifically, the rod-shaped cells of other organisms, though capable of growing and multiplying in the organic media, failed to change their shape to the spherical form.

The fact that transformation of the rod-shaped cells into spheres was readily reversible indicates that no genetic change took place. Within a few days after being transferred into proper medium, a great majority of cells (in some experiments nearly 100% of rod-shaped cells) were transformed into spherical shape or back from spheres into rods. The reversion of spherical cells into the original rod-shaped cells took place also without transfer of spheres into inorganic medium. After a prolonged time of keeping the transformed spheres in the organic medium, the regression took place automatically.

Morphological changes were accompanied by profound physiological and biochemical alterations. After transformation of rod-shaped cells into spheres and returning spheres back into rod shape, the capacity of cells to undergo repeated transformations was markedly affected. The growth rate of the regenerated cells was distinctly different for a long time from that of the rod-shaped cells which never experienced transformation into spheres. Distribution of the mechanisms involved in the building of cell walls was modified: the pattern of deposition of cell wall material only at the cell plate characteristic of the rod-shaped cells was changed into the uniform building of cell walls around the entire surface of each daughter cell and the activity of the wall building mechanisms was greatly increased. The activity and distribution of lytic enzyme involved in the digestion of cell walls in the process of cell division was profoundly affected: from the application of the lytic enzyme only to a narrow strip in the equatorial region in the rod-shaped cells to the digestion of the entire surface in the spherical cells.

The described transformations were readily reproducible though uniformity of the change, as indicated by the perfection of the newly evolved cell shape and the percentage of the transformed cells, varied from one experiment to another. Extracellular environment affects cellular mechanisms through changes in intracellular environment. Another factor which greatly affects the course of biochemical reactions and metabolic processes is the developmental status of cells. In the course of its growth-division cycle, a cell passes through a series of developmental stages characterized by specific morphological, physiological, and biochemical properties. The requirements for external factors for optimal function and development of the cell, as well as the reaction of cellular mechanisms to changing conditions, like those affecting transformation of the rod-shape into spherical form, also change. In a nonsychronized population of cells, the diversity of the developmental conditions of individual cells explains variations in the reactions of individual cells to the same external factors and to changes in these factors. With cell synchronization a much higher degree of uniformity is usually achievable.

References

Brachet, J. (1950). "Chemical Embryology." Wiley (Interscience), New York.

Calvayrac, R. (1970). Relation entre les substrates, la respiration et la structure mitochondriale chez *Euglena gracilis. Arch. Mikrobiol.* **73**, 308–314.

Cornutt, S. G., and Schmidt, R. R. (1964). Possible mechanisms controlling the intracellular level of inorganic polyphosphate during synchronous growth of *Chlorella pyrenoidosa. Exp. Cell Res.,* **36**, 102–110.

Frey-Wyssling, A. (1967). Gymnoplasts instead of "Protoplasts." *Nature London* **216**, 516.

Fritsch, F. E., (1965). "The Structure and Reproduction of the Algae," Vol. 1. Cambridge Univ. Press, London.

Herndon, W. (1958). Studies of chlorospaeracean algae from soil. *Amer. J. Bot.* **45**, 298–308.

Howard, A., and Pelc, S. R. (1953). Synthesis of deoxyribonucleic acid in normal and irradiated cells and its relation to chromosome breakage. *Heredity London* (Suppl.) **6**, 261–273.

Mitchison, J. M. (1957). The growth of single cells. I. *Schizosaccharomyces pombe. Exp. Cell Res.* **13**, 244–262.

Mitchison, J. M. (1971). "The Biology of the Cell Cycle." Cambridge Univ. Press, London.

Nihei, T., Sasa, T., Miyachi, S., Suzuki, K., and Tamiya, H. (1954). Change of photosynthetic activity of *Chlorella* cells during the course of their normal life cycle. *Arch. Mikrobiol.* **21**, 155–164.

Osafune, T., Mihara, S., Hase, E., and Ohkuro, T. (1972). Electron microscope studies on the vegetative cellular life cycle of *Chlamydomonas reinhardi* Dangeard in synchronous culture 1. Some characteristics of changes in subcellular structures during the cell cycle, especially in the formation of giant mitochondria. *Plant Cell Physiol.* **13**, 211–227.

Reid, A., Soeder, C. J., and Müller, I. (1963). Über die Atmung synchron kultivierter *Chlorella*. 1. Veränderungen des respiratorischen Gaswechsels im Laufe des Entwicklungscyclus. *Arch. Mikrobiol.* **45**, 343–358.

Sasa, T. (1961). Effect of ultraviolet light upon various physiological activities of *Chlorella* cells at different stages in their life cycle. *Plant Cell Physiol.* **2**, 253–270.

Schmidt, R. R. (1969). Control of enzyme synthesis during the cell cycle of *Chlorella. In* "The Cell Cycle," G. M. Padilla, G. L. Whitson, and T. L. Cameron, eds., pp. 159–177. Academic Press, New York.

Smith, G. M. (1950). "The Fresh-Water Algae of the United States," 2nd Ed. McGraw-Hill, New York.

Soeder, C. J., and Reid, A. (1967). Über die Atmung synchron kultivierter *Chlorella*. 11. Die Entwicklungsabhangigkeit der Veränderungen des respiratorischen Gaswechsels. *Arch. Mikrobiol.* **56**, 106–119.

Sorokin, C. (1957). Changes in photosynthetic activity in the course of cell development in *Chlorella. Physiol. Plant.* **10**, 659–666.

Sorokin, C. (1963a). On the variability in the activity of the photosynthetic mechanisms. *In* "Photosynthetic Mechanisms of Green Plants," pp. 742–750. Nat. Acad. Sci.–Nat. Res. Council, Washington, D.C.

Sorokin, C. (1963b). The capacity for organic synthesis in cells of successive developmental stages. *Arch. Mikrobiol.* **46**, 29–43.

Sorokin, C. (1964). Organic synthesis in algal cells separated into age groups by fractional centrifugation. *Arch Mikrobiol.* **49**, 193–208.

Sorokin, C. (1965). Photosynthesis in cell development. *Biochim. Biophys. Acta* **94**, 42–52.

Sorokin, C., and Corbett, M. K. (1975). Autospore formation in a *Stichococcus*-type alga. *Amer. J. Bot.* (submitted for publication).

Sorokin, C., and Myers, J (1954). Characteristics of a high-temperature strain of *Chlorella. Carnegie Inst. Washington Yearb.* **53**, 177–179.

Sorokin, C., and Myers, J. (1957). The course of respiration during the life cycle of *Chlorella* cells. *J. Gen. Physiol.* **40**, 579–592.

Sorokin, C., and Nishino, S. (1973). Transformation of rod-shaped algal cells into spherical cells. *Amer. J. Bot.* **60**, 907–914.

Sorokin, C., Corbett, M. K., and Nishino, S. (1972). Helical chloroplasts in a *Stichococcus*-type alga. *J. Phycol.*, **8**, 152–156.

Spizizen, J. (1962). Preparation and use of protoplasts. *Methods Enzymol.* **5**, 122–134.

Stefanelli, A. (1937). A new form of micro-respirometer; with a note on the effect of cleavage on the respiration of the egg of *Rana. J. Exp. Biol.* **14**, 171–177.

Talbert, D. M., and Sorokin, C. (1971). Respiration in cell development. *Arch. Mikrobiol.* **78**, 281–294.

Tamiya, H., Iwamura, T., Shibata, K., Hase, E., and Nihei, T. (1953). Correlation between photosynthesis and light-independent metabolism in the growth of *Chlorella. Biochim. Biophys. Acta* **12**, 23–40.

Tulasne, R., Minck, R., Kirn, A., and Krembel, J. (1960). Delimitation de la notion de formes L des bactéries: protoplastes, sphéroplastes et formes L. *Ann. Inst. Pasteur* **99**, 859–874.

Weibull, C. (1958). Bacterial protoplasts. *Annu. Rev. Microbiol.* **12**, 1–26.

Zeuthen, E. (1946). Oxygen uptake during mitosis. Experiments on the eggs of the frog *Rana platyrrhina. C. R. Trav. Lab. Carlsberg* **25**, 191–228.

Effect of Light Intensity on Dinoflagellate Growth and Photosynthesis

Olga v. H. Owens and H. H. Seliger

Department of Biology,
The Johns Hopkins University
Baltimore, Maryland

Introduction

In recent years, in extensive studies of phytoplankton ecology, investigators have attempted to describe and define the limits of algal communities. In the estuarine environment, the communities are constantly changing due to shifts in the environment, such as salinity, temperature, nutrients, presence of predators, and shading by other pigmented organisms. In addition, most of the algae are motile and so the definition of a phytoplankton community becomes extremely complex. We are attempting to describe some of the characters of these communities in terms of the physiology of the individual species, in much the same way that some of the other contributors of this volume examined the adaptation of the organism by studying its adaptive enzymes.

In this chapter, we are concerned with the characterization of these planktonic algae in order to develop some new and rapid optical methods for assessing their physiological state. To calibrate any new method, it is essential that we be able to determine the state of the cells by conventional and reliable techniques.

We know that two fundamental gas exchange reactions of plant cells, respiration and photosynthesis, vary widely with environmental condi-

tions. The studies reported here are concerned with the effect of light
intensity on these reactions.

In field experiments during the summer months high rates of CO_2
fixation are found routinely from phytoplankton samples from the Chesapeake Bay. On a chlorophyll basis, these rates are about five times
higher than saturating rates found in laboratory cultures of commonly
grown photosynthetic green and blue-green algae. Since dinoflagellates
are occasionally dominant in Chesapeake Bay samples, we asked whether the dinoflagellates have photosynthetic rates regulated by the same
factors that regulate photosynthesis in the smaller green algae.

To compare dinoflagellate photosynthesis to green alga photosynthesis it was necessary to have two of these organisms which would
grow in the same medium and under the same light conditions. Of the
several organisms we have in culture, two were chosen for comparison
because they represent two extremes in size and chlorophyll concentration. One was *Dunaliella* sp., a small, <10 μm green flagellate and the
other was *Gymnodinium splendens,* a large, 80 μm long photosynthetic,
naked dinoflagellate, colored reddish brown with carotinoid pigment,
presumably peridinin. Both are found in Chesapeake Bay. The *Gymnodinium* is one of the organisms that forms dark reddish-brown blooms
during the summer months.

We have attempted to study these organisms at cell concentrations
approximating the conditions under which the cells are found in nature.
These concentrations are much lower than normally used in laboratory
experiments. The minimum concentrations used were determined by the
sensitivity of our oxygen electrode.

Materials and Methods

Both organisms were grown in the same medium, f/2 of Guillard and
Ryther (1962), modified by using seawater diluted to half-strength with
distilled water but with other ingredients the same. This medium had a
total alkalinity within the range of that found in the Chesapeake Bay.
The cells were grown in flasks placed on a translucent, plastic shelf over
a bank of four 40 W cool white fluorescent tubes. Various intensities
were produced with screens and translucent paper under the flasks.
Light flux was measured with a thermopile at the surface of the table.
The temperature was 28° ± 1° at the surface of the shelf.

Chlorophyll concentrations were determined fluorometrically by the
method of Loftus and Carpenter (1971). Cell counts were made with
standard counting chambers. Oxygen exchange was measured with a

Clark type electrode calibrated with air saturated medium. CO_2 fixation was determined by the method of Steeman-Nielsen (1952). In earlier experiments rates were measured at several exposure time intervals to ensure linearity, then 10 min was adopted as the standard exposure time.

Results

Because *Dunaliella* seemed to resemble *Chlorella*, we first compared these two organisms. Table 1 shows various physiological parameters for *Dunaliella*, compared to those obtained for *Chlorella* by Myers and Graham (1971). Since both organisms are subject to wide variations in these values depending on the cultural conditions, the data were selected on the basis of the growth rate; that is, the table shows values for the two organisms when they are growing at nearly equal rates. They are shown to be remarkably similar in spite of different media. We concluded from these data that *Dunaliella* is a "conventional" photosynthetic organism, comparable to the well-known, classical *Chlorella*.

In the first experiments we grew *Dunaliella* and *Gymnodinium* at four different intensities of cool white fluorescent light, from 0.1×10^4 to 1.1×10^4 ergs $\cdot$ cm^{-2} $\cdot$ sec^{-1} until they were adapted. Then we made quantitative inocula and cell counts over a period of days for *Dunaliella* and weeks for *Gymnodinium* until we established the growth constants at each intensity. Figure 1 shows these constants. It is apparent that the small *Dunaliella* grew on a cell basis, six to eight times faster than the large *Gymnodinium*. Both organisms had their growth in number saturated at about 0.6×10^4 ergs $\cdot$ cm^{-2} $\cdot$ sec^{-1}. At the lowest intensity *Gymnodinium* grew at one-half its saturating rate, while *Dunaliella* grew at two-thirds its saturating rate.

Table 1 Physiological Parameters for *Dunaliella* and *Chlorella*

Parameter	Chlorella[a]	Dunaliella
$k \cdot$ day^{-1} (doubling time, hr)[b]	1.8 (9.25)	2.0 (8.45)
Cell volume, μm^3	49[c]	60[d]
pg chl/cell	0.359	0.34
Max. rate observed[e]		
(μmoles $\cdot$ mg chl^{-1} $\cdot$ hr^{-1})	205 (O_2)	210 (CO_2)

[a]Data of Myers and Graham (1971).
[b]k is growth rate constant.
[c]Calculated from packed cell volume.
[d]Estimated from microscope measurements.
[e]O_2 evolution and CO_2 fixation.

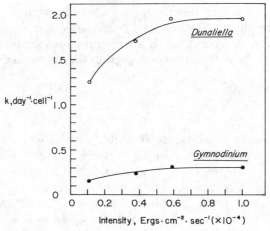

Figure 1 Growth rate versus light intensity for *Dunaliella* (o) and *Gymnodinium* (●) cultures.

The CO_2 fixation rates for the two organisms as functions of light intensity are shown in Figure 2. The two organisms had similar rates on a chlorophyll basis. *Gymnodinium* had a lower rate of CO_2 fixation at lower intensities, and appeared from these data not to be saturated at the higher intensity. Figure 3 shows a separate experiment with *Gymnodinium* in which no saturation was observed. Thus *Gymnodinium,* at an ambient light intensity sufficient to saturate the growth rate, did not show saturation in rate of CO_2 fixation. These data indicate instead that

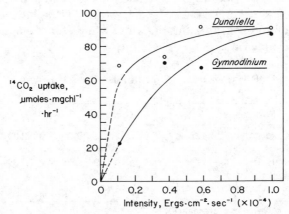

Figure 2 CO_2 fixation rate versus ambient light intensity for *Dunaliella* (o) and *Gymnodinium* (●) cultures.

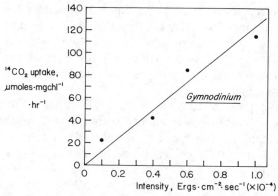

Figure 3 CO_2 fixation rate versus ambient light intensity for *Gymnodinium*.

Gymnodinium maintained a high rate of CO_2 fixation at high light intensities.

Although it is not valid to compare the energy fluxes directly because of the different spectral distributions, the intensities we used were low compared to direct sunlight which has a maximum of about 40×10^4 ergs $\cdot$ cm^{-2} $\cdot$ sec^{-1}. At least we can assume that we were not using extreme intensities to produce abnormally bleached cells. The range of intensities was only 10-fold but as shown in Figure 4, *Gymnodinium* adapted to these four intensities. Rates of CO_2 fixation versus light in-

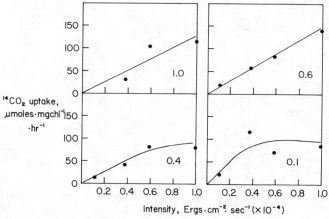

Figure 4 CO_2 fixation rate versus light intensity for *Gymnodinium* cultured at four intensities. The number in the lower right of each graph indicates the ambient intensity in ergs $\cdot$ cm^{-2} $\cdot$ sec^{-1} ($\times 10^{-4}$)

tensity are plotted for each of four cultures adapted to 0.1, 0.4, 0.6, and 1.0×10^4 ergs $\cdot$ cm^{-2} $\cdot$ sec^{-1} of cool white continuous light, respectively. Cultures grown at low ambient light intensity (two lower curves) saturated both at low rates and at low intensities. Cultures grown at relatively high ambient intensity (two upper curves) showed no saturation over the same intensity range.

The relative rates of oxygen exchange for *Dunaliella* are shown in Figure 5. Photosynthesis was about 20 times dark respiration. In low light the curve approaches linearity and the light intensity for saturation is at about 25% relative intensity. Light compensation is at less than 1% relative intensity. Figure 6 shows the results for *Gymnodinium* obtained under the same conditions. Only at above 45% relative intensity did the net production of oxygen exceed the dark oxygen uptake. Again no saturation was observed. It has been shown that at low intensity the rate of oxygen production is directly proportional to intensity. Any deviation from linearity in intact cells is caused by changes in oxygen uptake due to respiration. Figure 6 indicates that *Gymnodinium* has a high rate of dark respiration relative to photosynthesis. The abrupt change in slope that occurred at about 20% relative intensity indicates that dark respiration was probably inhibited by low intensity light (Owens and Hoch, 1963).

Table 2 shows the results of our attempts to establish an accounting between CO$_2$ fixation data and the overall cell energy budget. *Dunaliella* and *Gymnodinium*, each grown at the two extremes of light intensities, are compared.

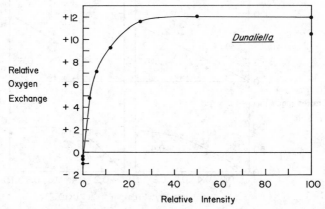

Figure 5 Oxygen exchange versus relative light intensity for *Dunaliella*. The positive values indicate relative oxygen production, above light compensation. The negative values indicate relative oxygen uptake, below light compensation.

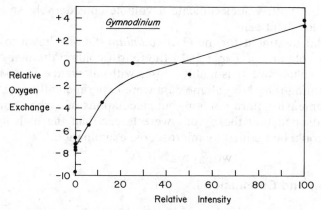

Figure 6 Oxygen exchange versus relative light intensity for *Gymnodinium* (see Figure 5 for explanation).

The first column shows that the CO_2 fixation rate experimentally determined in low light closely approximates the rate calculated from the measured doubling time and the formula of Mullin *et al.* (1966). This formula relates the carbon per cell to cell volume. The two values are in close agreement although the calculated rate should differ from the measured rate by an amount equal to the respiration rate.

In the second column the measured rate was used to calculate the carbon per cell and the cell volume. The value for cell volume is small compared to values based on estimates from microscopic measurements

Table 2 Carbon Dioxide Fixation in *Gymnodinium* and *Dunaliella* in Relation to Carbon Content and Growth Rate at Two Ambient Intensities

Parameter measured	*Dunaliella*		*Gymnodinium*	
	0.1×10^4 [a]	1.1×10^4 [a]	0.1×10^4 [a]	1.1×10^4 [a]
k · day⁻¹ (doubling time, hr)	1.26 (13.2)	1.97 (8.4)	0.227 (73.2)	0.367 (45.3)
Cell volume, μm^3	189[b]	27.8[c]	126,000[c]	70,000[d]
pg chl/cell	2.4	0.7	201	59.8
pg C/cell	27.6[c]	6.4[e]	3880[e]	2460[c]
Rate CO_2 fixation (μmoles · mg chl⁻¹ · hr⁻¹)				
Measured	69	91	22	87
Calculated	73[f]			61[f]

[a] Intensity in ergs · cm⁻² · sec⁻¹.
[b] Measured in Coulter counter in laboratory of Dr. W. R. Taylor.
[c] Calculated using formula of Mullin *et al.* (1966).
[d] Measured from displacement by proportional clay model.
[e] Calculated from CO_2 fixation rate, doubling time, and chlorophyll per cell.
[f] Calculated from carbon per cell, doubling time, and chlorophyll per cell.

(Table 1) but both values indicate a volume considerably smaller than that of the low light cells.

A similar treatment for the *Gymnodinium* data is shown in the third and fourth columns of Table 2. In the fourth column the measured and calculated values are reasonably close, with allowance for a relatively high respiration rate. No volume data were experimentally determined at the lower intensity, third column, but calculations of carbon content and volume indicated that these cells were larger than the high light cells. This fact could be verified by microscopic examination.

Discussion and Conclusions

We have attempted in these studies to evaluate the photosynthetic characteristics of these two very different cell types both of which grow in the estuarine environment. *Dunaliella* appears to be very much like other small green algae which have already been studied extensively, but *Gymnodinium splendens* seems to have some properties which differ from those of *Dunaliella*. These are (1) a high rate of dark respiration, and (2) a lack of a clearly defined light saturation of CO_2 fixation and oxygen production. These are properties of "sun" plants. Extensive studies of "sun" and "shade" higher plants have been made by Björkman *et al.* (1972). Others, notably Schmid and Gaffron (1967) for tobacco mutants, Myers and Graham (1971) and Reger and Krauss (1970) for *Chlorella*, Jørgensen (1964a,b) and Steeman-Nielsen and Jørgensen (1968) for diatoms have assessed the effects of light intensity. Sun plants have a low chlorophyll content and do less photosynthesis per unit of chlorophyll in low light, but thrive in bright sun. Yentsch and Lee (1966) reported very much higher saturation of CO_2 fixation for tropical phytoplankton than for a small, green, laboratory-grown flagellate.

The chloroplasts of sun plants have less chlorophyll and few or no grana, that is, the lamellae do not form stacks. Electron micrograph studies of dinoflagellates by Messer and Ben-Shaul (1972) for a species of *Peridinium* showed that grana appeared only when cultures reached the stationary phase of growth and a study by Dodge and Crawford (1969) of *Gymnodinium fuscum*, a species similar to our *G. splendens*, also showed a lack of grana. Thus we conclude that *G. splendens* easily becomes a "sun" plant at relatively low intensities and as a consequence has a low rate of photosynthesis in low light but a much higher rate in bright summer sun.

There are several factors which we have not yet studied but which must be considered. We did not increase our light to anywhere near that of sunlight and we have not yet seen the very high rates of CO_2 fixation observed in the field but our data predict that these rates are possible. Zelitch (1971) has made extensive studies of photorespiration and reports that losses of carbon of up to 50% of photosynthetic fixation can occur. So, while in weak light dark respiration may be inhibited (Hoch et al., 1963), in strong light photorespiration can occur. Bunt (1965) has attempted to assess the extent of the effects of light activated respiration in an antarctic diatom and offered a criticism of the ^{14}C technique.

The measurement of the ^{14}C uptake rate is a convenient experimental simplification for assessment of growth of a phytoplankton community. Similarly in nutritional studies the half-saturation constants for uptake are assumed to be the same as those for growth. However, we have shown that for G. splendens the growth rate can saturate while the ^{14}C uptake rate continues to increase with light intensity. One must be careful, therefore, in the use of ^{14}C uptake rate measurements for estimating the response of phytoplankton communities to changing environmental conditions.

We have not considered the role of accessory pigments. Mann and Myers (1968) have shown that the fucoxanthin of diatoms is an accessory pigment but the roles of chlorophyll c and peridinin of dinoflagellates have not been determined. We expect to continue these studies with this and other estuarine organisms.

Acknowledgments

The authors acknowledge with thanks Mr. N. Niren for help in some of the experiments, Mrs. C. Eisner for chlorophyll determinations, and Mr. S. Storms of Dr. W. R. Taylor's laboratory for the Coulter counter determination. The work was supported in part by AEC Contract AT(30-1)3278 and a research grant under NSF-RANN to the Chesapeake Research Consortium. Publication No. 802 of the Department of Biology, The Johns Hopkins University.

References

Björkman, O., Ludlow, M. M., and Morrow, P. A. (1972). Photosynthetic performance of two rainforest species in their native habitat and analysis of their gas exchange. *Annu. Rep. Director, Dept. Plant Biol. 1971–1972* (Carnegie Inst. Stanford, California), pp. 94–107.

Bunt, J. S. (1965). Measurements of photosynthesis and respiration in a marine diatom with the mass spectrometer and with carbon-14. *Nature, London* **207,** 1373–1375.

Dodge, J. D., and Crawford, R. M. (1969). The fine structure of *Gymnodinium fuscum* (Dinophyceae). *New Phytol.* **68,** 613–618.

Guillard, R. R. L., and Ryther, J. H. (1962). Studies on marine planktonic diatoms I. *Cyclotella nana* Hystedt and *Detonula confervacea* (Cleve) Gran. *Can. J. Microbiol.* **8,** 229–239.

Hoch, G., Owens, O. v. H., and Kok, B. (1963). Photosynthesis and respiration. *Arch. Biochem. Biophys.* **101,** 171–180.

Jørgensen, E. G. (1964a). Adaptation to different light intensities in the diatom *Cyclotella meneghiniana* Kütz. *Physiol. Plant.* **17,** 136–145.

Jørgensen, E. G. (1964b). Chlorophyll content and rate of photosynthesis in relation to cell size of the diatom *Cyclotella meneghiniana. Physiol Plant.* **17,** 407–413.

Loftus, M. E., and Carpenter, J. H. (1971). A fluorometric method for determining chlorophylls *a, b,* and *c. J. Marine Res.* **29,** 319–338.

Mann, J. E., and Myers, J. (1968). Photosynthetic enhancement in the diatom *Phaeodactylum tricornutum. Plant Physiol.* **43,** 1991–1995.

Messer, G., and Ben-Shaul, Y. (1972). Changes in chloroplast structure during culture growth of *Peridinium cinctum* Fa. *westii* (Dinophyceae). *Phycologia* **11,** 291–299.

Mullin, M. M., Sloan, P. R., and Eppley, R. W. (1966). Relationship between carbon content, cell volume and area in phytoplankton. *Limnol. Oceanogr.* **11,** 307–311.

Myers, J., and Graham, J. (1971). The photosynthetic unit in *Chlorella* measured by repetitive short flashes. *Plant Physiol.* **48,** 282–286.

Owens, O. v. H., and Hoch, G. (1963). Enhancement and de-enhancement effect in *Anaceptis nidulans. Biochim. Biophys. Acta* **75,** 183–186.

Reger, B. J., and Krauss, R. W. (1970). The photosynthetic response to a shift in the chlorophyll *a* to chlorophyll *b* ratio of *Chlorella. Plant Physiol.* **46,** 568–575.

Schmid, G. H., and Gaffron, H. (1967). Light metabolism and chloroplast structure in chlorophyll-deficient tobacco mutants. *J. Gen. Physiol.* **50,** 563–582.

Steemann-Nielsen, E. (1952). The use of radioactive carbon (C^{14}) for measuring organic production in the sea. *J. Cons.* **18,** 117–140.

Steeman-Nielsen, E., and Jørgensen, E. G. (1968). The adaptation of plankton algae I. General Part. *Physiol. Plant.* **21,** 401–413.

Yentsch, C. S., and Lee, R. W. (1966). A study of photosynthetic light reactions and a new interpretation of sun and shade phytoplankton. *J. Mar. Res* **24,** 319–337.

Zelitch, I. (1971). Photosynthesis, photorespiration, and plant productivity. Academic Press, New York.

The Biochemical Adaptations of Algae to Environmental Change

Raymond A. Galloway

University of Maryland
College Park, Maryland

Until about 20 years ago, little attention was given to mechanisms by which the metabolic control of reactions and of biochemical pathways in living systems were exerted. Much groundwork had first to be done with respect to our understanding of cell chemistry. The present level of comprehension of the biochemical nature of organisms permits some unraveling of this perhaps more sophisticated and subtle realm of physiology.

In the laboratory at the University of Maryland, our favorite organisms include several of the unicellular algae. Whereas higher plants are not flexible with respect to their organic composition because of their elaborate structural elements, this so-called simple group of plants is well known for its versatility and maleability with regard to response to changes in environment. Therefore they make excellent subjects for the study of physiological adaptation. This paper deals with the results of several such investigations. The work includes studies concerned with all of the primary environmental parameters of plants, viz. light, temperature, and the composition of the substrate or medium, especially nutrient and O_2 concentration, and the presence of heavy metals, antibiotics, or other chemicals which affect metabolism.

Galloway and Krauss (1959a,b), in the course of an examination of the inhibition of growth of green algae by the antibiotic polymyxin b, made the following observations: the antibiotic did not interfere with the growth and metabolism of *Chlorella vulgaris*, but at low concentrations caused death of *Chlorella pyrenoidosa* grown heterotrophically on glucose (Figure 1). It was demonstrated by means of Lineweaver-Burk type experiments (Figure 2) that the site of inhibition was at the level of phosphoglucose isomerase. When galactose was supplied as the carbon source, however, growth of *C. pyrenoidosa* was normal in the presence of polymyxin. Since the known pathway for galactose utilization by the Waldenase reaction leads to the formation of glucose-1-phosphate, the implication was clear that another pathway must be employed in the presence of the metabolic block to explain the observed differential sensitivity. When galactose is used as the sole carbon source, both galactose-1-phosphate and galactose-6-phosphate are found in the cell. Putting these facts together, the scheme shown in Figure 3 was generated to explain how the block was bypassed. It would seem that in naturally resistant organisms, the rerouting of glucose into galactose may account

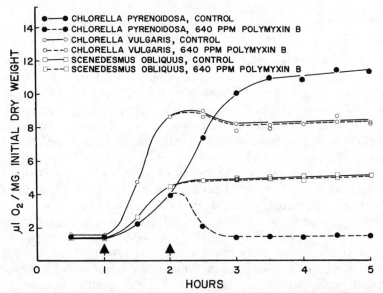

Figure 1 The effect of polymyxin B on endogenous and glucose respiration rates of *Scenedesmus obliquus*. The effect on glucose respiration both with and without magnesium is shown. (Arrows indicate additions of substrate and polymyxin B.) (From Galloway and Krauss, 1959a.)

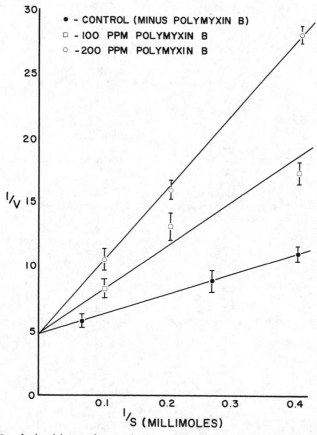

Figure 2 A double-reciprocal plot of the effect of polymyxin B on the activity of phosphoglucose isomerase obtained from rabbit muscle. The reaction mixture consisted of 0.1 ml of enzyme preparation which had been diluted 1 to 4000 with double-distilled water, and 0.4 ml of buffer solution, 0.06 *M* Sigma 7–9, adjusted to a pH of 7.0. Incubation was performed at 6°C for 35 min. $1/v =$ inverse of the optical density of the product of the reaction, fructose-6-phosphate, assayed according to the method of Roe. $1/S =$ inverse of the concentrations of the substrate, glucose-6-phosphate. Each point is an average of four determinations (from Galloway and Krauss, 1959b).

for their resistance, and the inability to make that conversion accounts for the sensitivity seen in other species.

Another example of a case in which the presence of an inhibitor revealed an otherwise cryptic pathway is seen in the work of Sherald and

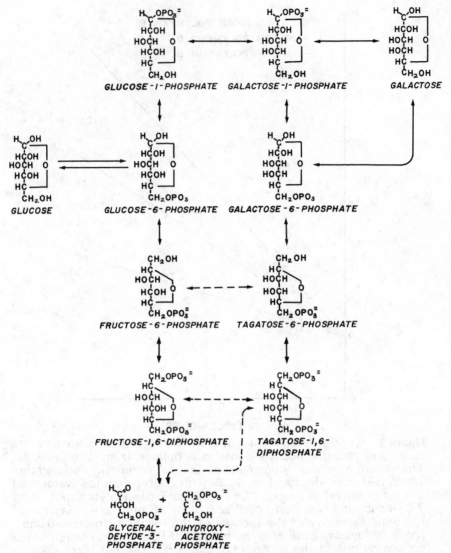

Figure 3 The sequence of hexose intermediates of an alternate pathway in relation to the classical glycolytic scheme (from Galloway and Krauss, 1959b).

Sisler in 1972. They happened to be using sporidia of *Ustilag maydis* and conidia of *Ceratocystic ulmi*, but the principle illustrated here is seen in many places in the phycological and mycological world. They found that both antimycin A and sodium azide blocked the normal course of terminal oxidation, but that another electron transport pathway became operative upon its inhibition. The respiration rate under these circumstances was 1.5–2.0 times the usual rate. A lowered affinity for O_2 indicated different terminal oxidases in the two sequences.

Sherald and Sisler also determined that several inhibitors interfere with the new sequence, including benzohydroxamic acid and hydroxyquinoline. However they have little effect on the normal pathway. Figure 4 depicts the pathways involved at the points of inhibition. Work is currently underway on the identification of the enzymes involved in the newly discovered pathway. It is suggested by these workers that this pathway may represent an earlier method for oxidative phosphorylation that has been evolutionarily improved. Whatever its origin may be, in both of the cases discussed here so far, we may see that the organisms are equipped with means to circumvent any natural inhibition of two different vital pathways. The alternative pathways are not as efficient as the "normal," but they could be of great survival value.

A somewhat less clearly understood, but most intriguing example of

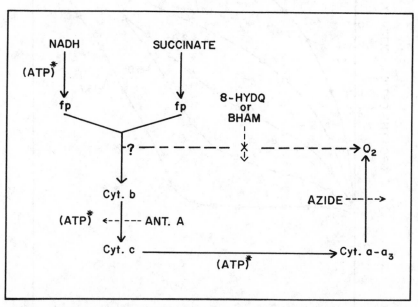

Figure 4 Schematic representation of primary (—) and alternate (---) respiratory pathways in sporidia of *Ustilago maydis* indicating the sites of action of antimycin A (ANT. A), AZIDE, 8-hydroxyquinoline (8-HYDQ), and benzohydroxamic acid (BHAM). Phosphorylation sites (ATP*); flavoprotein (fp), point of bifurcation (?) (from Sherald and Sisler, 1972).

adaptation was demonstrated by Gross in 1967. Reports of the toxicity of mannose are known from a very wide range of animals and plants. Working with *Chlorella infusionum*, var. *acetophila*, the author demonstrated mannose sensitivity, but unlike the situation in other organisms, the toxicity could be overcome. As may be seen from Figure 5, if one places *C. infusionum* in the presence of low levels of mannose, after a lag of some days the culture will begin to grow again. During the lag, most of the cells die, and a small percentage survive to produce a new

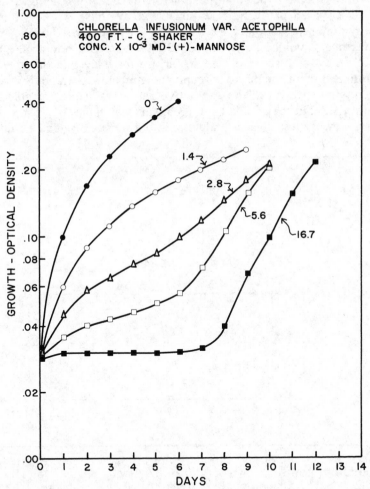

Figure 5 Growth of *Chlorella infusionum* var. *acetophila* shaken in cotton-plugged test tubes in the light as a function of increasing concentrations of D-mannose (from Gross, 1967).

mannose-resistant culture. This strain is unable to utilize carbohydrate as the sole source of carbon, including glucose and other sugars which had previously served as sources. Several compounds other than mannose, such as glucosamine and deoxyglucose, gave similar results, that is caused toxicity which was overcome in time, yielding strains of *Chlorella* which were incapable of heterotrophic growth.

The mannose-resistant strain cannot be restored to mannose sensitivity by simply removing mannose. It will apparently remain in its changed form indefinitely. But on the other hand, it can be converted to what would seem to be exactly its original mannose-sensitive, glucose-utilizing state if it is exposed for a long time (4 – 6 weeks) to glucose.

The original mannose-sensitive strain and the mannose-resistant strain were compared in a number of ways and little differences were revealed except for substrate utilization. They grew at the same rate autotrophically, and were largely affected the same way by various modifications of the medium. They produced cells of the same size and morphology. One difference was that in cultures of the original strain, grown heterotrophically on glucose, there were about 0.5% of the cells with gelatinous sheaths, and two to four times that many in the light. Mannose resistant cultures had approximately 95% such cells. The sheath may be seen by adding India ink to a drop of the culture on the slide. A study of five enzymes from the two strains showed no change in activity for hexokinase, 6-P-gluconate dehydrogenase, glucose-6-P-dehydrogenase and mannose-6-P-isomerase, but phosphatase activity was significantly higher in the sensitive strain.

The mechanism for resistance to mannose toxicity was indicated by the author to be either the presence of the sheath (acting simply as a physical barrier), the increased phosphatase activity, or most likely both. Mannose taken up and phosphorylated by the resistant strain would be immediately dephosphorylated and released as free sugar, as would glucose as well. The nature of the original toxicity to mannose is only hinted at by the author, but the point to be observed here is the remarkable change in the physiology of an organism brought about by an environmental change.

As early as 1949, Spoehr and Milner, in a pioneer paper of great importance, spoke of wide variation in the protein, lipid, and carbohydrate ratios in *Chlorella pyrenoidosa* as reflected by changes in the medium. They showed, among other things, that lipid content can vary from 4.5 to 85.6% of the dry weight. Later, in experiments designed to explore mechanisms to enhance the sterol content of algae, *Scenedesmus obliquis* was shown by Krauss and McAleer (1953) to respond positively to high light intensities. Von Witsch and Harder (1953; Figure 6)

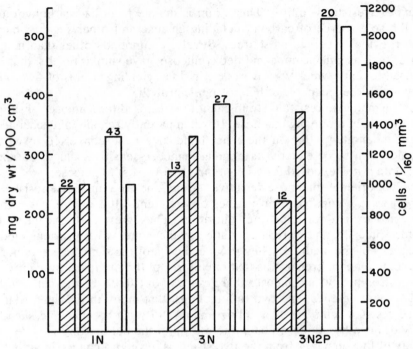

Figure 6 Influence of concentration of nitrogen and phosphorus in a culture medium on yield of dry matter and cell count of *Chlorella pyrenoidosa*. Ordinate on left gives dry weight, corresponding to wide bars; number at top of each wide bar gives percentage of fat in dry matter. Ordinate on right gives cell count, corresponding to narrow bars. Numbers at base give relative concentrations of nitrogen and phosphorus in culture medium, the one at left being the usual solution with respect to both nitrogen and phosphorus. For each concentration, yield and cell count are given after 14 days (crosshatched bars) and after 28 days (solid bars) (from von Witsch and Harder, 1953).

showed that generally in older cultures, (i.e., those no longer growing exponentially), there were higher fat concentrations than those in exponential growth, and that increasing nitrogen and phosphorus concentrations above "normal" levels decreased total fat concentration markedly. Since then, a closer examination in our laboratory has demonstrated some of the quantitative and qualitative changes in lipids which occur in algae as a result of environmental manipulation, specifically with respect to CO_2 concentration, temperature, cation levels in the nutrient medium, and light.

In 1969, Dickson, Galloway, and Patterson, working with *Chlorella fusca*, showed that fatty acids were qualitatively and quantitatively markedly affected by CO_2 concentrations ranging from 1% in air to 40%. Expressed as percent dry weight, total lipids range from 12.7% at 1% CO_2 to 17.7% at 40% CO_2. Figure 7 shows total fatty acid versus CO_2 concentration. Comparing this to growth rate, it would seem that after the environmental stress has reached the point where the production of new protoplasm and cell division have been badly affected, carbon assimilation continues, and the carbon can only accumulate as reserve products such as triglycerides.

The authors point out that one may expect to find inhibition of acetyl–CoA production under high CO_2 concentrations, and therefore con-

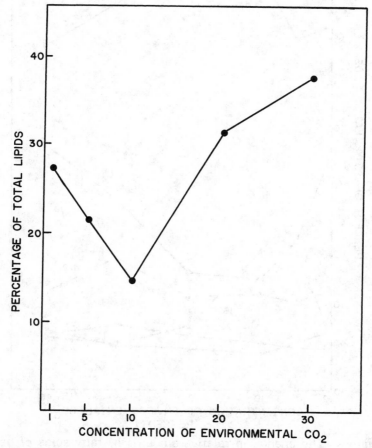

Figure 7 The change in total fatty acids a percent of total lipids of heterotrophic (dark) cultures of *Chlorella fusca* as a function of the concentration of environmental CO_2 (from Dickson, Galloway, and Patterson, 1969).

comitant reduction in fatty acid concentration would be anticipated. That this is the situation in going from 1 to 10% CO_2 supports this idea, but then the trend is sharply reversed. One may conclude that a new source of the precursor is established, or that a different precursor comes into play under these circumstances. Dickson *et al.* (1969) hy-

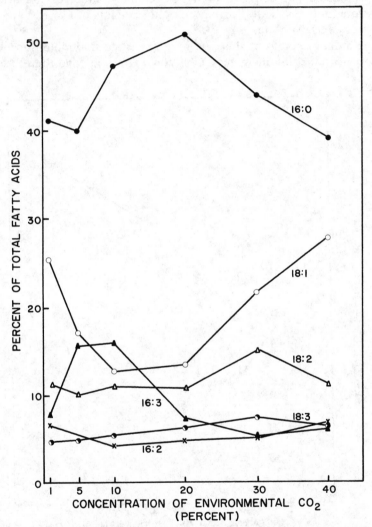

Figure 8 The change in relative amounts of fatty acids of heterotrophic cultures of *Chlorella fusca,* as a function of the concentration (%) of environmental CO_2 (from Dickson, Galloway, and Patterson, 1969).

pothesize that a likely candidate for such a role is glycolic acid. There is no evidence yet to choose between these possibilities for the control of this metabolic pathway. Figure 8 shows the changes in the important individual fatty acids. Here we see that the total change is not simply the sum of the parts, and that the effect is manifested differently on the various fatty acids. Those most affected are the ones in largest concentration, namely 16:0, 18:1, and 18:2.

In a personal communication from D. Orcutt, preliminary experiments seem to indicate that the fatty acid composition of a diatom, *Nitzschia closterium,* is strongly affected, both in quantity and quality, by light. He has shown over 100% difference in the total lipid content by high and low light.

Remarkable response has been seen by Patterson (1969) in the fatty acids of *Chlorella sorokiniana* with regard to culture temperature. This is a high temperature species with 39° as its optimum. Patterson tested responses at seven temperatures, from 14° to 38°. (As you may know, the organism cannot tolerate temperatures much above its optimum, which is why he stopped at 38°.) The effect of temperature on the degree of saturation is marked, as may be seen in Figure 9. Patterson showed that the predominate fatty acids at 38°, 22°, and 14°, respectively, were saturated (46%), triunsaturated (40%), and diunsaturated (47%). Increasing temperature from 14° to 22° resulted in an increase in the degree of unsaturation, and from there to 38° increasing temperature had the opposite effect. Increasing temperature, over this range, always resulted in fatty acids with a lower average chain length, as may be deduced from Figure 10. The C-16, C-18 acids together, each either saturated or with 1,2, or 3 double bonds, accounted for over 95% of the total fatty acids under all conditions. Total fatty acid production was highest at the extremes of the temperature range and lowest in the middle, at 26°. The total fatty acids, expressed as percent dry weight, were as follows: at 14°, 5.8%; 18°, 6.1%; 22°, 2.6%; 26°, 1.3%; 30°, 2.0%; 34°, 3.6%; 38°, 6.1%. Since chain length and the degree of unsaturation both increase going from 22° to 14°, the fatty acids of *C. sorokiniana* do not have an increasingly lower melting point with lower temperatures, which one may have expected. Looking only at these data, it would appear that increasing protoplasmic viscosity would result, but the entire lipid picture must be known before that is certain. At any rate, the effect of temperature is pronounced.

Finally, I'd like to give but a few examples of many such pieces of information obtained recently by MacCarthy (1972) in our laboratory. Again she was working with *C. sorokiniana* examining the effects of cation concentration in the medium on growth and biochemistry. In Figure

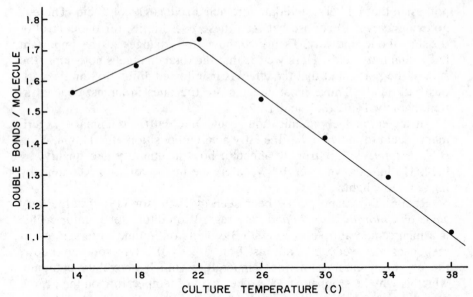

Figure 9 Effect of culture temperature on degree of unsaturation (double bonds per molecule) of *C. sorokiniana* fatty acids (from Patterson, 1969).

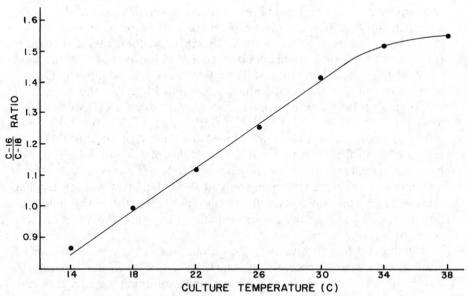

Figure 10 Effect of culture temperature on the C_{16}/C_{18} ratio of *C. sorokiniana* fatty acids (from Patterson, 1969).

11 we see the effect of the concentration of potassium, magnesium, and of calcium on the ratio of unsaturated to saturated fatty acids. In general she found that calcium was without effect on the organism except at toxic levels. Obviously, this is not true for potassium and magnesium. Looking at the same cell fraction, in Figure 12 we see that the effect of concentration levels of one element is very much a function of concen-

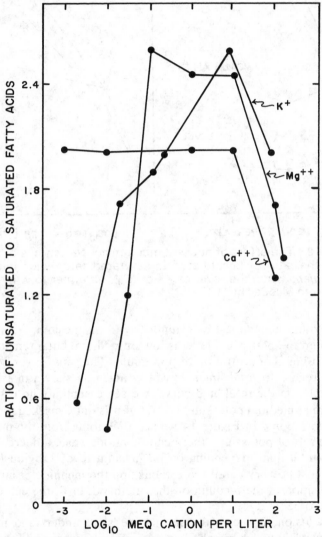

Figure 11 The effect of nutrient medium concentrations of Mg^{2+}, K^+, and Ca^{2+} on the ratio of unsaturated to saturated fatty acids of *Chlorella sorokiniana* in the series experiment (from MacCarthy, 1972).

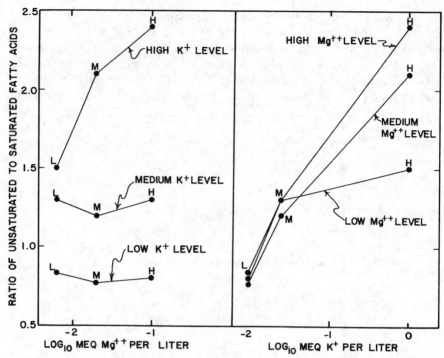

Figure 12 The effect of nutrient medium concentrations of Mg²⁺ and K⁺ on the ratio of unsaturated to saturated fatty acids in *Chlorella sorokiniana* when the level of K⁺ or Mg²⁺ is either low, medium, or high (from MacCarthy, 1972).

tration of other elements. For example, with magnesium, we see no response when the potassium level is low or medium, but a remarkable response in a high concentration of potassium. The same sort of effect occurs with regard to total lipids and fatty acids as shown in Figure 13. For example, on the total lipid curve, we see essentially no response to magnesium at medium potassium level, but it is quite marked at high and low concentrations. In Figure 14 we see that going from the medium to the high levels of potassium, there can be an increase, a decrease, or no change in total lipid, depending on magnesium level. Obviously, in nature one must be very careful in establishing the meaning of analyses of the composition of the medium on the one hand, or of the cell composition on the other.

In conclusion, it seems to me that we shall understand more and more the ways in which metabolic patterns can be warped or changed by environmental parameters in the years ahead. Such studies can serve

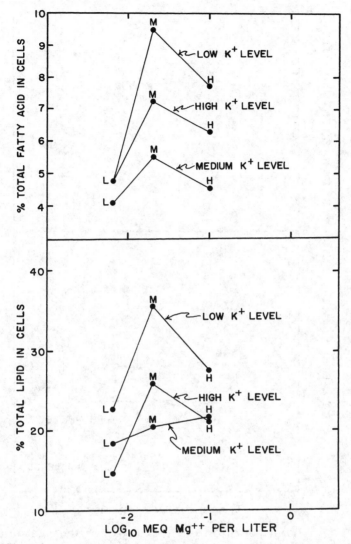

Figure 13 The effect of different Mg²⁺ levels on the total fatty acid and total lipid composition of *Chlorella sorokiniana* when the K⁺ level is either low, medium, or high (from MacCarthy, 1972).

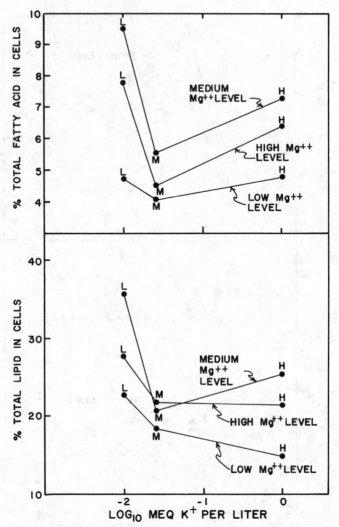

Figure 14 The effect of different K+ levels on the total fatty acid and total lipid composition of *Chlorella sorokiniana* when the Mg²⁺ level is either Low, Medium, or High (from MacCarthy, 1972).

two very useful purposes: (1) they are likely to enhance our understanding of cell chemistry in general; and (2) from a very practical point of view (something not to be taken lightly in these difficult days of grantsmanship) one may well be able to increase the usefulness of an organism to mankind, as a food source, as a producer of some desirable compound or class of compounds or for whatever purpose, by intelligent manipulation of the environment.

References

Dickson, L. G., Galloway, R. A., and Patterson, G. W. (1969). Environmentally-induced changes in the fatty acids of Chlorella. *Plant Physiol.* **44,** 1413–1416.

Galloway, R. A., and Krauss, R. W. (1959a). The differential action of chemical agents, especially polymyxin B, on certain algae, bacteria, and fungi. *Amer. J. Bot.* **46,** 40–49.

Galloway, R. A., and Krauss, R. W. (1959b). Mechanisms of action of polymyxin B on *Chlorella* and *Scenedesmus. Plant Physiol.* **34,** 380–389.

Gross, R. E. (1967). Species stability and the mechanisms of toxicity of D-mannose and certain derivatives in the genus *Chlorella* Beij. Doctoral dissertation, Dep. Bot., Univ. of Maryland, College Park, Maryland.

Krauss, R. W., and McAleer, W. J. (1953). Growth and evolution of species of algae with regard to sterol content. *In* "Algal Culture from Laboratory to Pilot Plant," (by John S. Burlew, ed.) *Carnegie Inst. Washington Publ.,* **600,** 316–325.

MacCarthy, J. J. (1972). The effect of nutrient medium cation levels on the biochemistry of *Chlorella.* Doctoral dissertation, Dep. Bot. Univ. of Maryland, College Park, Maryland.

Patterson, G. W, (1969). Effect of temperature on fatty acid composition of *Chlorella sorokiniana. Lipids* **5,** 597–600.

Sherald, J. L., and Sisler, H. D. (1972). Selective inhibition of antimycin A-insensitive respiration in *Ustilago maydis* and *Ceratocystic ulmi. Plant Cell Physiol.* **13,** 1039–1052.

Spoehr, H. A. and Milner, H. W. (1949). The chemical composition of *Chlorella;* effect of environmental conditions. *Plant Physiol* **24,** 120–149.

von Witsch, H., and Harder, R. (1953). Stoffproducktion durch grunalgen and diatomeen in masskultur. *In* "Algal Culture from Laboratory to Pilot Plant," (John S. Burlew, ed.). *Carnegie Inst. Washington Publ.* **600,** 154–165.

Locomotor Responses to Environmental Variables by Sharks and Teleosts

H. Kleerekoper

*Department of Biology,
Texas A&M University
College Station, Texas*

In quantitative studies of locomotor responses of fishes to environmental variables, it is essential to establish criteria by which the responses can be verified and measured. Generally, physiological, particularly electrophysiological, responses to such variables by individual peripheral receptors are unequivocal and acceptable as reliable criteria for perception in properly controlled experimental conditions.

On the other hand, the locomotor and orientation responses of the unrestrained whole organism are frequently obscure and difficult to analyze since they result from the integration and assessment of many continuously varying bits of information with which the environment bombards the animal incessantly. Only in the most favorable situations the resulting locomotor response may be clear and its analysis "simple." The recently described response of ripe male channel catfish (*Ictalurus punctatus*) to a sex pheromone exuded by ripe females of the species (Timms and Kleerekoper, 1972) is a good example of such a response (Figure 1).

However, in the course of many experiments done in the author's laboratory over several years it has become clear that the directness and clarity of the spectacular response of *Ictalurus punctatus* is exceptional. Rather, locomotor responses to environmental variables, even to those

383

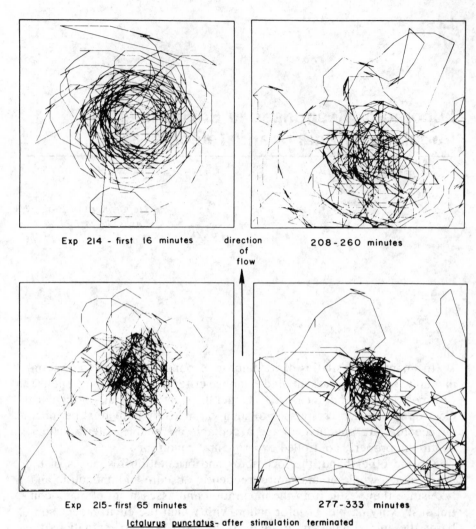

Exp 214 - first 16 minutes   direction   208-260 minutes
                                         of
                                        flow

Exp 215- first 65 minutes   277-333 minutes

Ictalurus punctatus- after stimulation terminated

Figure 1 Two experiments demonstrating the response of male _Ictalurus punctatus_ to lingering traces of a sex pheromone exuded by a female of the species during the breeding season (from Timms and Kleerekoper, 1972).

of great biological import, are often subtle, not readily discernible, and difficult to analyze quantitatively.

A good example of such a situation is illustrated in Figure 2 which represents a plot of the locomotor tract of a nurse shark _(Ginglymostoma cirratum)._ This plot represents the animal's "response"

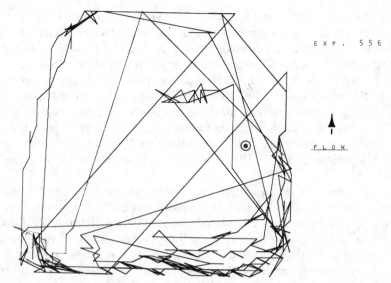

EXP. 556

FLOW

Figure 2 Initial response of *Ginglymostoma cirratum* to an odor (shrimp extract). ⊙ point source of stimulus.

to fresh, filtered extract of the food source (shrimp) to which the animal was accustomed. (Kleerekoper *et al.*, unpublished observations). The extract was introduced at a discrete locus in the floor of the monitor tank. Only during a very short period at the beginning of the release of the extract was there a suggestion of localization of the source. Such a "result" is both unconvincing and unsatisfactory since, one would conclude from the evidence of the plot that chemical stimulation by a food source does not evoke locomotor response. This is contrary to other available evidence regarding not only the species but even the same individual. Instances like this in a variety of experimental conditions have been frequent in our laboratory; they point at the need for additional criteria by which the locomotor behavior in response to environmental variables may be studied quantitatively and in depth.

In the formulation of such criteria the following considerations seemed valid. Locomotion may be quantitatively described by the spatial and temporal distribution of frequency, direction, and magnitude of turns, steps between turns, and velocity (Kleerekoper *et al.*, 1970). Once these variables are known and their mathematical relationships are established, an accurate, quantitative picture can be developed of the locomotor behavior of a fish or any other organisms. The significance of such knowledge is bound to be considerable and may be instrumental in the analysis of fundamental problems, such as the nature of the mechanisms

which control orientated locomotor behavior. However, in the context
of this presentation, it is proposed that a quantitative comparison of the
variables of locomotor behavior during a control period with those resulting from subsequent exposure to environmental changes may provide a sensitive tool for the assessment of responses to the environment
too subtle to be discerned by direct observation or even in tracking records. Some recent experimental results will now be presented in support
of this thesis. Although the two monitor techniques by which the per-
taining data were collected have been described earlier in various papers
(e.g., Kleerekoper, 1967, 1969), a short outline of the methods seems
indicated.

In one method the movements of the fish are monitored in round
tanks, made of acrylic material or stainless steel, 210 cm in diameter, 40
cm deep, and located in chambers under constant lighting. Hollow di-
viders, radially oriented from the periphery, incompletely divide the tank
into 16 compartments, leaving an open area in the center 100 cm in diameter. A central standing pipe serves as an overflow. Each alternate
divider contains a stabilized 6 V light source that, by means of stops,
produces two vertical, adjustable columns of light. Adjustable mirrors
deflect one column to the right and the other to the left, through the
transparent walls of the divider, into the water. Each remaining divider
contains two banks of photoconductive cells, one bank being oriented
toward the light projected from the left, the other toward that from the
right. Thus, each one of the 16 compartments is guarded by a vertical,
eight-cell photoelectric gate, which is triggered by the passage of the
fish. The increase in resistance, which results from the interception of
the light projected onto the photocells, affects an electronic circuit located outside the experimental chamber. The data, representing the number
of the gate and the time of entry or departure, are punched on paper tape
and transposed to magnetic tape for computer processing.

In the second method monitoring of movements is achieved in a
square tank which measures 5.0 by 5.0 by 0.5 m; a square matrix of
1936 photoconductive cells on 10-cm centers is embedded in its bottom.
Interception by the fish of light, projected by a collimated field from a
suspended ceiling above the tank, produces in the photocell affected an
increase in resistance which forms the input to an electronic interface
with an online computer. The latter is programmed to establish the ad-
dress of the photocell in the x, y matrix and the elapsed time from the
start of the experiments. These data are recorded on magnetic tape and
stored on memory disks for the subsequent computation and analysis of
a variety of parameters which characterize locomotor behavior.

In each of the 16 compartments of the multiple choice, round monitors, different chemical and physical conditions can be created to study preference or avoidance behavior in response to single or a wide range of combinations of variables. The locomotor analysis is programmed to supply information on frequency of entries and of time of sojourn in each compartment, the sequence of pathways taken by the fish as it moves between specific compartments, the orientation of that pathway in reference to the compartment of departure, and the time required to move from the compartment of departure to that of destination. Since the monitors can be rotated, geographic and topograhic bias in the movements can be accounted for statistically. All the operations are automated, including the durations of various phases of an experiment either on a time or activity basis.

Recordings of detailed locomotor patterns and of their constituent variables are obtained in the large, square monitor tank which offers no impediments to free, spontaneous locomotion within its boundaries. The flow of water across this monitor is almost perfectly laminar so that chemical conditions can be created in well-defined zones with the large mass of water of this tank. In addition, 200 blunt needles, implanted flush with the floor of the tank in a square matrix, allow for the infusion of chemical stimuli in single or multiple loci to form "trails" in desirable patterns variously oriented with reference to the direction of water flow.

By submitting 17 different locomotor variables to time series and auto regressions analyses, most promising insight has already been obtained into the behavior and interdependence of these variables in the goldfish (Matis *et al.*, 1974 a,b) which was further expanded recently (Matis *et al.*, unpublished).

Some of these techniques were applied to the data of the before-mentioned nurse shark experiment for which the plot of the animal's locomotor track is pictured in Figure 2. Although the locomotor track did not reveal response to the infusion of the shrimp extract, a time series analysis of the distance travelled, carried out by Dr. J. Matis and Mr. D. Childers, yielded clear and significant results. Figure 3 represents the mean distance traveled based on pooled data collected in the monitor tank as a whole, for successive 15-min periods. The arrows indicate the start and finish of the infusion of the extract at the point indicated in Figure 4. Although response of the animal to the stimulus is suggested, it is not conclusive. However, when the data are broken down so as to represent the animal's behavior in four equal quadrants of the monitor tank (Figure 4), significant results are obtained which not only demonstrate response but also reflect effects of the experimental conditions prevailing in these quadrants. Figure 5 clearly illustrates the differences in behavior in the four quadrants of which 1 and 2 are upstream, 3 and 4

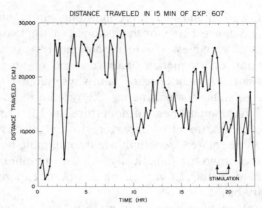

DISTANCE TRAVELED IN 15 MIN OF EXP. 607

Figure 3 Time series analysis of the distance traveled by *Ginglymostoma cirratum* in the monitor tank as a whole during 24 hr. Arrows indicate the period of release of food odor at a point source in
the floor of the tank.

downstream of the stimulus source. This analytic technique is now being
used to ascertain the accuracy with which the animals are able to locate
the source of the stimulus as a function of the interaction between flow
and chemical stimulus.

Notable is a prolonged initial exploratory phase following the introduction of an animal into the monitor tank. In this and all other shark
experiments, to be reported elsewhere, this phase lasts between 5–6 hr,
whereas in the goldfish this initial phase is very much shorter

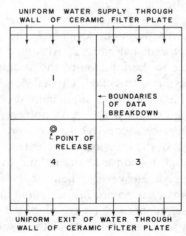

UNIFORM WATER SUPPLY THROUGH
WALL OF CERAMIC FILTER PLATE

Figure 4 ◎ Point of release of the food odor in relation to the direction of water flow.

% DISTANCE TRAVELED IN 15-MIN INTERVALS OF EXP. 607 QUADRANTS

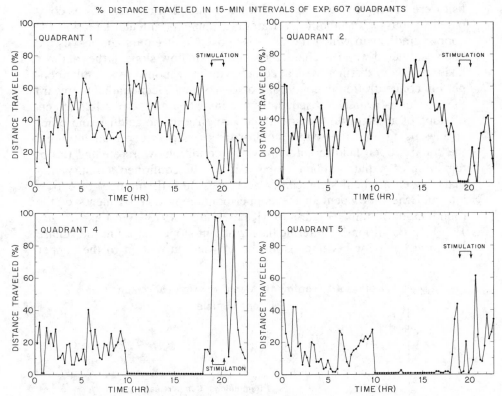

Figure 5 Time series analysis of the data of Figure 3 broken down for the four quadrants of the tank shown in Figure 4.

(Kleerekoper *et al.*, 1974). Attention is drawn here to this phenomenon since all available evidence points to the strong effect of the exploratory phase on locomotor characteristics and to the great likelihood that during this phase locomotor response to environmental variables may be quite different from that during later periods. The characteristics of exploratory behavior in sharks continues to be investigated in this laboratory.

Further complexities in our studies on locomotor response to various environmental conditions were found in the much neglected area of interaction of stimuli. In various recent papers we reported on the orientated response of some teleosts to subacute concentrations of copper ions. Our initial findings (Kleerekoper *et al.*, 1972), from experiments done in the square monitor tank, seemed at variance with results previously reported by others in that in free choice, open field situations, the fish were "attracted" to a mass of water containing copper ions as compared to masses of laboratory water. In our experimental situation the copper gradient to which the fish is exposed as it enters and leaves the copper-affected water is characterized by a shallow slope. Other authors had found very distinct avoidance behavior in response to a similar copper ion concentration in conditions of very sharp, steep gradients toward the laboratory water. Subsequently, we investigated the possible effects of slope of gradient on the orientated response in the goldfish and other species using both the round monitor tank (sharp, steep gradients) and the square, open field monitor in which conditions were created to obtain an intermediate gradient slope. The results confirmed our suspicion that a steep gradient significantly decreases both the number of entries into and the time spent in the copper-containing compartments of the round monitor tank (Figure 6) (Kleerekoper, 1973; Westlake *et al.,* 1974). In conditions of intermediate gradient slope, set up in the square tank, the behavior became again one of weak attraction to the copper

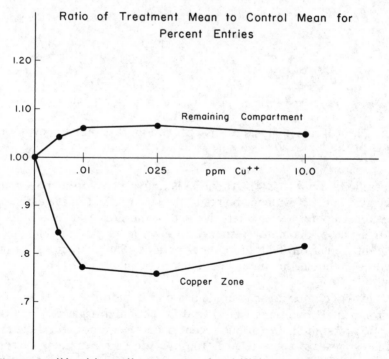

Figure 6 "Avoidance" response of goldfish to copper ions at various concentrations forming steep gradients with the surrounding mass of "clean" water (from Westlake *et al.,*1974).

zone. It is obvious that much more attention should be paid to these ubiquitous environmental variables of water flow and chemical stimulations as interacting stimuli.

I should like to terminate this presentation with still another recent example of the complexities of our problem. We just saw that a copper containing mass of water is avoided by goldfish and other species provided that the gradient of the copper ion concentration is steep. However,

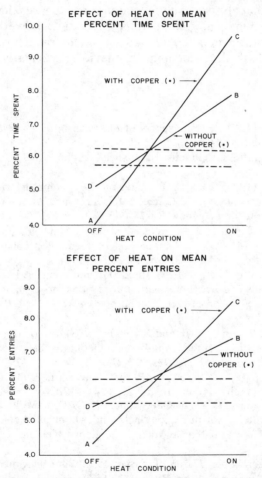

Figures 7 and 8 The effect of the interaction of temperature and copper ions on the orientation behavior of goldfish. Copper ions alone are avoided (A) but a concurrent elevation of the temperature of the water by 0.4°C produces strong attraction (C) (from Kleere-koper *et al.*, 1973).

a slight increase in temperature, from 21.0° to 21.4°C, turns the originally repulsive mass of copper water significantly attractive although the temperature increase alone, that is, in the absence of the copper ion, is only slightly more attractive than the surrounding laboratory water at 21.0°C. The interaction of the two variables is rather spectacular (Figures 7 and 8; Kleerekoper *et al.*, 1973). It is concluded from the preceding examples that the quantitative assessment of the variables which together characterize locomotor behavior may constitute a valuable tool for the recognition and analysis of subtle locomotor responses, including orientation, to environmental stimuli. It is imperative, however, that much more precise information be gathered on the interaction of environmental variables as stimuli for locomotor behavior, particularly orientation.

References

Kleerekoper, H. (1967). Some aspects of olfaction in fishes, with special reference to orientation. *Amer. Zool.* **7,** 385 – 395.

Kleerekoper, H. (1969). "Olfaction in Fishes." Indiana Univ. Press. Bloomington, Indiana.

Kleerekoper, H. (1973). Effects of copper on the locomotor orientation of fish. Ecological Research Series. Office of Research and Monitoring. U.S. Environmental Protection Agency, R3-73-045.

Kleerekoper, H., Timms, A. M., Westlake, G. F., Davy, F. B., Malar, T., and Anderson, V. M. (1970). An analysis of locomotor behavior of goldfish *(Carassius auratus).* *Anim. Behav.* **18,** 317 – 330.

Kleerekoper, H., Westlake, G. F., Matis, J. H., and Gensler, P. J. (1972). Orientation of goldfish *(Carassius auratus)* in response to a shallow gradient of a sublethal concentration of copper in an open field. *J. Fish. Res. Bd. Can.* **29,** 45 – 54.

Kleerekoper, H., Waxman, J. B. and Matis, J. (1973). Interaction of temperature and copper ions as orienting stimuli in the locomotor behavior of the goldfish *(Carassius auratus).* *J. Fish. Res. Bd. Can.* **30,** 725 – 728.

Kleerekoper, H., Matis, J., Gensler, P., and Maynard, P. (1974). Exploratory behaviour of goldfish. *Anim. Behav.* **22,** 124 – 132.

Matis, J. H., Childers, D., and Kleerekoper, H. (1973). Multivariable multilag models of fish behavior in an open field under controlled conditions. Biometrics Society, Western North America Regional Meeting, U. Utah. *Biometrics* **29,** 611.

Matis, J. H., Kleerekoper, H., and Gensler, P. (1974a). Nonrandom changes in orientation of goldfish. *Anim. Behav.* **22,** 110 – 117.

Matis, J., H. Kleerekoper, and P. Gensler. (1974b). A time series analysis of some aspects of locomotor behavior of goldfish *(Carassius auratus).* J. Interdiscipl. *Cycle Res.,* **4,** 145 – 158.

Timms, A. M., and Kleerekoper, H. (1972). The locomotor responses of male

Ictalurus punctatus, the channel catfish, to a pheromone released by the ripe female of the species. *Trans. Amer. Fish. Soc.* 302–310.

Westlake, G. F., Kleerekoper, H., and Matis, J. (1974). The locomotor response to a steep gradient of copper ions by the goldfish. *J. Water Resourc. Res.* **10,** 103–105.

Respiratory Adaptations of Aquatic Animals

John L. Roberts

Department of Zoology
University of Massachusetts
Amherst, Massachusetts

Introduction

I find it refreshing as a comparative physiologist to occasionally read again the old reviews of G. S. Carter, August Krogh, and A. S. Pearse on respiratory adaptations (1931, 1941, 1950, respectively). When I do this, I begin to wonder again how we are doing since their times in answering the why, when, and how questions about respiratory mechanisms and their role in "the emigration of animals from the sea."

Professor Carter's comment of 1931 still is pertinent;

> the respiratory organs of animals are fundamentally all built on the same plan. In all, the surface of an epithelium is brought into contact with the medium, and, whenever the animal possesses a respiratory circulation, a rich supply of the blood is brought very close to the surface of this epithelium, either in capillaries or in intercellular spaces. The respiratory exchange is carried out across the thin layer separating the blood from the surrounding medium. So far lungs and gills are similar, but it is when the conditions outside the surface of the epithelium are considered that the differences in the physiology of the two organs become apparent.

These differences, as Carter recognizes, have come about through

the "cut and try" processes of evolution to protect the respiratory surface, and the animal, from desiccation, and to provide ventilation for the
respiratory surfaces of the more advanced and active animals at the least
possible metabolic cost. He also notes that whether the respiratory epithelium is damp from a covering film of water as is true of lungs or is
washed by a respiratory current as at gill surfaces, the same process of
gaseous exchange down partial-pressure gradients in a solution governs
both. It means that rates of oxygen delivery at the wet exchange surface
of the respiratory organs are the same for respiratory streams of air-saturated water and air, despite the large absolute differences in amounts of
oxygen present per unit volume of air and water.

The practical problem of maintaining a specific metabolic rate differs
greatly, however, between an animal breathing in air and one breathing
water. For example, the amphibious shore crab *Carcinus maenus* must
ventilate a far larger volume of water through its gill chambers when
below tidal level to obtain a milligram of oxygen than the volume of air it
needs to ventilate when scrabbling about on the rocks above tidal level.
Expressed as a ratio, the availability of oxygen to this crab in air versus
air-saturated seawater at 20°C is 15:1.

Having set the scene, it is plain for at least the reason already stated:
ventilation of gills in water must be a laborious activity compared to
breathing in air. Other functions, such as water and ion regulation,
blood-gas transport, anaerobiosis, nitrogen excretion, and reproduction,
have also been intimately tied to the respiratory adaptations under consideration, but these will only be touched lightly as the space limitations
permit. I will not attempt to trace very far the succession in respiratory
remodeling that has led some arthropods, gastropods, and higher vertebrates to forsake aquatic life for a life on land. Yet, I shall point out now
that "relief" from the respiratory work load of aquatic life must have
been a potent stimulus to niche-selection processes in terrestrial colonization as exemplified here for the decapod crustaceans and fish.

Many of the topics that will be covered have been reviewed by Ballintijn (1972), Bliss (1968), Edney (1960), Hughes (1963, 1972), Hughes
and Shelton (1962), Johansen (1970, 1971), Randall (1970), Shelton
(1970), Steen (1971), and Wolvekamp and Waterman (1960).

Properties of Respiratory Fluids

At any one moment in the life of an animal when it is actively respir-
ing by propelling a fluid (air or water) over its respiratory surfaces, most
all of its effort expended appears as frictional losses. Some energy is also

dissipated as losses due to acceleration and absorption in elastic elements. The latter two kinds of energy loss probably are small for gill breathers in water or air because the gill sieve typically is a through-flow system with stops, restarts, and coughs that ordinarily do not sum to more than 10% of a respiratory period or cycle. On the other hand, energy losses to elastic elements in tidal ventilation of lungs assumes an importance equal to frictional losses, partly because air is much less dense and viscous than water, and partly because a large mass of tissue is stretched by lung inflation (Hildebrandt and Young, 1965).

The magnitude of difference in the respiratory energetics of moving air versus water and the physical properties of the two media suggest at first sight that gill respiration in water is an impossible task. For example, at 20°C the diffusion rate of oxygen in air is about 300,000 times faster than in water. Water density is higher than air by about 900 times, and water is about 56 times more viscous. How was the problem solved by the "cut and try" engineering processes of evolution? One answer is that it took time, something like 500 million years. The best answer for the diffusion problem at the moment is that it has been solved by assurance in design, of a very intimate contact between the active respiratory surfaces of the gill and the respiratory current (Steen and Berg, 1966). The sieve pores or spaces between exchange surfaces, the secondary lamellae, are no wider in many fish than 0.02 mm (Hughes, 1966), and the diffusion path through the epithelium between the water and the blood may be as short in some tunas as 0.5 μm (Hughes, 1970).

Several years ago G. M. Hughes and I discussed the physical properties of water in terms of positive and negative interactions with the increasing metabolic needs of rainbow trout, *Salmo gairneri*, warmed from 5° to 25°C (Hughes and Roberts, 1970). This same analysis shown in Figure 1 should be equally valid for the aquatic gill respiration of other animals. On balance, the drop in viscosity of water is the only change in physical parameters that can significantly offset the increasing metabolic load as the temperature rises. We know that blood viscosity changes in a like fashion to water as temperature changes (Burton, 1965) so a positive relief to the cardiac workload should occur as well (Jones, 1971). The two "opposites" shown in Figure 1, diffusion rate and the absorption coefficient of oxygen in water (α), more or less cancel out as the temperature changes. Their product, the permeation coefficient, changes very little. It is this term that is the more useful to describe the availability of oxygen to animals and its transport to their cells.

When what is known and not known about physical parameters is considered along with the tendency of animals to integrate changes in their physical environments with the different accommodations available

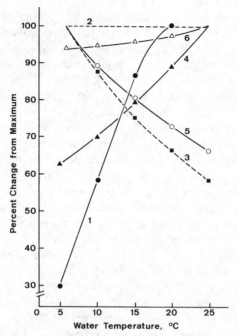

Figure 1 Effects of temperature change on the respiration rate of the brook trout, *Salvelinus fontinalis,* and several properties of water given as percentages of maximal values and numbered: (1) trout respiration rate; (2) density; (3) viscosity; (4) oxygen diffusion rate in water, *D;* (5) oxygen absorption coefficient in water, α; (6) oxygen permeation coefficient, *D'*, the product of $\alpha \times D$. (Redrawn from Hughes and Roberts, 1970.)

to them, the comprehensive evaluation of any one factor is difficult. The balance sheet for the thermal effects and interactions described is still incomplete (see also Hills and Hughes, 1970; Rahn, 1966; Randall, 1970; Steen, 1971).

Gill Structure

Decapod Crustaceans

Gills generally do not adapt well for aerial respiration. It is not surprising for the gill structure, which can be either filamentous (decapods) or lamellate (decapods, fish), is designed as a fragile water sieve with a very large surface area presented to the respiratory stream, but a very small volume (Figure 2). When gill-breathing animals are lifted out of

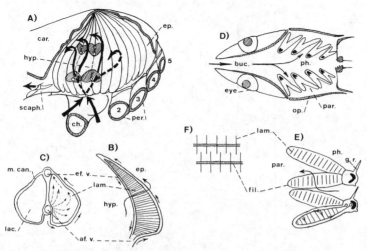

Figure 2 The circulatory patterns of water and blood through the gills of a decapod crustacean *(Carcinus maenus)* (A–C), and an idealized fish (D–F). Details of phyllobranch structure are given in frontal view (B), and in cross section along the axis to show the lateral lamellae (C), and the lamellar circulation. Similar details are shown for two gill arches (E), and the demibranch stacks of filaments bearing the lamellae (E, F). Abbreviations are: car., carapace (shown partially dissected); ch. bases; per. 2, 3, 4, 5, pereiopod bases; scaph., scaphognathite; ep. and hyp., epi- and hypobranchial chambers; lam., lamellae; af. v. and ef. v., afferent and efferent blood vessels; m. can., marginal canal; lac., intralamellar lacunae (blood spaces); buc. and ph., buccal and pharyngeal chambers; op., operculum; par., parabranchial chamber; g. r., gill raker. Counter flow patterns of water and blood occur at the lamellar exchange surfaces in both crabs and fish. (Redrawn from Alexander, 1970; Drach, 1930; Hughes *et al.,* 1969.)

water, the gills of most slump due to capillarity and their own water-sodden weight. Thus the exchange surface is at once reduced and unsatisfactory for aerial respiration.

Some crabs and a few fish show gill modifications that partially protect the gills from collapse when they emerge from water and resort to aerial breathing (crabs, Wolvekamp and Waterman, 1960; fishes, Steen, 1971). The cuticular structure of the gills in amphibious crabs has been claimed to be more rigid (Raffey, cited by Krogh, 1941). But, the general trend among the semiterrestrial decapods has been a reduction in the gill number and gill surface area, and the adoption of a variety of conservative alternatives of not very remarkable character (Carter, 1931; Edney, 1960). Comparisons of the branchial adaptations for a selected group of

Table 1 Habits and Gill Surface Areas of Various Crabs and Fish[a]

Species (family, and common name)	Gill area (cm² · g⁻¹)	Habits	Respiratory modifications
Crabs (Decapoda)			
Callinectes sapidus (Portunidae), blue crab	13.67	Aquatic, burrowing open sea, estuarine, very active	
Libinia emarginata (Inchidae), spider crab	5.66	Aquatic, benthic, open sea, sluggish	
Panopeus herbstii (Xanthidae), mud crab	8.74	Amphibious, burrowing, oyster beds, crevices, moderately active	
Uca pugilator (Ocypodidae), sand fiddler crab	6.24	Amphibious, burrowing, sandy beaches, very active	Branchial troughs for water retention; branchial wall vascularization
Uca minax (Ocypodidae), fiddler crab	5.13	Amphibious, burrowing, salt marsh banks, very active	Branchial troughs for water retention; branchial wall vascularization
Ocypode albicans (Ocypodidae), ghost crab	3.25	Terrestrial, burrows in dunes, night, active	Spongy masses for water retention in branchial wall; branchial vascularization

Fishes			
Euthynnus pelamis (Scombridae), skipjack tuna	13.20	Aquatic, open ocean very active, pelagic	Ram ventilator and obligate swimmer
Coryphaena sp. (Coryphaenidae), dolphin	3.70	Aquatic, open ocean, very active, pelagic	
Stenotomus crysos (Sparidae), scup	5.06	Aquatic, midwater, open ocean, active	Ram ventilator
Pleuronectes platessa (Pleuronectidae), plaice	4.33	Aquatic, benthic, sandy bottom, active	
Callionomus lyra (Callionymidae), dragonet	2.92	Aquatic, benthic, open ocean, moderately active	Opercular tube, directs excurrent respiratory stream upward
Opsaunus tau (Batrachoididae), oyster toadfish	2.14	Aquatic, benthic in oyster beds, sluggish	Withstands low P_{O_2} habitats at low tide exposure, respiratory conformer
Anabas testudineus (Anabantidae), climbing perch	1.50	Amphibious, wet season migratory, moderately active	Air labyrinth, gulps air, CO_2 eliminated via gills

[a]References: Gray (1957); Hughes (1970); Hughes and Gray (1972).

crab and fish species are given in Table 1 along with comments on their habits and dependence upon free water. Source references are listed in table footnotes.

The adaptive modifications seen in crabs are of three sorts (Carter, 1931): avoidance of gill desiccation by special means to retain branchial chamber water; elaboration of the vascularized branchial epithelium in the form of complex folds and tufts to compensate for gill reduction; and airflow facilitation by expansions of the epibranchial parts of the gill cavities, and formation of special incurrent openings posteriorly (also hinging up the posterior carapace margin when in air; Wolvekamp and Waterman, 1960). Clearly, most of the respiratory adaptations in crabs center on protection against water loss (also see Bliss, 1968). No detailed studies on gill morphometrics that have been as useful to the study of gill function in fishes are available at present for any of the decapods.

Fishes

When most fish are lifted out of water, they suffer all of the problems of a "fish out of water." Yet a small number of species are able to make use of aerial respiration when stranded during a dry season or when the P_{O_2} in eutrophic ponds and swamps drops and the P_{CO_2} rises to intolerable levels. Johansen (1970, 1971) and Steen (1971) identify four categories for the respiratory adaptations found in these amphibious fishes. These follow as listed by Steen:

1. *Mouth breathers* with increased vascularization of mouth and pharynx,
2. *Intestinal breathers* with increased vascularization of the gastrointestinal tract,
3. *Bladder breathers* with a swim bladder supplied with postbranchial blood, and
4. *Lung breathers* with a lung supplied with prebranchial blood.

Modifications of the general type of the first group are the most diverse and most commonly encountered (Johansen, 1970). Special alternating arrangements of gill filaments and shaping of the gill lamellae that serve to reduce the slump effect in air are found in a few species (Carter and Beadle, cited by Johansen, 1970). The best known fish of this group is the electric eel, *Electrophorus electricus*. Its gills are so reduced as to be essentially useless (Johansen, 1970).

Comparisons of the respiratory techniques exploited by the mouth breathing fish and the amphibious crabs reveals a striking convergence in function and morphology just as does a comparison between gill breathing fish generally, and the more active higher invertebrates that utilize active gill ventilation (Johansen *et al.*, 1970). As among the air breathing decapods, the development of aerial respiration by fish seems to have evolved in niche selection as a means to escape oxygen lack in poor quality respiratory environments and also to avoid desiccation.

Reduction in the exchange surface area of gills is an identifiable trend in the air-breathing fish as well (Johansen, 1970). On the other hand, expansion of the available exchange surface seems to have followed with the evolution of fishes adapted to high-speed swimming (Table 1). In fact, the progression of increase in gill surface per unit body weight directly relates to the metabolic demands of activity in different habitats, from lowest to highest in the order: benthic, midwater, pelagic (Hughes, 1970; Hughes and Gray, 1972). Morphologically, the surface area is a function of gill filament and lamellar spacing as well as the lengths of individual lamellae, and the total surface is inversely related to body size within a species (Hughes, 1966, 1970; Steen and Berg, 1966). Other area-related progressions in the structural design of gills also are apparent. The detailed morphometric observations of Hughes and of Steen and Berg have shown that structural elements of the lamellae separating the blood and water tend to thin out as the effective gaseous exchange area increases. This factor too follows the several trends relating habitat selection and activity as illustrated in Figure 3. A marked divergence in respiratory adaptations also followed penetration of fishes into oxygen-poor waters. The climbing perch (*Anabas* sp., Figure 3) has a very thick lamellar epithelium in common with other amphibious fish equipped with accessory air-breathing organs (Johansen, 1971). Most species that have remained aquatic seem to have maintained a short diffusion barrier between water and blood. The toadfish gill with very thick lamellae is exceptional, but the toadfish also happens to be a respiratory conformer (Hughes and Gray, 1972).

The result of Hughes' analyses of gill structure in sluggish to active fishes shows that very active pelagic life (e.g., Scombridae) has required a compromise that follows the need for large-area gills, low resistance to flow of the respiratory stream, and space limitations in the branchial chambers of a fish with a compact body of optimal hydrodynamic shape. The gills of scombrids are large, but do offer a high resistance to flow. Yet the lamellae are dimensionally smaller than those of less-active species on that the sieve pores are both smaller in cross-sectional area and shorter (Hughes, 1970). Whether or not another compromise has occurred in the scombrids, namely, acceptance of a high water pressure to overcome the greater calculated gill resistance to flow, is an unresolved question. Calculations by Brown and Muir (1970) show that the respira-

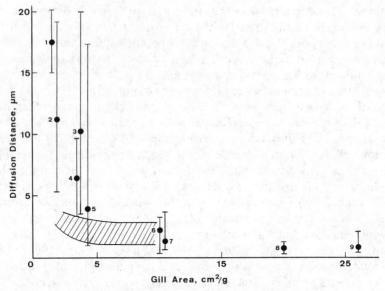

Figure 3 Total gill area per unit body weight (cm² · g⁻¹) and estimated diffusion distance through lamellar tissue between water and blood for fish with differing niches. Means and ranges measured from gill electronmicrographs. Cross-hatched area represents the relations known for other teleost and elasmobranch species. Numerical identifications are: 1, climbing perch, *Anabas* sp.; 2, spotted dogfish, *Scyliorhinus* sp.; 3, piked dogfish, *Squalus acanthias;* 4, trout; 5, plaice, *Pleuronectes platessa;* 6, horse mackerel, *Trachurus* sp.; 7, mackerel, *Scomber* sp.; 8, yellowfin tuna, *Thunnus albacares;* 9, skipjack tuna, *Euthynnus pelamis.* (From Hughes, 1970.)

tory needs of the skipjack tuna *Katsuwonus pelamis* can be met conservatively when swimming by conversion to ram ventilation (see later section). Their estimate indicates that the across-gill pressure required for basal-speed swimming maintenance need be no higher than that measured in other, actively ventilating fish at rest.

Respiratory Functions of Gills

General Comments

The single best indicator that the metabolic load imposed by breathing water versus air is, of course, the absolute volume difference of oxygen in these two media as earlier mentioned. Critical to the argument is the ventilation efficiency of handling air as opposed to water. Pump mechanics for tidal ventilation of air in and out of vertebrate lungs, and branchial ventilation of water through the gills of crabs and fish, suggest that both systems are nearly ideal for pumping at low velocities and pressure heads. Slippage losses should be minimal on the basis of design, in one case for moving a low-density, low-viscosity fluid, and in the other, for pumping a fluid of relatively high density and viscosity. The energy loss due to slippage by the scaphognathite propellers of crabs has not been analyzed, but I would expect these devices to be poor-quality pumps for propelling air in a crab out of water. However, their main function in air may be to maintain air and water turbulence in the branchial chambers, to throw water over the gills, and allow gaseous diffusion around the open margins of the carapace (see also Wolvekamp and Waterman, 1960).

Ventilation-Perfusion Ratios

Another indicator of the work of ventilation is the ventilation-perfusion ratio. It is of more direct physiological interest because it is an expression of the ratio between volumes of respiratory medium ventilated and the blood flow past the respiratory epithelium per unit of time. The perfusion ratio for man and most mammals at rest is 1:1. Ratios established for a few fish are much larger, usually not less than 10:1. The only value that has been reported for a decapod crustacean is 21:8 (Johansen *et al.*, 1970). An interesting case is the antarctic icefish *Chaenocephalus aceratus*. It is a hemoglobinless fish, but only subject to the small temperature variations that occur in the antarctic seas, from − 0.8° to 1.6°C. Holeton (1970) found a resting perfusion ratio of only 3:1 or considerably less than ratios established for other fish. The explanation based on Rahn's arguments (1966), is straightforward. If a high perfusion ratio is characteristic of aquatic gill breathers, the only way the ratio could be dropped significantly would be for the rate of blood circulation to be somehow increased. Holeton reports that these fish have unusually large hearts, lower than usual systolic blood pressures, large stroke volumes, and they have much reduced the vascular resistance to flow through the gill lamellae. All of these observations do indeed favor the conclusion that the low perfusion ratio is an adaptation for fast circulation of a blood with a low oxygen-carrying capacity.

Extraction Efficiency of Gills

Clearly, the main function served by the well-known counter flows of the respiratory stream and the blood past the diffusion barrier that constitutes the total respiratory surface, is the exchange of oxygen and carbon dioxide. The ventilation-perfusion ratio is one index, but another is needed if the overall degree of success in gas transfer to the blood is to be calculated. This is the percent utilization of oxygen present in the respiratory medium. Functionally, percent utilization is the ratio of the P_{O_2} measured in the incurrent and excurrent respiratory streams. However, it is not a precise statement about oxygen transfer to the blood at any one site on a respiratory surface; nor, does it give adequate information about the dynamic efficiency of loading the respiratory pigment. This is the reason that water flow within the gill chamber and gill perfusion by blood are processes complicated by turbulence, nonuniform flow and by shunting (bypass flow). Further, these factors are importantly conditioned by branchial morphology and by body size. The percent, utilization is relatively easily monitored and has great utility for deriving other terms. of use to the respiratory physiologist by application of the Fick principle (see also Hughes, 1972; Johansen et al., 1970; Randall, 1970; Steen, 1971).

Gill systems of fish usually have higher extraction efficiencies than lung systems of other vertebrates at rest. For man, the figure is about 25% at rest, but it improves with exercise as the ventilation-perfusion ratio sharply rises (Guyton, 1966). The gill system of fish contrasts dramatically, in that relatively high percent utilizations, ranging from 40 to 80% have been determined for resting fish, but the figures fall rapidly as activity levels increase (Ballintijn, 1972; Hughes, 1964, 1966; Rahn, 1966; Shelton, 1970). The reasons for the decline in efficiency of gill systems have been well considered by Hughes (1966) and more recently by Ballintijn (1972). The consequence, however, is clear: as activity increases gill ventilation imposes an increasingly heavy metabolic load upon the life of a gill breather.

The Work Load of Gill Ventilation

Estimations of how large a work load gill ventilation adds to the metabolic budget of a fish have been subject to much disagreement (Alexander, 1970; Ballintijn, 1972; Cameron and Cech, 1970; Johansen, 1971; Jones, 1971; Shelton, 1970). No one disputes the view that the work load of ventilation increases out of proportion with the energy load of swimming. The estimates range widely for the resting condition, and it should be pointed out that even the approximation for man, about 2%, is in doubt (Hildebrandt and Young, 1965). The low resting estimate for fish is 0.5% (Alexander, 1970) and almost certainly, it is too low to be given serious consideration (Ballintijn, 1972). Other estimates range from 18 to 43% (Schumann and Piiper, 1966), and from 5 to 15% (Cameron and Cech, 1970). Ballentijn estimates the resting cost of ventilation to metabolism of fish versus the cost to man to range from 3.5 to 9 times. Recall that both the ventilation-perfusion ratio and the percent

utilization values for fish greatly exceed those for man and, further, that
an unfavorable oxygen volume ratio exists between air and water. The
fact then becomes more obvious that the gill breather has a very efficient
respiratory mechanism just as long as activity is kept minimal.

Evidence suitable for estimating the work of breathing in invertebrates is scanty. Newell *et al.* (1972) have reported that the respiration
of the shore crab *Carcinus maenus* is about 16% less in air than in water.
Most of the difference probably can be attributed to the ventilation-perfusion work expenditure in aquatic respiration. Another study by Johansen *et al.* (1970) indicates that the ventilation-perfusion ratio of the large
aquatic crab *Cancer magister* is about 22 and the percent utilization
about 18. Allowing for the less efficient ventilatory system of a crab
(Hughes *et al.*, 1969), the approximation of 16% cost of ventilation to
the resting metabolic budget of a crab seems reasonable. The studies of
Arudpragasam and Naylor (1964) and Hughes *et al.* (1969) both have
revealed an oxygen extraction efficiency of 10–20% in the branchial
chambers of inactive *Carcinus*.

Compensations for Ventilation Work Load and Habitat

General Comments

If the activity behavior of marine fish is examined along with the design and function of the branchial apparatus, my contention that niche
selection has been influenced by the high metabolic cost of gill ventilation gains additional support. Benthic fish typically depend largely on the
opercular phase of ventilatory cycles (Hughes, 1960). In animals, like
the sculpin *Myoxocephalus octodecimspinosus* or the toadfish *Opsanus
tau*, the opercular aspiration phases may approach 90% or better of single cycles when the fish are quiet and left undisturbed. Ventilation in
pelagic fish contrasts markedly for they either depend largely on the
buccal force pump to overcome gill resistance to flow or, like most midwater fish, they rely on the balanced action of both pumps. The aspiration function of the opercular pump in benthic species is greatly facilitated by extensive development of the branchiostegal apparatus that bal-
loons out during opercular aspiration to allow the peribranchial spaces to
expand many times over their volume at the beginning of the opercular
phase. Only remnants of the branchiostegal rays remain in association
with the opercular doors of fast midwater and pelagic species
(McAllister, 1968). Figure 4 illustrates another functional difference related to activity of the respiratory pumps. Resting respiratory cycles
range in frequency as might be expected for fish in different environments: the longest cycles are found in benthic species and the shortest in

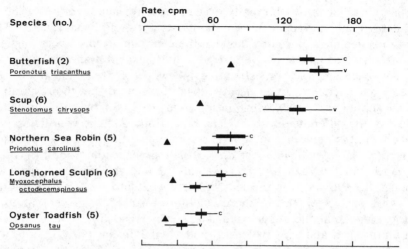

Figure 4 Comparisons of cardiac (c) and opercular ventilation (v) rate of marine fishes with differing niches. The rate functions were recorded via indwelling ECG electrodes from resting fish after recover from anesthesia. Triangles (▲) represent means of the lowest ventilation rates visually recorded from undisturbed fish in the display tanks, Aquarium, National Marine Fisheries Service, Woods Hole, Massachusetts. Means (thin vertical lines) are shown with ± S.D. (thin horizontal lines) and ± 2 S.E. (thick horizontal bars). (From Sister Mary Arthur Logan and J. L. Roberts, unpublished.)

midwater and pelagic fishes (see also, Hughes, 1960, 1963). Cardiac rates show the same trend but, proportionately, the difference in the range of cardiac frequencies is not as large so that heart rates of benthic species at rest generally are faster than their opercular rates.

Active and Passive Gill Ventilation

A compromise in the selection of the life habits of fishes may have been necessitated by the low efficiency of gill ventilation at such a time when a fish becomes active and swims at moderate to high velocities. This is the transition from active ventilation to passive or ram ventilation that is now known to occur when many marine fish reach a swimming velocity that will generate sufficient pressure at the open mouth to ventilate the gills (Roberts, 1970). This "different" mode of ventilation was first experimentally verified by Hall in 1931 (see Heath, 1973; Johansen, 1971). He found the Atlantic mackerel, *Scomber scombrus*, which were retarded in swimming by towing Erhlenmeyer flasks, could not load their hemoglobin to normal levels. He surmised, in part from visual observations, that adult mackerel are unable to survive while standing "dead in the water" or at slow swimming speeds because the active ventilation mode has somehow been "lost" by this continuous swimmer. Other scombrid fishes, the tunas, also seem only to use passive ventilation routinely for they too are obligate swimmers under usual circumstances (Brown and Muir, 1970; Magnuson, 1970).

Muir and Buckley (1967) added to the growing list of fish known to ram ventilate, with their description of the very unusual habits of the small shark sucker *Remora remora*. It ram ventilates only when "hitching" a ride on a porpoise, shark, or other convenient, large passer-by (Figure 5). The shark sucker begins to drop its ventilation rate as the water velocity reaches 50 cm · sec^{-1}. All remoras tested by Muir and Buckley completed the transition between modes by the time the water flow in their swimming tunnel reached 80 cm · sec^{-1}.

My own experiments have added three more species of fish to the list of ram ventilators, but not one of the striped mullets *Mugil cephalus* that were used gave any indication of conversion to ram ventilation at the maximum velocity attainable in my apparatus. The results are shown in

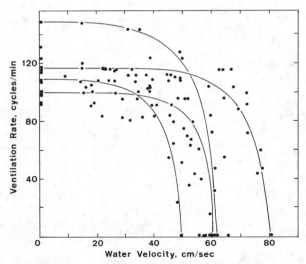

Figure 5 Ventilation rates recorded from shark suckers *Remora remora* attached to the sides of a Plexiglas water tunnel as the water flow was increased from 0 to 80 cm · sec^{-1}. Scatter data from six fish on one or several days. Eye-fitted curves represent patterns of rate change (drop-out of single cycles) for four fish with the highest and lowest resting rates, and the highest and lowest final velocities for the completion of the transition from active to passive ventilation. (Redrawn from Muir and Buckley, 1967.)

Figure 6 with velocity ranges and median values for the ventilatory transitions to the passive mode. Other features dealing with the possible control for the inhibition of rhythmic ventilation are to be considered elsewhere, but I should point out that the four species of ram ventilators shown, unlike the *Remora*, must be swimming for the transition to occur. Bypass flow at a velocity adequate to support passive ventilation does not induce the transition in any of the species listed in Figure 6 unless they are swimming.

The advantage gained by ram ventilational most certainly is a reduction in the metabolic cost of ventilation. It is also likely, but as yet not directly verified, that the buccal-opercular pump system, as it has evolved in teleosts, fails in its basic design concept to meet the metabolic needs of the high-speed swimmers among pelagic fishes. According to Magnuson (1970), scombrid fish must swim at speeds exceeding requirements for ram ventilation just to maintain hydrostatic equilibrium once they attain a body size of about 20 cm fork-length. The reason is simple. They are negatively buoyant because their swim bladders are reduced or

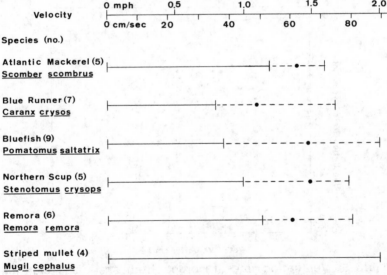

Figure 6 Mean values and ranges (dashed line) for completion of active to passive transitions in gill ventilation of various mid-water and pelagic fishes (number of individuals observed). The striped mullet showed no drop-out of single respiratory cycles when swimming (usually indicative of conversion to ram ventilation) at the maximum flow-velocity attainable. (From Roberts, unpublished data; *Remora* data from Muir and Buckley, 1967.)

absent, so in a sense, challenging the design concept is an academic argument for the scombrids. But the case is that some midwater and inshore pelagic fish like the scup, small bluefish, and the blue runner, also can make use of the passive mode once they attain a swimming speed of about 1 mph.

Ram ventilation is not without metabolic cost, but the gain is clear. Brown and Muir (1970) have calculated that the additional drag added to swimming by passive ventilation for a 44-cm skipjack tuna *Katsuwonus pelamis* swimming at a basal speed of 66 cm · sec^{-1} is about 7% of the total drag. When they derived the metabolic cost, a value from 1 to 3% resulted. The advantage to be gained by conversion to passive from active ventilation should be obvious to any fish.

Summary

Niche selection by gill breathing animals has resulted in a few very different redesigns of gill structure and functional modes of mechanical ventilation to minimize the metabolic load of ventilation, and to allow (1) occupancy of habitats requiring high activity levels for survival, as exemplified for life on beaches and mud flats, for terrestrial life in general, and for life as midwater and pelagic predators; and (2) partial escape from O_2-deficient waters by resorting to aerial respiration in, for example, eutrophic estuaries, marshes, swamps, and seasonal ponds.

Decapod crustaceans and some fish have managed to strengthen the gill structure with a parallel loss in gill area, but with the addition of accessory respiratory surfaces to facilitate amphibious life. Yet, since these "amphibians" are still tied to periodic returns or access to water to avoid desiccation, their distribution is limited to river banks, beach strands or humid regions. The vertebrate line succeeded in complete emancipation from amphibious life only with the adoption of the lung as an entirely new device and the development of a watertight skin.

Quite another approach has been adopted by some midwater and pelagic fish to minimize the metabolic load of aquatic gill ventilation. The performance of rhythmic gill ventilation degrades seriously as a fish becomes active; just when it must meet the increased oxygen demands for cruise and burst swimming. The solution seems to have been simple, namely open-mouth swimming and suppression of cyclic ventilation movements. If present calculations are correct, the metabolic savings for conversion from active to passive gill ventilation are dramatic as swimming speeds increase. The gain in elimination of energy losses due to rhythmic contractions of the branchial musculature clearly offsets the added drag to swimming presented by the resistance of the gill sieve to water flow.

The simplicity of the ram-ventilation tactic is only apparent, however, for morphological modifications are not obvious in these fish. Fascinating problems remain to be resolved. These center on neural adaptations that permit some of these fish to switch between active and passive ventilation modes, regardless of size and according to swimming speed (about 1 mph). It is a "choice," however, that may be lost to many scombrids which become obligate swimmers once a body size is reached when maintenance of hydrostatic equilibrium requires them to swim at speeds that exceed the velocity minimums necessary to support ram gill ventilation.

Acknowledgment

Parts of the research reported in this review were supported by NSF Research Grant GB 8022.

References

Alexander, R. McN. (1970). "Functional Design in Fishes." Hutchison, London.

Arudpragasam, K. D., and Naylor, E. (1964). Gill ventilation volumes, oxygen consumption and respiratory rhythms in *Carcinus maenus* (L.). *J. Exp. Biol.* **41**, 309–321.

Ballintijn, C. M. (1972). Efficiency, mechanics and motor control of fish respiration. *Resp. Physiol.* **14**, 125–141.

Bliss, D. E. (1968). Transition from water to land in decapod crustaceans. *Amer. Zool.* **8**, 355–392.

Brown, C. E., and Muir, B. S. (1970). Analysis of ram ventilation of fish gills with application to skipjack tuna *(Katsuwonus pelamis)*. *J. Fish. Res. Bd. Can.* **27**, 1637–1652.

Burton, A. C. (1965). Hemodynamics and the physics of the circulation. *In* "Physiology and Biophysics," (T. C. Ruch, and H. D. Patton, eds.), pp. 523–542. Saunders, Philadelphia, Pennsylvania.

Cameron, J. N., and Cech, J. J., Jr. (1970). Notes on the energy cost of gill ventilation in teleosts. *Comp. Biochem. Physiol.* **34**, 447–455.

Carter, G. S. (1931). Aquatic and aerial respiration in animals. *Biol. Rev.* **6:** 1–35.

Drach, P. (1930). Etude sur le système branchial des Crustacés Décapodes. *Arch. Anat. Microsc.* **26**, 83–133.

Edney, E. B. (1960). Terrestrial adaptations. *In* "The Physiology of Crustacea," (T. H. Waterman, ed.), Vol. I, pp. 367–393. Academic Press, New York.

Gray, I. E. (1957). A comparative study of the gill area of crabs. *Biol. Bull.* **112**, 34–42.

Guyton, A. C. (1966). "Textbook of Medical Physiology." Saunders, Philadelphia, Pennsylvania.

Hall, F. G. (1930). The ability of the common mackerel and certain other marine fishes to remove dissolved oxygen from sea water. *Amer. J. Physiol.* **93,** 417–421.

Heath, A. G. (1973). Ventilatory responses of teleost fish to exercise and thermal stress. *Amer. Zool.* **13,** 491–503.

Hildebrandt, J., and Young, A. C. (1965). Anatomy and physics of respiration. *In* "Physiology and Biophysics," (T. C. Ruch and H. D. Patton, eds.), pp. 733–760. Saunders, Philadelphia, Pennsylvania.

Hills, B. A., and Hughes, G. M. (1970). A dimensional analysis of oxygen transfer in the fish gill. *Resp. Physiol.* **9,** 126–140.

Holeton, G. F. (1970). Oxygen uptake and circulation by a hemoglobinless antarctic fish (*Chaenocephalus aceratus* Lonnberg) compared with three red-blooded antarctic fish. *Comp. Biochem. Physiol.* **34,** 457–471.

Hughes, G. M. (1960). A comparative study of gill ventilation in marine teleosts. *J. Exp. Biol.* **37,** 28–45.

Hughes, G. M. (1963). "Comparative Physiology of Vertebrate Respiration." Harvard Univ. Press, Cambridge, Massachusetts.

Hughes, G. M. (1964). Fish respiratory homeostasis. *Symp. Soc. Exp. Biol.* **18,** 81–107.

Hughes, G. M. (1966). The dimensions of fish gills in relation to their function. *J. Exp. Biol.* **45,** 177–195.

Hughes, G. M. (1970). Morphological measurements on the gills of fishes in relation to their respiratory function. *Folia Morphologica (Prague),* **18,** 78–95.

Hughes, G. M. (1972). Morphometrics of fish gills. *Resp. Physiol.* **14,** 1–25.

Hughes, G. M., and Gray, I. E. (1972). Dimensions and ultrastructure of toadfish gills. *Biol. Bull.* **143,** 150–161.

Hughes, G. M., and Roberts, J. L. (1970). A study of the effect of temperature change on the respiratory pumps of the rainbow trout. *J. Exp. Biol.* **52,** 177–192.

Hughes, G. M., and Shelton, G. (1962). Respiratory mechanisms and their nervous control in fish. *Advan. Comp. Physiol. Biochem.* **1,** 275–364.

Hughes, G. M., Knights, B., and Scammell, C. A. (1969). The distribution of P_{O_2} and hydrostatic pressure changes within the branchial chambers in relation to gill ventilation of the shore crab *Carcinus maenas* L. *J. Exp. Biol.* **51,** 203–220.

Johansen, K. (1970). Air breathing in fishes. *In* "Fish Physiology," (W. S. Hoar, and D. J. Randall, eds.), Vol. IV, pp. 361–411. Academic Press, New York.

Johansen, K. (1971). Comparative physiology: Gas exchange and circulation in fishes. *An. Rev. Physiol.* **33,** 569–612.

Johansen, K., Lenfant, C., and Mecklenburg, T. A. (1970). Respiration in the crab, *Cancer magister. Z. Vergl. Physiol.* **70,** 1–19.

Jones, D. R. (1971). Theoretical analysis of factors which may limit the maximum oxygen uptake of fish: the oxygen cost of the cardiac and branchial pumps. *J. Theor. Biol.* **32,** 341–349.

Krogh, A. (1941). "The Comparative Physiology of Respiratory Mechanisms." Univ. of Pennsylvania Press, Philadelphia, Pennsylvania.

Magnuson, J. J. (1970). Hydrostatic equilibrium of *Euthynnus affinis,* a pelagic teleost without a gas bladder. *Copeia 1970* **1,** 56 – 85.

McAllister, D. E. (1968). Evolution of branchiostegals and classification of teleostome fishes. *Nat. Mus. Can. Bull. 221, Biol. Ser.* 77.

Muir, B. S., and Buckley, R. M. (1967). Gill ventilation in *Remora remora. Copeia 1967,* **3,** 581 – 586.

Newell, R. C., Ahsanullah, M., and Pye, V. I. (1972). Aerial and aquatic respiration in the shore crab *Carcinus maenus* (L.). *Comp. Biochem. Physiol.* **43,** 239 – 252.

Pearse, A. S. (1950). "The Emigrations of Animals From the Sea." Sherwood Press, Dryden, New York.

Rahn, H. (1966). Aquatic gas exchange: theory. *Resp. Physiol.* **1,** 1 – 12.

Randall, D. J. (1970). Gas exchange in fish. *In* "Fish Physiology," (W. S. Hoar, and D. J. Randall, eds.), Vol. IV, pp. 253 – 292. Academic Press, New York.

Roberts, J. L. (1970). Gill ventilation in swimming fish. *Amer. Zool.* **10,** 516.

Schumann, D., and Piiper, J. (1966). Der Sauerstoffbedarf der Atmung bei Fischen nach Messungen an der narkotisierten Schleie *(Tinca tinca). Pfluegers Arch. Gesamte. Physiol.* **288,** 15 – 26.

Shelton, G. (1970). The regulation of breathing. *In* "Fish Physiology, (W. S. Hoar, and D. J. Randall, eds.), Vol. IV, pp. 293 – 359. Academic Press, New York.

Steen, J. B. (1971). "Comparative Physiology of Respiratory Mechanisms." Academic Press, New York.

Steen, J. B., and Berg, T. (1966). The gills of two species of haemoglobin-free fishes compared to those of other teleosts, with a note on severe anaemia in an eel. *Comp. Biochem. Physiol.* **18,** 517 – 526.

Wolvekamp, H. P., and Waterman, T. H. (1960). Respiration. *In* "The Physiology of Crustacea," (T. H. Waterman, ed.), Vol. I, pp. 35 – 100. Academic Press, New York.

Part V
Adaptive Value of Biological Time Measurements

Adaptive Significance of Circannual Rhythms in Birds

E. Gwinner

Max Planck Institut für Verhaltensphysiologie,
Seewiesen und Erling-Andechs/Obbs.

Introduction

The environment of most plants and animals is not constant but rather is subject to considerable temporal variations. In order to understand more fully how an organism is adapted to its environment, it is necessary to investigate how it is adapted to temporal environmental changes. The most obvious temporal variations to which individual organisms are exposed result from the rotation of the earth about its own axis, from the rotation of the earth about the sun, and from the rotation of the moon about the earth. These movements give rise to tidal, daily, lunar, and annual rhythms in the environment which provide challenges and opportunities for evolutionary adaptation comparable to those provided by spatial environmental diversity. As a consequence, many organisms have become adapted morphologically, physiologically, and behaviorally to these temporal patterns in the environment in a manner similar to that in which they have become adapted to spatial patterns in the environment. This is most apparent from the fact that many biological activities are performed at specific times, namely at those phases of the tidal, daily, lunar, and annual cycle at which they are most likely to be successful.

Such temporal adjustment to external periodicities is achieved in many organisms by simple stimulus – response systems in which particular activities are directly promoted by an environmental variable. Control of many biological functions by temperature or photoperiod provide obvious examples. However, in many other instances adjustment to the temporal structure of the environment is accomplished by another type of mechanism, developed by many organisms as an adaptation to any of the four main environmental periodicities. Many plants and animals have evolved endogenous rhythms with periods approximating those of the environmental cycles. These endogenous rhythms, normally synchronized to the environmental cycles, provide for an appropriate timing of biological functions relative to temporal environmental change. Most ubiquitous and best investigated are circadian rhythms: endogenous oscillations which match the daily environmental cycles. However, comparable circatidal, circalunar, and circannual rhythms are known to exist as well. This chapter focuses on the adaptive value of *circannual* rhythms. It considers how animals (particulary birds) utilize circannual rhythms for the appropriate timing of their various biological activities relative to the external annual cycle and relative to each other.

The Endogenous Nature of Annual Cycles in Animals

The existence of endogenous annual rhythms has been suggested for a long time, but it was not until some 10 years ago that circannual rhythms were first rigorously demonstrated. Pengelly and Fisher (1963), working on the control of hibernation in ground squirrels, observed that the annual rhythms of torpor and body weight persisted for several years even in animals kept under seasonally constant conditions. In the years following this discovery, circannual rhythms have been demonstrated not only in other mammals but also in mollusks, arthropods, reptiles, and birds (see Gwinner, 1971, 1974 for reviews). Figure 1 shows the circannual rhythm of hibernation in 23 golden-mantled ground squirrels, *Citellus lateralis*, kept for about 4 years under constant conditions of photoperiod and temperature. These animals continued to hibernate about once a year despite the fact that they were deprived of all annual environmental information. Most importantly the periods of these hibernation rhythms deviated from exactly 1 year. This is more obvious in Figure 2 in which some of these data are presented in a different way. Here, each symbol indicates the date at which hibernation began in individual animals in successive years of the experiment. It is clear that most animals entered hibernation earlier each year than the previous year, indicting that under such seasonally constant conditions the period of the annual hibernation rhythm was shorter than 12 months. In other words,

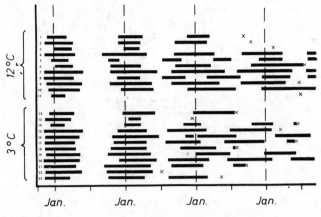

Time (months, years)

Figure 1 Circannual rhythm of hibernation in the golden-mantled ground squirrel *Citellus lateralis*. Animals were kept for about 4 years under a constant 12-hr photoperiod. Temperature was either 12°C (upper 11 animals) or 3°C (lower 12 animals). Black bars indicate periods of hibernation. × animal died (from Pengelly and Asmundson, 1969).

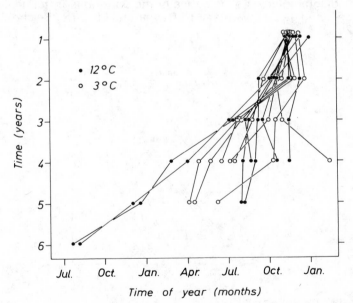

Time of year (months)

Figure 2 Onset of hibernation of individual *Citellus lateralis* from Figure 1 which survived more than three hibernation periods. Successive onsets of hibernation of each individual animal are connected by a line. Closed symbols: animals kept at 12°C. Open symbols: animals kept at 3°C (after Pengelly and Asmundson, 1969).

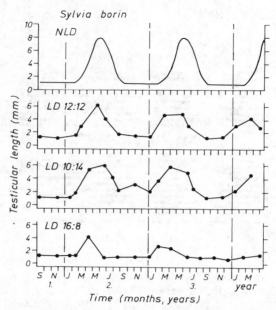

Figure 3 Circannual rhythm of testicular size in three garden warblers, *Sylvia borin*, kept for about 32 months under constant 12-, 10-, and 16-hr photoperiods, respectively (lower three diagrams). The upper diagram shows schematically the variations in testicular size in free-living garden warblers. NLD = natural LD (after Berthold *et al.*, 1972b).

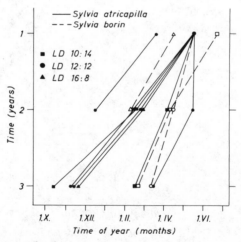

Figure 4 Progressive yearly change in the time of maximum testicular size in garden warblers, *Sylvia borin*, and blackcaps, *S. atricapilla*, kept for as long as 32 months under constant 10-, 12-, and 16-hr photoperiods, respectively (after Berthold *et al.*, 1972b).

420

the squirrels' subjective year deviated under constant conditions from the true objective year: the endogenous annual clock "ran fast" in most animals.

Another example of a circannual rhythm is shown in Figure 3 which depicts the rhythm of testicular size in three individual garden warblers, *Sylvia borin,* kept for about 32 months under a constant 12-, 10-, or 16-hr photoperiod. It is clear that these birds go through a pronounced testicular cycle about once each year, and that this rhythm is essentially indistinguishable from that of free-living conspecifics. The only major difference between the behavior of experimental and free-living birds is, again, found in the period length of the rhythms. In all three experimental birds testicular growth starts earlier each year than the previous year. This shortening of the period is more clearly shown in Figure 4; it is, again, obvious that the rhythms free-run with a period shorter than 12 months.

This deviation of the biological period from the environmental period found in these and in other experimental studies is of significance for two reasons. On the one hand, these findings definitely exclude the possibility that the observed rhythms were induced by some unknown annual environmental factors which might have penetrated the experimental chambers; if this were the case, the rhythms would have shown a period of exactly 1 year. On the other hand, these findings imply that there must be annual cycles in the environment which synchronize the circannual rhythms with the natural year in free-living animals. Unfortunately, whereas the synchronizing agents or *Zeitgebers* entraining circadian, circatidal, and circalunar rhythms have been studied in some detail (Enright, this volume; Neumann, this volume), almost nothing is known so far about the way in which circannual rhythms are synchronized with the natural year (see Gwinner, 1971, 1973 for discussion). This ignorance is, of course, a serious drawback in the discussion of the adaptive value of circannual rhythms. Nevertheless, a few points can be made and in the following paragraphs emphasis will be laid on the discussion of three well-investigated functions of circannual rhythms in birds.

Timing in an Unpredictable Environment

There are organisms which are dependent on an accurate seasonal timing of annual events even though they are exposed during an extended part of the year to environmental conditions deficient in reliable temporal cues. This is the situation in migratory birds which breed in the temperate zones but winter in regions close to the equator. Figure 5

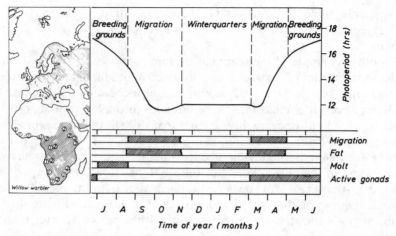

Figure 5 Left, Annual distribution of the willow warbler, *Phyllosco-pus trochilus*. Numbers refer to the breeding and wintering areas of different races. Right, upper figure, Photoperiod experienced in the course of a year by individuals which winter close to the equator; lower figure, schematic representation of the occurrence of various annual events. See text for further explanations. (Distribution map after Dementiew and Gladkow, 1954.)

shows on the left side a map depicting the annual distribution of the willow warbler, *Phylloscopus trochilus*, a common Palaearctic passerine bird. The breeding grounds of the western races are in central and northern Europe, but the wintering areas are in tropical and central Africa. The upper curve shows the photoperiodic conditions experienced in the course of a year by such individuals which winter close to the equator. It is clear that these birds are exposed to pronounced photoperiodic changes only while they are in their temperate zone breeding grounds, and during parts of their migrations, but that they are exposed to a constant photoperiod of about 12 hr from the beginning of October to the end of March. Moreover, in many of these tropical regions other environmental factors such as temperature or precipitation vary greatly from year to year, in a quite irregular and unpredictable way so that all factors known or suggested as annual timing cues in birds are of no use for these animals while they are in their winter quarters. Nevertheless, several annual activities are carried out at precise times during that period, as is indicated schematically in the lower section of this diagram. A complete molt takes place in January and February; gonadal growth is initiated in the winter quarters or shortly after the beginning of homeward migration and most significantly spring migration and the fattening associated with migration commence from year to year at precisely the same species-specific time (Gwinner, 1968a).

In an extended series of experiments we showed that all these events are controlled (in this and in several other species with similar migratory habits) by an endogenous circannual rhythmicity and, hence, are largely independent of environmental cues (Gwinner, 1968a, 1971; Berthold *et al.*, 1972a,b), Figure 6 (lower section) shows the behavior of nine willow warblers which were transferred in late September (a time at which free-living conspecifics cross the Sahara Desert on their fall migration), from the natural photoperiodic conditions of their breeding grounds to a constant 12-hr photoperiod. For comparison, the upper two graphs show the behavior of two representative control birds kept over the whole period of observation under the natural photoperiodic conditions of their breeding grounds. It is clear that the experimental birds behave essentially like the control birds: all birds molt in winter at about the appropriate time and all birds initiate spring migratory restlessness in February or March, the time at which free-living conspecifics begin homeward migration. Moreover, the four birds kept for 2 years under experimental conditions also showed summer molt and autumnal migratory restlessness in the second year at approximately the appropriate time. We have shown in other individuals that these annual rhythms of molt and migratory restlessness continue under constant conditions for as many as three cycles (Gwinner, 1968a; Berthold *et al.*, 1972a). Hence, there is no doubt that in this species the whole complex of molt, migratory activity and, to some extent, that of body weight, is preprogrammed in the bird's endogenous circannual organization.

These findings suggested that the need for a proper timing of annual events in an environment which does not provide reliable temporal cues may have given rise to the evolution of circannual rhythms. This hypothesis is supported by comparative studies of closely related species which inhabit environments differing with regard to the adequacy of temporal environmental cues. In our own investigations we have compared the willow warbler with its closest relative, the chiffchaff, *Phylloscopus collybita*. These two species are very similar in appearance, breeding biology, habitat preferences, etc. The chiffchaff, however, differs markedly from the willow warbler in that its winter quarters are in the Mediterranean area and in northern Africa (Figure 7). Hence in this species the annual cycles of molt and migration could be controlled directly by environmental cues, because these birds are exposed throughout the year to regular changes in photoperiod and climatic factors. Moreover, there are good reasons to believe that it might be even more advantageous for this species to depend mainly on external rather than on internal timing cues.

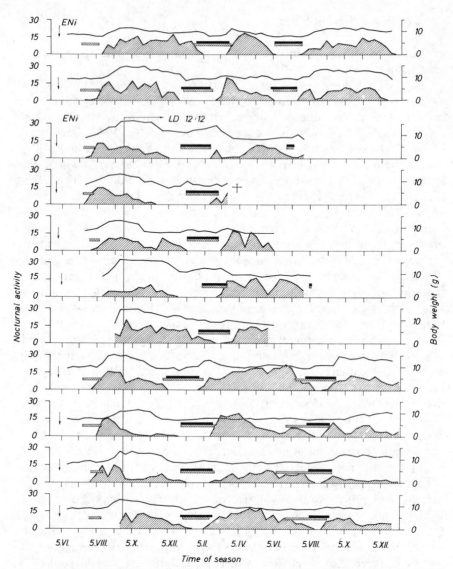

Figure 6 Seasonal variations in migratory restlessness, body weight and molt in willow warblers, *Phylloscopus trochilus*. Upper two diagrams (ENi = Erling, natural light conditions, indoors): data from birds kept for 19 months under the natural photoperiodic conditions of their breeding grounds. Lower nine diagrams: data from birds kept from late September (vertical line) in a constant 12-hr photoperiod. ↓, Date of hatching. Shaded area, Nocturnal migratory restlessness given in number of ½ hr intervals during which a bird was active each night; mean values of successive thirds of a month are plotted. Solid bars, Molt of the large wing and tail feathers. Shaded bars, Molt of body feathers. −, Body weight. †, Bird died (after Gwinner, 1971).

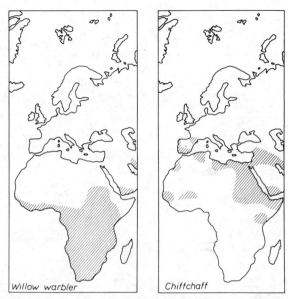

Willow warbler

Chiffchaff

Figure 7 Wintering distribution of the willow warbler, *Phylloscopus trochilus,* and of the chiffchaff, *P. collybita* (after Dementiew and Gladkow, 1954).

The chiffchaffs leave their northern breeding grounds much later in autumn than the willow warblers and return again to the north much earlier in spring than the willow warblers. As a consequence the chiffchaffs are often confronted with unfavorable weather conditions at the time of migration, and it is, therefore, of vital importance to these birds to be responsive to the prevailing weather conditions.

The circannual control of annual rhythms is, indeed, much less rigid in the chiffchaffs than in the willow warblers. Figure 8 shows the results of an experiment in which chiffchaffs have been kept under exactly the same constant conditions as the willow warblers in the experiment described before. It is clear that the annual rhythms in this species become highly disorganized under such conditions. *Zugunruhe*, initially patterned like that of control birds kept in natural light conditions, becomes increasingly irregular. Molt is extremely prolonged in some birds and interrupted or reduced to a partial body molt in others, and changes in body weight are almost entirely absent in these birds. A few chiffchaffs which we have kept for as long as 27 months under a constant 12-hr photoperiod became aperiodic with regard to all measured annual functions by the end of the first year of the experiment (Gwinner, 1971).

These results suggested that a circannual rhythmicity may be strong-

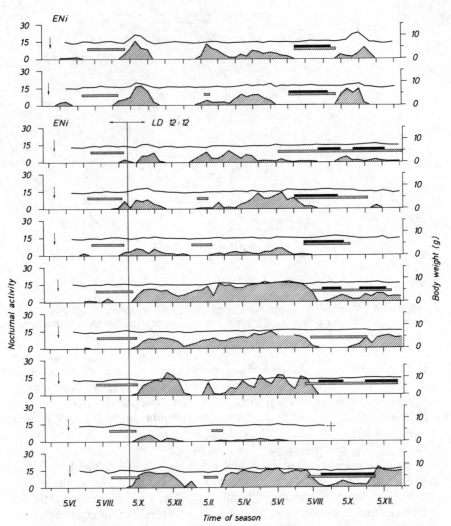

Figure 8 Seasonal variations in migratory restlessness, body weight, and molt in chiffchaff *Phylloscopus collybita*. Upper two diagrams (ENi = Erling, natural light conditions, indoors): data from birds kept for 19 months under the natural photoperiodic conditions of their breeding grounds. Lower eight diagrams: data from birds kept from late September (vertical line) in a constant 12-hr photoperiod. See Figure 6 for explanations (after Gwinner, 1971).

ly involved in the control of annual events in species which are dependent on a precise timing of their annual functions even under environmental conditions deficient in reliable environmental cues. In contrast, a circannual rhythmicity may be only weakly involved, or not at all, in species for which reliable environmental cues are available and for which it is advantageous to be responsive to prevailing environmental conditions. This hypothesis is supported by results obtained from a comparative study on two species of another genus of migratory song birds (genus *Sylvia*). We found a relationship between the pattern of migration and the extent to which a circannual rhythmicity is involved in the control of annual events similar to that in *Phylloscopus* warblers discussed above (Berthold *et al.*, 1972a,b). The hypothesis is further supported by the results of Pengelly and Kelly (1966) and of Heller and Poulson (1970) with various species of ground squirrels *(Citellus)* and chipmunks *(Eutamias)*. Among these various squirrels, species differ widely in the extent to which a circannual rhythmicity controls hibernation, body weight, gonadal development, and other functions and there is, again, a negative correlation between the rigidity of endogenous control mechanisms and the extent to which an animal has to be responsive to unpredictable environmental changes. In summary, then, all the results presented so far suggest that one of the factors which might have led to the evolution of circannual rhythms in animals is the need for a correct timing of seasonal events relative to the annual environmental cycles.

Programming of Temporal Patterns

In migratory birds, circannual rhythmicity appears to be significant not only for the adjustment of migration to temporal aspects of the environment but also for the adjustment of migration to the appropriate spatial migratory course.

Many field observations indicate that the average daily migratory speed of many European long-distance migrants on their fall migrations is not constant, but rather varies as a function of latitude. In willow warblers migratory speed is low both at the beginning of migration in Europe and near the end of migration in central and southern Africa, but it is high during the time at which these birds cross the Mediterranean Sea and the Sahara Desert. This is not surprising considering the inhospitable physical conditions of these latter areas which provide almost no opportunity for a bird to rest. However, the increased migratory performance during that part of migration is imposed upon the birds not only directly by the adverse external conditions but also appears to be preprogrammed, at least in part, in the bird's endogenous organization. The temporal pattern of migratory restlessness in captive willow warblers follows closely the temporal pattern of actual migration in free-living conspecifics. Furthermore, the period during which these birds exhibit the most intense nocturnal activity coincides with the period during which free-living conspecifics cross the Mediterranean Sea and the Sahara Desert at their highest daily migration rates (Gwinner, 1968a,b).

There is evidence that such an endogenous program might in addition determine the total distance covered by a particular species during fall migration. This is suggested, for instance, by the fact that closely related species, migrating different distances on their fall migrations, show pronounced differences in the duration and in the total amount of fall migratory restlessness if kept under identical conditions. As can be seen in Figure 9, willow warblers exhibit much more migratory restlessness during their fall migratory period and stay longer in migratory condition than chiffchaffs. These differences correspond generally to the differences in the migratory distances between these two species (Figure 7). A similar relationship between migratory restlessness and migratory distance was found in six species of warblers of the genus *Sylvia*. Figure 10 indicates that the total amount of migratory restlessness exhibited in fall by these various species is proportional to the distance between breeding grounds and winter quarters. Additional evidence suggesting that these endogenous programs controlling fall migratory restlessness are organized in

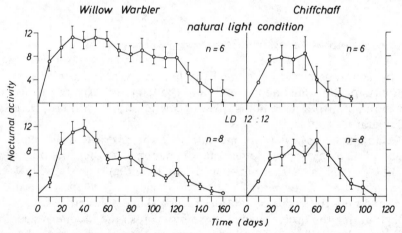

Figure 9 Variations in fall migratory restlessness in two groups of willow warblers, *Phylloscopus torchilus,* and chiffchaffs, *P. collybita,* respectively. Birds were kept either under the natural photoperiodic conditions of their breeding grounds over the whole period of observation or they were transferred from such conditions to a constant 12-hr photoperiod. Time of transfer for willow warblers was between days 50 and 80; for chiffchaffs between days 0 and 30. Vertical bars represent standard errors. For further explanation see Figure 6 (from Gwinner, 1968b).

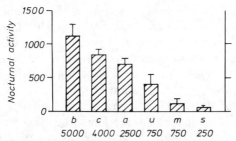

Figure 10 Duration of fall migratory restlessness (expressed as the total number of ½-hr intervals during which nocturnal activity was registered over the entire fall migratory season) in six warbler species of the genus *Sylvia*. Mean values and ± standard errors of the means are given for the six to nine individuals which comprised an experimental group in each species. Birds were kept under photoperiodic conditions approximating those of their respective breeding grounds. Numbers at the bottom of each column give the approximate distance (in kilometers) over which the various species migrate a = *Sylvia atricapilla*, b = *S. borin*, c = *S. cantillans*, m = *S. melanocephala*, s = *S. sarda*, u = *S. undata* (after Berthold, 1973).

such a way as to produce just enough migratory activity to reach the winter quarters has been presented elsewhere (Gwinner, 1972). In summary, the results mentioned in this paragraph indicate that in warblers the temporal pattern of migration is endogenously controlled not only with regard to the times of beginning and end, but also with regard to the amount of migratory performance during migration.

Maintenance of the Appropriate Temporal Sequence of Successive Annual Events

If one investigates the adaptive significance of endogenous annual rhythms, one should not only ask how a particular activity is timed relative to the external world, but also how different activities are timed relative to one another. There are annual functions which under natural conditions are necessarily mutually exclusive, for instance, reproduction and migration. Other functions are dependent on one another; migration, for instance, can only be successful if it is preceded by fattening. Obviously, the proper temporal relationship between various annual functions is of adaptive significance, and the question arises, how is it achieved?

The rigid temporal sequence in which annual events occur in many animals even under constant environmental conditions has given rise to

the hypothesis that the successive activities are somehow physiologically dependent on one another. Mrosovsky (1970) has even suggested
that circannual rhythms might result from "a sequence of linked stages,
each taking a given amount of time to complete and then leading into the
next, with the last stage linked back into the first again." Such a possibility has also been discussed by Enright (1970).

There are now data which argue against such a hypothesis. The
strongest evidence against it comes from the observation in warblers
that under constant environmental conditions the different annual functions may drastically change their phase relationships with one another
(Gwinner, 1968a; Berthold et al., 1972a,b). An example of this phenomenon is depicted in Figure 11. Here, the upper graph shows schematically the normal temporal relationship between the molt and the testis
cycle of garden warblers under natural photoperiodic conditions. The
period of increased testis size is preceded by prenuptial molt and followed by postnuptial molt. The two lower graphs show that this sequence may become disorganized under constant photoperiodic conditions. This is particularly obvious if one compares the testicular cycle
with that of postnuptial molt. In the case of the bird kept in LD 12:12,

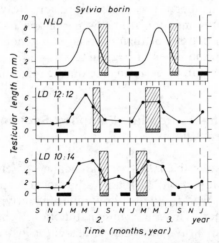

Figure 11 Dissociation of the circannual rhythms of testicular size
and molt in two garden warblers, *Sylvia borin,* kept for 32 months
under constant 12- and 10-hr photoperiods, respectively (lower two
diagrams). The upper diagram shows schematically the normal temporal relationship between the testis and molt cycles in free-living
individuals. Solid bars: prenuptial molt; shaded bars with shaded
columns on top: postnuptial molt. For further explanations see text
(after Berthold *et al.,* 1972b).

the first postnuptial molt, takes place at about the normal time relative to the testis cycle, that is, shortly before the testes have regressed. The second postnuptial molt, in contrast, sets in much earlier relative to the testis cycle, i.e., shortly before the testes reach maximal size. Indeed, the bird molts at a time when it is in optimal breeding conditions, a phenomenon which would never occur in nature. This effect is even more conspicuously shown by the bird kept in LD 10:14, in which the interval between two successive summer molts is so short, that the second postnuptial molt actually begins near the beginning of testis growth.

We have observed similar changes in the phase relationship between other functions as well. In some animals different functions have drifted out of phase relative to one another by more than half a year. Hence, these data suggest that the different functions are rather independent of one another and possibly controlled by different circannual rhythms, which under constant conditions may become entirely uncoupled from each other.

The physiological implications of such a conclusion have been discussed elsewhere (Gwinner, 1968a, 1974; Berthold et al., 1972a,b). In the present chapter the significance of these findings for the interpretation of one important aspect of temporal adaptation should be mentioned. It is well known from many bird species, including warblers, that under natural conditions there may be differences from one population to another in the phase relationship between successive seasonal activities. In young willow warblers, for instance, fall migration begins at an earlier age and earlier relative to the preceding postjuvenile molt in northern populations than in southern populations (e.g., Gwinner et al., 1972; Berthold et al., 1975). This difference is of adaptive significance since birds from northern populations hatch later in the year than birds from southern populations, but they leave their breeding grounds at almost the same time of year as southern populations to avoid unfavorable fall weather conditions. These differences are probably due, at least in part, to genetic differences between populations. This is suggested by the results of the experiment summarized in Figure 12. In this experiment willow warblers from the northern race *acredula* and the southern race *trochilus* were kept from an age of about 9 days under the same constant 18-hr photoperiod. It is clear that the characteristic differences known from free-living individuals of these populations persist under these constant conditions; the northern race initiates migratory restlessness at an earlier age and earlier relative to postjuvenile molt than the southern race.

Hence, these results suggest that changes in the phase relationship between different activities occur in birds kept under constant environ-

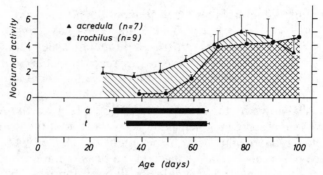

Figure 12 Fall migratory restlessness (shaded areas) and postjuvenile molt (solid bars) in willow warblers of the northern race *acredula*
(a) and of the southern race *trochilus (t)* kept from an age of 9 days
under a constant 18-hr photoperiod. For further explanations see text
(after Gwinner *et al.,*1972).

mental conditions, and furthermore, that such variation in the temporal
relationship of annual events may have evolved as a strategy for adaptation to different environmental conditions. If it is true that different overt
annual functions are controlled by different endogenous circannual
rhythms, such interpopulation variation in the phase relationship could
be interpreted as the result of genetic differences in the mechanisms
which couple the various rhythms to one another.

References

Berthold, P. (1973). Relationships between migratory restlessness and migration
   distances in six *Sylvia* species. *Ibis* **115**, 594–599.
Berthold, P., Gwinner, E., and Klein, H. (1972a). Circannuale Periodik bei
   Grasmücken. I. Periodik des Körpergewichts, der Mauser und der Nach-
   tunruhe bei *Sylvia atricapilla* und *S. borin* unter verschiedenen konstanten
   Bedingungen. *J. Ornithol.* **113**, 170–190.
Berthold, P., Gwinner, E., and Klein, H. (1972b). Circannuale Periodik bei
   Grasmücken. II. Periodik der Gonaden bei *Sylvia atricapilla* und *S. borin*
   unter verschiedenen konstanten Bedingungen. *J. Ornithol.* **113**, 407–417.
Berthold, P., Gwinner, E., and Querner, U. (1975). Vergleichende Untersuch-
   ung der Jugendentwicklung südwestdeutscher und südfinnischer Garten-
   grasmücken *Sylvia borin. Ornis. Fenn.* (in press).
Dementiew, G. P., and Gladkow, N. A. (1954). Die Vögel der Sowjetunion.
   Sovetskaya Nauka, Bd. 6, Moscow.
Enright, J. T. (1970). Ecological aspects of endogenous rhythmicity. *Annu. Rev.
   Ecol. System.* **1**, 221–238.
Gwinner, E. (1968a). Circannuale Periodik als Grundlage des jahreszeitlichen

Funktionswandels bei Zugvögeln. Untersuchungen am Fitis *(Phylloscopus trochilus)* und am Waldlaubsünger *(P. sibilatrix). J. Ornithol.* **109,** 70–95.

Gwinner, E. (1968b). Artspezifische Muster der Zugunruhe bei Laubsängern und ihre mögliche Bedeutung für die Beendigung des Zuges im Winterquartier. *Z. Tierpsychol.* **25,** 843–853.

Gwinner, E. (1971). A comparative study of circannual rhythms in warblers. *In* "Biochronemetry," (M. Menaker, ed.), pp. 405–427. Academy of Sciences, Washington, D.C.

Gwinner, E. (1972). Endogenous timing factors in bird migration. *In* "Animal Orientation and Navigation," (S. R. Galler, K. Schmidt-Koenig, G. J. Jacobs, and R. E. Belleville, eds.), pp. 321–338. NASA, Washington, D. C.

Gwinner, E. (1973). Circannual rhythms in birds: their interaction with circadian rhythms and environmental photoperiod. *J. Reprod. Fert.* (Suppl. 19), 51–65.

Gwinner, E. (1974). Endogenous organization of annual rhythms in birds. *In* "Circannial Clocks," (E. T. Pengelly, ed.). Academic Press, New York.

Gwinner, E., Berthold, P., and Klein, H. (1972). Untersuchungen zur Jahresperiodik von Laubsängern. III. Die Entwicklung des Gefieders, des Gewichts und der Zugunruhe südwestdeutscher und skandinavischer Fitisse *(Phylloscopus trochilus trochilus* und *Ph. t. acredula). J. Ornithol.* **113,** 1–8.

Heller, H. C., and Poulson, T. L. (1970). Circannian rhythms II. Endogenous and exogenous factors controlling reproduction and hibernation in chipmunks *(Eutamias)* and ground squirrels *(Spermophilus). Comp. Biochem. Physiol.* **33,** 357–383.

Mrosovsky, N. (1970). Mechanisms of hibernation cycles in ground squirrels: Circannian rhythm or sequence of stages. *Pa. Acad. Sci.* 44:172–175.

Pengelly, E. T., and Asmundson, S. M. (1969). Free-running periods of endogenous circannian rhythms in the golden-mantled ground squirrel, *Citellus lateralis. Comp. Biochem. Physiol.* **30,** 177–183.

Pengelly, E. T., and Fisher, K. C. (1963). The effect of temperature and photoperiod on the yearly hibernating behavior of captive golden-mantled ground squirrels *(Citellus lateralis tescorum). Can. J. Zool.* **41,** 1103–1120.

Pengelly, E. T., and Kelly, K. H. (1966). A "circannian" rhythm in hibernating species of the genus *Citellus* with observations on their physiological evolution. *Comp. Biochem. Physiol.* **19,** 603–617.

Circadian Rhythms in Animal Orientation

Klaus Hoffmann

Max Planck Institut für Verhaltensphysiologie
Erling-Andechs

Introduction

Time-compensated orientation with reference to celestial bodies is one of the classical fields in which the adaptive significance of biological clocks is obvious. Its discovery has not only stimulated work on the adaptive significance of timing mechanisms in other functions, but has also given new impetus to the study of the physiology of endogenous rhythms (Pittendrigh, 1954).

Direction finding with the help of celestial cues was discovered in 1911 by Santschi. By some simple, ingenious experiments he was able to prove that ants could use the sun to find their direction back to the nest. In the following years a similar mode of orientation was found in a vast variety of arthropods, gastropods, and polychaetes. The animals were able to find and maintain a direction by using the sun or moon, or, as in most experimental demonstrations, an artificial light source. This mode of orientation became known as the light compass reaction.

Such a simple way of orientation may suffice for short periods of time when the movement of the sun or moon is negligible; for instance, maintaining the same direction for several minutes, or in the case of ants, returning to the nest fairly rapidly following departure. It would be misleading, however, if several hours elapsed between departure and return, or if the same direction had to be kept for several hours as in migrating birds. This difficulty could be overcome if the animals were able to make allowance for the time elapsed, and to correct their direction according-ly. Such a possibility was mentioned by Santschi in 1913, and later for birds by Wachs (1926). However, these ideas did not receive much con-sideration, especially since experiments in ants (Brun, 1914) and bees (Wolf, 1927) seemed to directly contradict them.* It was not until 1949 that time-compensated sun orientation was discovered simultaneously and independently by Gustav Kramer in starlings and by Karl v. Frisch in honeybees.

Direction Finding by the Sun

In the fall of 1949 Kramer observed that European starlings, kept in outside aviaries with a clear view of the sky, showed migratory restless-ness which was oriented in the direction corresponding to the normal migratory direction of the local population. He was able to obtain the same performance in small circular cages, and in a series of elegant ex-periments he demonstrated conclusively that the sun was the orienting stimulus (Kramer, 1950a,b, 1952). Since the birds maintained the same direction over extended periods of time, and at different times of day, Kramer concluded that they must be able to compensate for the sun's movement.

This capacity could be most clearly shown in birds that were trained to obtain food in a certain compass direction (Kramer and v. St. Paul, 1950; Kramer, 1952). Figure 1 shows a later experiment with a starling trained to the east at Wilhelmshaven and later retrained and tested in the arctic. As can be seen, the bird roughly seeks his food in the same com-pass direction during all hours of the day, while keeping very different angles with the sun at the different times. Experiments like these firmly established that starlings are able to find directions with the help of the sun, and to compensate for its motion. Additional confirmation came from experiments under an artificial sun (Kramer, 1952).

Further experimentation was aimed at a better understanding of the time mechanism underlying the compensation for the sun's motion. If trained starlings are exposed to artificial light–dark cycles out of phase with the natural day, and if this treatment is able to reset their clock,

---

*With improved methods Wolf's findings in the honeybee were later shown to have been erroneous (Meder, 1958). In ants, Jander (1957) found that these animals have to learn sun compass orientation, and hence their behavior in spring and in summer is dif-ferent.

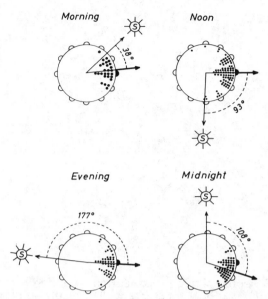

Figure 1 Directional choices of a starling trained to the east in the arctic at 68°21′ N in midsummer at different times of day. Each dot represents one critical choice. The semicircles on the circumference represent the 12 feeders, with the feeder the bird was expected to select being drawn solid. The thick arrow gives the mean direction. S, sun. Note that the angle with the sun is different at different times of day. (Adapted from Hoffmann, 1959.)

predictable deviations from the original training direction should result. Figure 2 gives the expected direction for a bird that was trained to the south and then exposed to an artificial light–dark cycle beginning 6 hr after local sunrise and ending 6 hr after local sunset. Figure 3 shows actual results of such an experiment. The birds behaved according to prediction. When they were again exposed to the natural light conditions, the direction of their food choices again corresponded to the original training direction. Such experiments showed that the clock underlying compensation for the changing position of the sun could be readily reset by shifted light schedules (Hoffmann, 1953, 1954).

Additional experiments demonstrated that by such treatment the clock is not shifted abruptly, but is gradually drawn into phase with the new light schedule, as evidenced by the gradual shift of the direction chosen. An example is given in Figure 4 for starlings whose clock was advanced for 6 hr. The direction chosen shifted gradually from the original training direction to the new direction which had not yet been reached after 3 days in the artificial light schedule. In a further set of

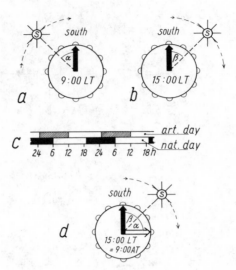

Figure 2 Expected change of direction of a starling trained to look for food in the south, if its clock has been shifted 6 hr backward by exposing it to an artificial light–dark cycle 6 hr behind the natural day as indicated in (c). The expected angle with the sun before (a, b) and after shifting (d) is indicated. The black and hatched areas in (c) indicate darkness. S, sun; LT, local time; AT, artificial time. Solid arrow, training direction; open arrow, direction expected after shift of clock. (From Hoffmann, 1954.)

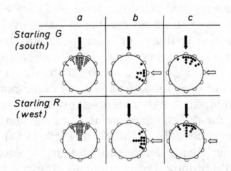

Figure 3 Change of direction in two starlings orienting by the sun. A, Critical tests during training in natural day; b, after 12–18 days in artificial day, 6 hr behind local time (see Figure 2); c, 8–17 days after return into the natural day (outside aviary). Note change of direction in (b), and return to original direction in (c). For further explanation see Figures 1 and 2. (After Hoffmann, 1954.)

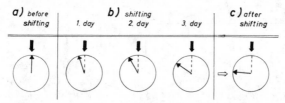

Figure 4 Change of direction in starlings after abrupt shift of light cycle 6 hr forward. Mean directions before (a), during (b–d), and after (e) shift of clock are indicated by the centrifugal arrows. Experiments with three birds combined. (Adapted from Hoffmann, 1954.)

experiments trained starlings were exposed to constant illumination, and their perch-hopping activity was continuously recorded (Figure 5, left). Locomotor activity showed a clear-cut circadian rhythm with a period shorter than 24 hr. When, under these conditions, the directional choice of the birds was tested, it deviated from the original training direction (Figure 5, right) corresponding in direction and in degree to the state of their circadian clock as indicated by the activity rhythm. When the artificial light regime corresponding to the natural day was reestablished, the starlings' clocks became resynchronized, and the birds again headed in the old training direction (Figure 5c).

These findings clearly show that the clock underlying time compensated direction finding with the sun has the same properties, and seems to be identical with the clock underlying other circadian rhythms. It is entrained by the external light cycle, can be reset by a phase-shift of this cycle, and continues to run under constant conditions with a period that can deviate from exactly 24 hr. With the help of this clock, the movement of the sun is compensated for and thereby the finding of definite compass directions independent of time of day is possible; therefore this type of orientation is now generally called sun compass orientation.

In the same fall in which sun compass orientation was discovered in starlings, the compensation for the changing position of the sun was also demonstrated in the honeybee (Frisch, 1950). A simple orientation by the sun had already been demonstrated in 1927 (Wolf, 1927). As Frisch (1965, p. 335) writes, he had considered this possibility "too fantastic" and therefore deferred the decisive experiment again and again. It was finally performed on September 24, 1949. On the eve of that day bees were trained to a feeding place west of the hive, and the next morning the stock was moved to another site with completely different surroundings. When the behavior of the bees was tested, it was found that they were now searching in the correct compass direction, although they had to fly away from the sun instead of flying toward it as during training

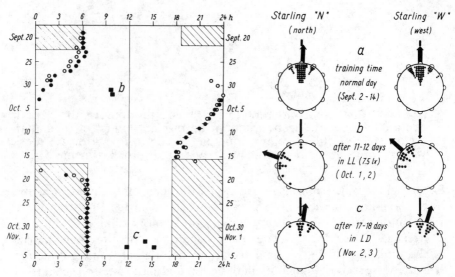

Figure 5 Rhythm of locomotor activity (left) and direction finding (right) of two starlings kept in constant light and temperature. Note that the rhythm of activity advances about ½ hr per day in constant light, and that the direction in (b) is changed correspondingly. Left, Hatched areas indicate darkness; onsets of activity are given by open (starling N) or solid (starling W) circles; the black squares mark the test times corresponding to (b) and (c) at the right. Right, Tests on orientation during training (a), after 10–11 days in constant conditions (b), and in artificial day synchronous with natural day (c). LL, constant conditions; LD, light–dark cycle corresponding to natural day. Centrifugal arrows give mean direction of choices. For further explanation see Figure 1. (From Hoffmann, 1960.)

time the evening before. This and many other experiments conclusively demonstrated that the bees were able to compensate for the sun's movement (Frisch, 1965).

After sun compass orientation had been discovered in starlings and honeybees, it was found in other species of birds and insects, and in a still increasing number of arthropods and vertebrates. In nearly all cases in which an attempt was made, the underlying clock and thereby the direction taken could be readily shifted by a shift of the light regime. In several instances it was also shown that the clock continued running under constant light conditions and is independent of local time. An example is given in Figure 6 from experiments with the sandhopper *Talitrus saltator*. This animal lives in the littoral zone. If exposed to dry conditions it tries to escape in a compass direction which is perpendicular to its local shore line. To find this direction it can use sun compass

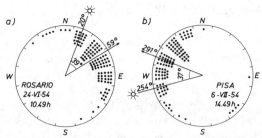

Figure 6 Escape directions of sand hoppers *(Talitrus saltator)* collected from a population near Pisa, Italy. (a) Animals tested at Rosario, Argentina, collected on July 10. (b) Animals tested near place of collection at the same universal time (i.e., 14149 GMT) at which experiment (a) was performed. Note that the angle with the sun is the same in both cases. Dates and official local times for the experiments at the two places are given. Each dot represents the position of one animal. The arrows give the mean escape directions (After Papi, 1955.)

orientation (Pardi and Papi, 1952). Papi (1955) collected such sandhoppers near Pisa in Italy and shipped them to Argentina. During transport they were kept in constant dark. When they were exposed to the sun in Argentina, the sandhoppers kept the same angle with the sun as did control animals tested near the place of collection at the same hour of universal time, in spite of the fact that the sun's altitude as well as its direction of motion was vastly different from that at home.

The function of sun compass orientation may vary, depending upon the species and the situation. In day-migrating birds it has been shown to be used for orientation during "migration" in caged situations. In bees it is part of the intricate orientation and communication system that allows the animals to signal and find promising feeding places. In several littoral arthropods the sun compass may be used if the animals are stranded in dry areas; it allows them to return to moist areas, thus escaping death from desiccation. In some frogs sun compass orientation has been shown to serve in finding the shoreline and thus to avoid predation by fish (Ferguson *et al.*, 1965).

Despite the diversity of its function, the basic components of sun compass orientation are the same in practically all cases examined; the circadian clock allows the animals to compensate for the changing position of the sun and thereby to find definite compass directions. It must be stressed that sun compass orientation is only one of the orientational mechanisms that are available to the animal. Its existence can usually only be shown in experimental conditions that rule out other possibilities.

Bicoordinate Navigation by the Sun?

In several wild bird species as well as in homing pigeons it has been demonstrated that these animals are able to home over large distances, regardless of the direction in which they have been displaced, and that they can head in the home direction soon after release at an unknown site (Kramer, 1961; Schmidt-Koenig, 1965; Wallraff, 1967; Matthews, 1968; Keeton, 1974). When sun compass orientation in starlings had been found, it was suggested that the sun might be used not only for direction finding, but also for the determination of the position of a site to which a bird had drifted by accident, or been transported by an investigator.

A complete hypothesis for true bicoordinate navigation by the sun was suggested by Matthews (1953, 1968). The hypothesis suggests that the birds are able to determine the sun's culmination altitude from seeing a very small part of the sun's arc, and by comparing the values thus obtained at the point of release with those last seen at home to determine their latitudinal displacement. The birds are also thought to be able to determine the time of the sun's culmination and thereby local time, and by comparison with their internal clock, still running on home time, to determine their longitudinal displacement. A modification of this hypothesis was introduced by Pennycuick (1960). He suggested that the birds are able to determine the altitude of the sun and its rate of change at the release site, and to compare these two values with those expected at home at that time according to their internal clock. The information thus obtained would be: if the sun is too low, fly toward it, if it is too high, fly away from it; if the rate of increase of sun altitude is higher than at home, fly to the left of the sun, if it is lower, fly to the right. The latter hypothesis is physiologically somewhat more plausible and avoids some theoretical objections that have been raised against Matthews' version, but the basic requirements on the perceptional abilities of the birds are practically the same. Therefore, both hypotheses will be treated together here.

These hypotheses require a very high resolution power of the sense organs involved in measuring the sun's altitude, combined with an extremely precise and rigid clock, as has been pointed out several times (Kramer, 1952; Hoffmann, 1965, 1972; Keeton, 1974). A clock which was 10 min early or late would, at a latitude of 45° lead to a deviation of only about 2.5° in sun compass orientation,* and the clock would be re-

---

*Six degrees under the most unfavorable conditions, i.e., at summer solstice around noon.

set by the following dusk and dawn. In traveling by sun navigation, however, such an error of the clock would lead a bird to a place more than 120 miles east or west of home, and no correction of the clock would be possible.

The sun navigation hypothesis has the indisputable merit that it stimulated a tremendous amount of research. In most cases the experiments involved homing pigeons. It seemed supported by repeated observations that birds oriented well under sunny conditions but showed random departures under overcast. It must be mentioned, however, that in some cases oriented departures were reported even under overcast conditions (see below).

Some experiments by Matthews also seemed to strongly support the hypothesis. The most convincing of these was based on the fact that around equinox the sun's declination and therefore its noon altitude changes rather rapidly from day to day. Matthews reasoned that if birds were prevented from seeing the sun for several days around autumnal equinox, and were then released some distance south of their home, they would experience a sun altitude that is lower than that last seen at home. Hence they would assume that they had been transported to the north and would head towards south instead of north. An experiment with homing pigeons seemed to support the hypothesis (Matthews, 1953); the majority of birds thus treated headed in a southernly direction (Figure 7 A). Since this experiment provided the best and nearly the only direct experimental evidence in favor of Matthews' hypothesis, several attempts were made to repeat it. However, all these attempts have failed so far (Figure 7 B – F), including one in which part of the pigeons came from the same stock as those used by Matthews (Figure 7 E). In all cases experimentals were indistinguishable from controls, and all headed roughly toward home. A corresponding experiment performed around vernal equinox also failed to give the results predicted by the sun navigation hypothesis (Keeton, 1974).

Matthews (1955) also performed a few experiments aimed at interfering with the chronometer assumed to underlie sun navigation. He reported that when he exposed homing pigeons to artificial light–dark cycles 3 hr in advance of the local day he observed no differences between experimentals and controls. But if he first gave the birds 4–5 days with an irregular schedule of light and dark, and then exposed them for 5–19 days to a light schedule 3 hr in advance or behind local time, he observed that the experimental birds headed roughly in the direction predicted by his hypothesis.

However, a massive bulk of similar experiments by Schmidt-Koenig (1961, 1965, 1972) and others (Graue, 1963; Keeton, 1974) gave com-

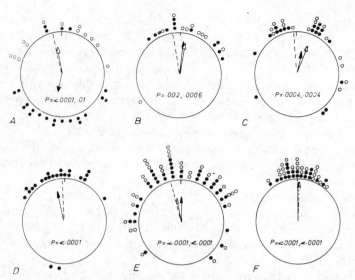

Figure 7 Departure directions of pigeons at autumnal equinox, released south of their home left. Experimentals that were prevented
from seeing the sun for several days before being released (solid
dots); controls that were allowed full view of the sun (open circles).
Open arrow heads, mean of controls; solid arrow heads, mean of
controls; solid arrow heads, mean of experimentals. Dashed line
gives home direction. p-values for controls (first value) and experimentals (second value) are given. (A, after Matthews, 1953; B, after
Rawson and Rawson 1955; C, after Kramer 1955; D, after Kramer,
1957; E, after Hoffmann 1958; F, after Keeton 1970.) Note that in
all cases except in (A) experimentals and controls head in the same
direction.

pletely different results. Birds that had been exposed to an artificial
light–dark cycle out of phase with the local day started neither in the
direction of the controls nor in the direction predicted by the sun navigation hypothesis. Instead they started in a direction that was to be predicted if the sun was only used as a compass, comparable to the experiments reported earlier in this chapter with starlings. Figure 8 gives the
departure bearings of pigeons whose clock had been advanced by 6 hr.
Regardless of whether the birds were released north, south, east, or west
of home, they started in a direction about 90° to the left of the home
direction, as is to be expected if the sun is not used for bicoordinate navigation, but only provides the compass contained in a two-step procedure. Such findings were made in practically all such experiments except those by Matthews mentioned above.

The same result was obtained even if the pigeons were allowed a full

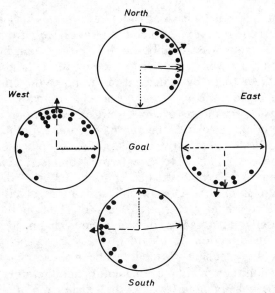

Figure 8 Departure directions of pigeons whose clocks had been shifted 6 hr in advance, released 30–80 km to the north, south, east, and west of the left. Each dot represents the departure bearing of one bird. The arrows on the periphery of the circle give the mean departure direction. Inside the circle solid arrows indicate the direction to be expected with bicoordinate navigation by the sun, dashed arrows give the direction to be expected if the sun is only used as a compass, and stippled arrows give the home direction. (After Emlen, 1975.)

view of the sky and the sun during the process of clock shifting in that part of each day when artificial and natural daylight overlapped (Alexander, 1973, quoted from Keeton, 1974). This suggests that during the time they did not get any useful information from the sun other than that it was daytime. Walcott and Michener (1971) and Schmidt-Koenig (1972) have recently also performed smaller time-shifts ranging from 5 to 120 min. The results again support the view that the sun is only used as a compass and not for bicoordinate navigation. In another experiment Walcott and Michener (1971) exposed pigeons first to an irregular light schedule for 9 days; during that time they also received 30% D_2O in their drinking water. D_2O has been shown to slow down circadian rhythms and other rhythmic phenomena in a variety of organisms (Bruce and Pittendrigh, 1960; Enright, 1971). The pigeons were then transported to a place about 265 miles west from their home loft where they were held in an open aviary with full view of the sun for 6–9 days. Thus they had ample time to reset their clocks to local time at this place. Finally, they were released from a place about 52 miles west from their home loft. The release spot was roughly on the line between home and the aviary in which they were exposed to the sun after the disruption and D_2O treatment. All these birds headed in the home direction as did the controls, as expected if the sun is only used as a compass.

The findings on the effects of clock shift experiments reported above would only be compatible with the sun navigation hypothesis if one assumes that the birds possess two clocks that are both used in orientation. One of these would have to be extremely precise and also very rigid and would have to be unaffected by shifts in the light–dark regime or by application of D_2O. This clock would then be involved in the determination of the coordinates of the release site. Then the bird would use the sun compass with its readily adjustable clock that need not be highly precise to find its direction. It is evident that such a use of two clocks does not seem very plausible. While it has been shown that the organism may contain a multitude of coupled oscillators and therefore the assumption of several clocks is quite feasible, the existence of a clock with the degree of precision and rigidity postulated for sun navigation seems highly unlikely in view of the present evidence.

Recently several other findings have been reported that are incompatible with navigation by the sun. In several cases home oriented de-

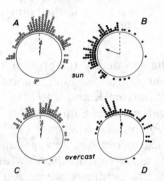

Figure 9 Departure directions of untreated pigeons (A and C) and of pigeons whose clock had been advanced for six hours (B and D). (A) and (B) under sunny conditions, (C) and (D) under overcast. (C) and (D) released from unfamiliar sites. Note that under overcast both groups head towards home, while under sunny conditions the birds whose clocks have been advanced vanish in a direction to the left of the home direction. Solid arrows, mean departure directions; dashed line, home direction. (From Keeton, 1974.)

partures were reported when pigeons were released under complete overcast (Schmidt-Koenig, 1965; Wallraff, 1966; Keeton, 1969, 1971). One could argue that in these cases the birds were able to exactly localize the sun even behind the cloud cover. Keeton (1971, 1974) trained pigeons to fly in inclement weather; under such conditions he found that birds whose clock had been shifted did not show the deviation typical for releases under sunny skies, but headed homeward as did the controls (Figure 9). When magnets were mounted on the pigeons, they were disoriented under overcast, but not under the sun. This suggests that the birds can also make use of the earth's magnetic field to find their direction. This is supported also by the finding (Merkel *et al.,* 1964; Wiltschko, 1968, 1972) that European robins are able to find their migratory direction with the help of the magnetic field when celestial cues are lacking. Both the magnetic field and the sun seem to give information on compass directions only. Normally both these would coincide, but in birds whose clock have been shifted they would conflict. Nevertheless, in all cases in which they were available the celestial cues were preferred. Presumably they are more precise and more easily accessible than the magnetic cues (for further discussion see Hoffmann, 1972; Keeton, 1974).

In view of the findings reported above I think the overall evidence against true bicoordinate navigation by the sun is so overwhelming that the search for the highly precise and rigid clock underlying it is unnecessary. The sun can take part in homing orientation, but it is only used as a compass. The compass can also be supplied by the earth's magnetic field. We are thus in the same situation as 20 years ago when Kramer (1953, 1957) developed his map-and-compass concept, assuming that goal orientation in birds might be composed of two fundamentally different steps: one, the map component for establishing the coordinates of the release site, the other, the compass component, for determining the direction of flight. Since then a new compass, the magnetic field, has been discovered, but for the map step, i.e., true bicoordinate navigation, no overall hypothesis exists at the moment (Keeton, 1974). The old hypotheses have been disproved and no convincing new ones have been proposed.

References

Bruce, V. G., and Pittendrigh, C. S. (1960). An effect of heavy water on the phase and period of the circadian rhythm in *Euglena. J. Cell. Comp. Physiol.* **56,** 25–31.

Brun, R. (1914). "Die Raumorientierung der Ameisen." Gustav Fischer, Jena.

Emlen, S. T. (1975). Migration: orientation and navigation. *In* "Avian Biology." (D. S. Farner and J. R. King, eds.), Vol. 5. Academic Press, New York.

Enright, J. T. (1971). Heavy water slows biological timing processes. *Z. Vergl. Physiol.* **72**, 1–16.

Ferguson, D. E., Landreth, H. F., and Turnipseed, M. R. (1965). Astronomical orientation of the Southern Cricket Frog, *Acris gryllus. Copeia 1965,* 58–66.

Frisch, K. von. (1950). Die Sonne als Kompass imLeben der Bienen. *Experientia* **6**, 210–221.

Frisch, K. von. (1965). "Tanzsprache und Orientierung der Bienen." Springer, New York.

Graue, L. C. (1963). The effect of phase shifts in the day-night cycle on pigeon homing at distances of less than one mile. *Ohio J. Sci.* **63**, 214–217.

Hoffmann, K. (1953). Experimentelle Änderung des Richtungsfindens beim Star durch Beeinflussung der "inneren Uhr." *Naturwissenschaften* **40**, 608–609.

Hoffmann, K. (1954). Versuche zu der im Richtungsfinden der Vögel enthaltenen Zeitschätzung. *Z. Tierpsychol.* **11**, 453–475.

Hoffmann, K. (1958). Repetition of an experiment on bird orientation. *Nature* **181**, 1435–1437.

Hoffmann, K. (1959). Die Richtungsorientierung von Staren unter der Mitternachtssonne. *Z. Vergl. Physiol.* **41**, 471–480.

Hoffmann, K. (1960). Experimental manipulation of the orientational clock in birds. *Cold Spring Harbor Symp. Quant. Biol.* **25**, 379–387.

Hoffmann, K. (1965). Clock mechanisms in celestial orientation of animals. *In* "Circadian Clocks," J. Aschoff, ed.), pp. 426–441. North-Holland, Amsterdam.

Hoffmann, K. (1972). Biological clocks in animal orientation and in other functions. *Proc. Int. Symp. Circadian Rhythmicity,* pp. 175–205, Pudoc, Wageningen.

Jander, R. (1957). Die optische Richtungsorientierung der roten Waldameise (*Formica rufa* L.). *Z. Vergl. Physiol.* **40**, 167–238.

Keeton, W. T. (1969). Orientation by pigeons: is the sun necessary? *Science* **165**, 922–928.

Keeton, W. T. (1970). Do pigeons determine latitudinal displacement from the sun's altitude? *Nature London* **227**, 626–627.

Keeton, W. T. (1971). Magnets interfere with pigeon homing. *Proc. Nat. Acad. Sci.* **68**, 102–106.

Keeton, W. T. (1974). The orientational and navigational basis of homing in birds. *Advan. Study Behav.* **5**, 47–132.

Kramer, G. (1950a). Orientierte Zugaktivität gekäfigter Singvögel. *Naturwissenschaften* **37**, 188.

Kramer, G. (1950b). Weitere Analyse der Faktoren, welche die Zugaktivität des gekäfigten Vogels orientieren. *Naturwissenschaften,* **37**, 377–378.

Kramer, G. (1952). Experiments on bird orientation. *Ibis* **94**, 265–285.

Kramer, G. (1953). Wird die Sonnenhöhe bei der Heimfindeorientierung verwertet? *J. Ornithol.* **94**, 201 – 219.

Kramer, G. (1955). Ein weiterer Versuch, die Orientierung von Brieftauben durch jahreszeitliche Änderung der Sonnenhöhe zu beeinflussen. Gleichzeitig eine Kritik des Versuchs. *J. Ornithol.* **96**, 173 – 185.

Kramer, G. (1957). Experiments on bird orientation and their interpretation. *Ibis* **99**, 196 – 227.

Kramer, G. (1961). Long distance orientation. *In* "Biology and Comparative Physiology of Birds," (A. J. Marshall, ed.), Vol. 2, pp. 341 – 371, Academic Press, New York.

Kramer, G., and v. St. Paul, U. (1950). Stare (*Sturnus vulgaris* L.) lassen sich auf Himmelsrichtung dressieren. *Naturwissenschaften* **37**, 526 – 527.

Matthews, G. V. T. (1953). Sun navigation in homing pigeons. *J. Exp. Biol.* **30**, 243 – 267.

Matthews, G. V. T. (1955). An investigation of the "chronometer" factor in bird navigation. *J. Exp. Biol.* **32**, 39 – 58.

Matthews, G. V. T. (1968). "Bird Navigation," 2nd Ed. Cambridge Univ. Press, Cambridge, Massachusetts.

Meder, E. (1958). Über die Einberechnung der Sonnenwanderung bei der Orientierung der Honigbiene. *Z. Vergl. Physiol.* **40**, 610 – 641.

Merkel, F. W., Fromme, H. G., and Wiltschke, W. (1964). Nicht-visuelles Orientierungsvermögen bei nächtlich zugunruhigen Rotkehlchen. *Vogelwarte* **22**, 168 – 173.

Papi, F. (1955). Experiments on the sense of time in *Talitrus saltator* (Montagu) (Crustacea – Amphipoda). *Experientia* **11**, 20.

Pardi, L., and Papi, F. (1952). Die Sonne als Kompass bei *Talitrus saltator* (Montagu), Amphipoda, Talitridae. *Naturwissenshaften* **39**, 262 – 263.

Pennycuick, C. J. (1960). The physical basis of astronavigation in birds: theoretical considerations. *J. Exp. Biol.* **37**, 573 – 593.

Pittendrigh, C. S. (1954). On temperature independence in the clock system controlling emergence time in Drosophila. *Proc. Nat. Acad. Sci* **40**, 1018 – 1029.

Rawson, K. S., and Rawson, A. M. (1955). The orientation of homing pigeons in relation to change in sun declination. *J. Ornithol.* **96**, 168 – 172.

Santschi, F. (1911). Observations et remarques critiques sur le mechanisme de l'orientation chez les fourmis. *Rev. Suisse Zool.* **19**, 303 – 338.

Santschi, F. (1913). A propos de l'orientation virtuelle chez les fourmis. *Bull. Soc. Hist. Natur. Afr. Nord*, **4-6**, 231 – 235.

Schmidt-Koenig, K. (1961). Die Sonne als Kompass im Heim-Orientierungssystem der Brieftauban. *Z. Tierpsychol.* **18**, 221 – 244.

Schmidt-Koenig, K. (1965). Current problems in bird orientation. *Advan. Study Behav.* **1**, 217 – 278.

Schmidt-Koenig, K. (1972). New experiments on the effect of clock shifts on homing in pigeons. *In* "Animal Orientation and Navigation," (NASA SP-262), pp. 275 – 282. U.S. Gov. Printing Office, Washington, D.C.

Wachs, H. (1926). Die Wanderungen der Vögel. *Ergeb. Biol.* **1**, 479 – 639.

Walcott, C., and Michener, M. C. (1971). Sun navigation in homing pigeons — attempts to shift sun coordinates. *J. Exp. Biol.* **54,** 291–316.

Wallraff, H. G. (1966). Über die Anfangsorientierung von Brieftauben unter geschlessener Wolkendecke. *J. Ornithol.* **107,** 326–336.

Wallraff, H. G. (1967). The present status of our knowledge about pigeon homing. *Proc. 14th Int. Ornithol. Congr.* 331–358.

Wiltschko, W. (1968). Über den Einfluss statischer Magnetfelder auf die Zugorientierung der Rotkehlchen *(Erithacus rubecula). Z. Tierpsychol.* **25,** 537–559.

Wiltschko, E. (1972). The influence of magnetic total intensity and inclination on directions preferred by migrating European robins *(Erithacus rubecula). In* "Animal Orientation and Navigation (NASA SP-262)," pp. 275–282. U.S. Gov. Printing Office, Washington, D.C.

Wolf, E. (1927). Über das Heimkehrvermögen der Bienen. II. *Z. Vergl. Physiol.* **6,** 221–254.

Lunar and Tidal Rhythms in the Development and Reproduction of an Intertidal Organism

Dietrich Neumann

Physiological Ecology Section
Department of Zoology
University of Cologne
Cologne

Introduction

In most species the time of reproduction is adapted to environmental situations: certain seasons, times of day, or phases of the tides. As has been recognized in a vast number of experimental studies, exact synchronization with the environment is in general the result of physiological timing mechanisms. Circadian clocks are the best known timers and are involved in the programming of daily behavior, in celestial orientation, as well as in the photoperiodic control of development. The following report deals with two adaptive aspects of biological time measurement: (1) the diversity of timing mechanisms that are utilized by intertidal organisms, e.g., endogenous lunar rhythms, circadian rhythms, and hourglass timers, and (2) the genetic adaptation of these timing mechanisms to different environmental conditions. Both aspects will be demonstrated in one and the same species, the intertidal midge *Clunio marinus*. Distributed on European coasts from temperate to arctic latitudes, *Clunio* exists as several geographic races, and the races exhibit noticeable differences in timing mechanisms. The lunar rhythm in development and reproduction will first be discussed.

Semilunar Periodicity of Reproduction in *Clunio*

As in other poikilotherms producing more than one generation a year, the length of a generation in *Clunio* depends on temperature. At Helgoland it ranges from 3–4 months for the summer generation, and 7–10 months for the hibernating generation (Figure 1). In winter, the larval instars become dormant and pupation is inhibited; apparently photoperiod has no influence (Neumann, 1966). With rising temperatures in the sea during late spring, emergence occurs every 15 days, at the time of full and new moon, resulting in a semilunar periodicity of reproduction. Figure 2 demonstrates in detail that the emergence times regularly occur shortly after the changes of the moon, at that very moment when the extremely low waters of the spring tides expose the *Clunio* habitat in the lower range of the intertidal zone, and only in the afternoon. Thus, throughout the year a specific tidal situation, such as the afternoon low water of spring tides, occurs at nearly the same time of day every 15 days; since the tidal cycle of 12.4 hr shifts nearly 0.8 hr each day, this amounts to 12 hr every 15 days.

Clunio marinus may serve as a model of lunar rhythms in other intertidal organisms. Such examples include the spawning of the famous *Palolo* in the Pacific Ocean (Caspers, 1951; Hauenschild *et al.*, 1968), the runs of the grunion at the California beach (Walker, 1949), and the sexual reproduction of the brown algae *Dictyota* (Bünning and Müller, 1961; Vielhaben, 1963). In all these cases a strong synchronization with a tidal situation occurring regularly every 15 or 30 days at about the same time of day was described.

The adaptive significance of this timing is self-evident in *Clunio*, for the *Clunio* imago is one of the most short-lived of all insects. Its life span is only about 2 hr. Copulation takes place immediately after emergence; 15 min later the females may start laying their eggs on algae in the exposed lower part of the intertidal zone. The synchronization of emergence with the low water of spring tides guarantees both a concen-

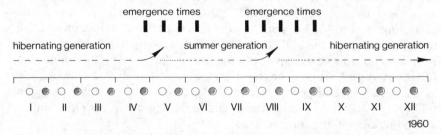

Figure 1 Time of emergence and reproduction (black rectangles) of a *Clunio marinus* population at Helgoland on the North Sea.

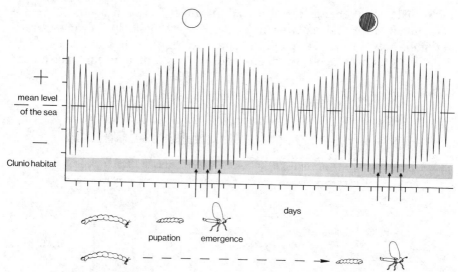

Figure 2 Relationship of emergence time to water level and phase of the moon during one month. The gray strip indicates the level of the *Clunio* habitat being exposed during extreme low waters.

tration of the short-lived adults, and a suitable environment for the off-spring.

What are the reliable cues of the environment which control the time of reproduction? What are the attributes of the corresponding timing mechanism? In *Clunio* populations with a semilunar periodicity, there are two points in the development of each specimen which are strictly time controlled: pupation and emergence. Because *Clunio* stays for only 3 – 5 days in the pupal stage, the semilunar periodicity of emergence corresponds to a semilunar periodicity of pupation, i.e., pupation is restricted to the days preceding full and new moon. Three to five days later, the emergence of the adult must be synchronized with the low water at a specific time of day. The following experiments will show that in the semilunar periodicity of reproduction there exists a semilunar and a daily timing mechanism (Neumann, 1966, 1968, 1969, and unpublished data in the "turbulence" experiments of Figures 3, 5 and 6). This combination allows the temporal coordination of reproduction with the optimum phases of the environmental cycle.

The Semilunar Timing Mechansim

When *Clunio* larvae were bred in a lighting schedule of 12 hr light and 12 hr dark (LD 12:12), the development time from hatching of the

first instar until emergence of the adult ranged between 7 and 12 weeks
(Figure 3, top) and emergence occurred arhythmically. Two separate
stimuli, however, could evoke a semilunar rhythm. If a dim moonlight
(0.4 lx) was provided for 3 nights each 30 days, then a semilunar emer-

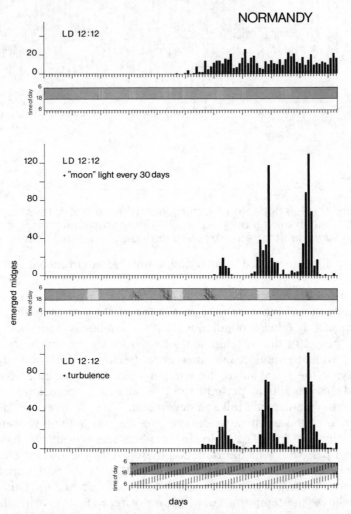

Figure 3 Entrainment of a semilunar rhythm in cultures of the Normandy population by artificial cycles of moonlight (middle) and tidal turbulence (below). The cultures started at the left side during the first instar. The schematic graph beneath each diagram represents the experimental conditions in LD 12:12. White: 12 hr light; dark gray: 12 hr night; light gray: 12 hr of dim light (0.4 lx) given every 30 days for four consecutive nights; vertical line: time of tidal turbulence.

gence pattern resulted (Figure 3, middle). A 12.4-hr tidal cycle of water turbulence superimposed on a 24-hr light–dark cycle was effective as well (Figure 3, bottom).

The moonlight experiment suggests that the semilunar rhythm is not controlled by a single stimulus–response system, because pupation always occurred near the moonlight period or about 2 weeks later. Evidence for an endogenous semilunar rhythm is given in Figure 4, where a free-running rhythm was evoked by a single stimulus and persisted for nearly four cycles until the cultures were exhausted. The endogenous rythym brings larvae into a state of readiness for pupation approximately every two weeks. The semilunar oscillator is an important link in the semilunar timing mechanism. In analogy to the "circadian clock" it may be called "circasemilunar" or "circasyzygical" clock (Neumann, 1969). Similarly, the synchronizing effect of moonlight on an endogenous lunar rhythm has been established in the polychaete *Platnereis* by Hauenschild (1956, 1960) and in the brown algae *Dictyote* by Bünning and Müller (1961) and Vielhaben (1963).

From a physiological point of view the oscillating mechanism of such biological clocks is without a doubt the chief problem. However, if we consider the adaptive significance of the timing mechanism as a whole, two further problems arise: (a) the entrainment of the clock by external *zeitgebers*, (b) the internal coupling of the clock with the rhythmic function in development or behavior. In the case of *Clunio* one can gain further insight into entrainment by observing two population specific adaptations.

As mentioned earlier, the Normandy population can be entrained by two different *zeitgebers:* moonlight and tidal turbulence. Figure 5 summarizes similar experiments with the Helgoland population. In contrast

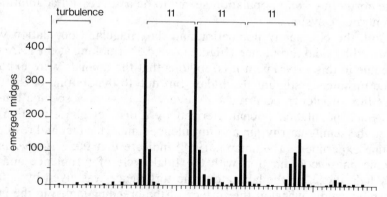

Figure 4 Free-running semilunar rhythms induced in a Helgoland population by water turbulence.

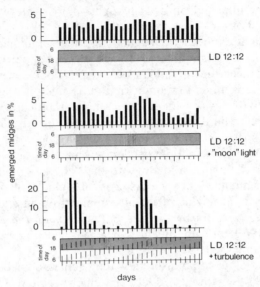

Figure 5 Effect of LD cycles (above), moonlight (middle), and water turbulence (below) on emergence of Helgoland populations.

to the Normandy stock, artificial moonlight had negligible influence. Helgoland (54° N) is situated farther north than Normandy and it is nearer to the fringe of temperate latitudes. One may suppose that at Helgoland a nocturnal dim light might be an unreliable *zeitgeber* during June and July, when the height of the full moon becomes extremely low, and dusk and dawn shorten the length of full darkness to a few hours (Neumann, 1966, 1968). The lack of effectiveness of moonlight in the more northern *Clunio* population seems to be a successful adaptation of the entraining system.

Both the Normandy population and the Helgoland population were entrained by tidal turbulence (Figures 4 and 5). Looking at the *zeitgeber* schedule in this experiment it is obvious that the animals were exposed to the turbulence stimulus each day, but due to the shifting of the tidal cycle the turbulence occurred only every 15 days at a specific time of day. Each population is characterized by a distinct phase relation between the semilunar rhythm and turbulence time. This fact and results of shifting experiments (Neumann, 1968) indicate that the *zeitgeber* has a specific phase coordination with the tidal cycle of turbulence and the daily light cycle. In the laboratory the turbulence was given by a small splashing paddle wheel at the surface of the breeding tanks; in the intertidal habitat this time cue is probably the mechanical stimulus given by wave action during flood tide.

Along the European coast spring tides occur on the same days of the lunar month, but the phase relation between the tides and the local time of day may differ by several hours. For example, tides at Normandy and Helgoland differ by nearly 150 min. Because the semilunar rhythm of both populations is synchronized in the field with the spring tides, the entrainment of the timing mechanism of each population has to be adapted to the local phase of the tides. Figure 6 demonstrates that under the same *zeitgeber* program the peaks of the semilunar rhythms of Normandy and Helgoland stock differ by nearly 3 days; this corresponds well with the difference between the tidal cycles at the two locations: 150 min, or 3 days in terms of the daily shifting of the tides by nearly 50 min.

The Normandy and Helgoland populations illustrate the genetic adaptation of the semilunar timing mechanism to local tidal conditions. Because of the many local differences in the tides, a great number of geographic races can be expected along the Atlantic coast of France, Spain, and England. Further analysis of the distinct phase relationship

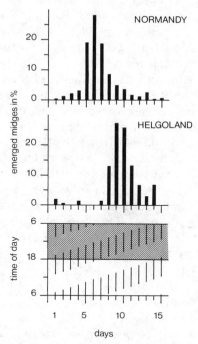

Figure 6 Relationship of emergence time to the tidal cycle of turbulence in Normandy and Helgoland populations.

between light cycle and tidal turbulence (or moonlight) will afford more information about the entraining system as well as the coupling system of the complex semilunar timing mechanism. This will be similar to photoperiodic time measurement (Bünning, 1967; Pittendrigh, 1972) if it can be shown that *Clunio* has a sensitive stage for turbulence or moonlight during a specific time of the night; the sensitive stage would then coincide with the tidal cycle every 15 days and with the moonlight cycle every 30 days.

The Daily Timing Mechanism

In the field, the semilunar emergence time of a *Clunio* population is restricted to a certain time of day which is correlated with the local time of low water of the spring tides. When *Clunio* is cultivated in artificial light cycles the imagos emerge at a population-specific time of day relative to the light cycle. The daily timing is characterized by two facts: (a) it is completely independent of the semilunar timing of the beginning of pupation, (b) it is determined by a circadian clock as in *Drosophila* (Bünning, 1967; Pittendrigh, 1966) and many other insects. The daily emergence time can be reset to any desired local time by altering the light program. Thus, the 24-hr light–dark cycle is the dominating zeitgeber of the daily timing mechanism.

Corresponding to the time-displacements of the tidal cycle along the coasts, one must expect that populations from different places will differ in their diurnal emergence times in the field and also in the laboratory. A population specific adaptation of the circadian timing mechanism was confirmed in laboratory studies (Figure 7). By means of cross-breeding experiments, genetic control was demonstrated. In the case of two French populations the experiments indicate that a difference of 4 hr in the mean emergence time is controlled by a few genes only (Figure 8). The curves of F_1, F_2, and backcross illustrate the segregation typical for quantitative characters. Presumably a control by a few genes has permitted beneficial gentic flexibility during the evolution of the two populations.

The Tidal Timing Mechanism

At the present time the *Clunio marinus* story comes to an end above the Arctic Circle. The populations of the fjords of northern Norway comprise a geographic race whose emergence time is controlled by an

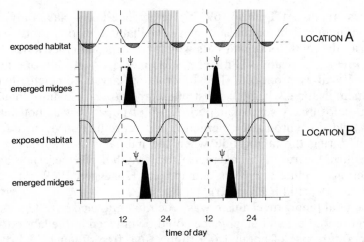

Figure 7 Schematic representation of emergence time in two populations of *Clunio* showing relationship to the water level at the site of origin as well as Ψ in artificial LD studies (after Neumann, 1966).

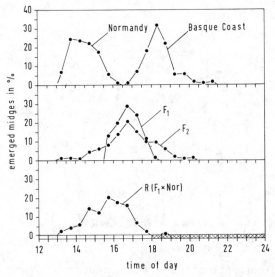

Figure 8 Crossbreeding between two populations which differ in their daily emergence time. Above: emergence time of parental stocks; middle and below: emergence time of F₁, F₂ and backcross (light, 0600–1800; dark, 1800–0600) (from Neumann, 1967).

hourglass timer. At Tromsö (69° N) emergence takes place only during the continuous light of midsummer. The habitat of this arctic race is primarily the midlittoral mud flats which are exposed twice a day by the tides. Field observations (Pflüger, 1973) indicate that only one generation per year is produced. The hibernating larvae complete their development in June, when the substrate temperatures rise more than 10°C during exposure. A semilunar periodicity of pupation was not detected in the field. Synchronized emergence and reproduction occurred every 12.4 hr during the falling tide when the habitat was resurfacing. This synchronization results in a precise tidal rhythm of emergence and reproduction (Remmert, 1965; Neumann and Honegger, 1969; Pflüger and Neumann, 1971; Pflüger, 1973).

The tidal timing mechanism was recently unraveled by Pflüger (1973, see Figure 9). Peaks of emergence could be induced in the laboratory by a temperature rise of about 1°C or more. No free-running tidal rhythm, however, could be observed in any experiment. There was always an immediate peak (direct response) and a second peak 11 – 13 hr later; this demonstrates the action of an hourglass timer which inhibits emergence for about 12 hr during a final phase of pupation. In the field the tempera-

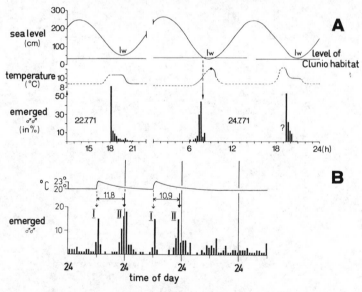

Figure 9 Emergence of the arctic population of *Clunio marinus* from Tromso, Norway. A, Tidal rhythm in the field in relation to tides and water temperature. B, Laboratory experiments in LL with brief temperature rises which immediately evoke a first peak (I) and a second (II) nearly 11 – 12 hr later (after Pfluger, 1973).

ture of the substrate regularly rises every 12.4 hr during exposure of the habitat so that a direct response is induced when the hourglass phase of the preceding tide ends. This superposition of an hourglass timing mechanism and a direct response guarantees a very good synchronization of the rhythm of reproduction with the tides.

Tidal timing mechanisms of other kinds have been observed in crustaceans, snails, mussels, and fish; many examples concern the control of locomotory behavior (Enright, 1963b; Naylor, 1958; Zann, 1973; Gibson, 1970). In most of these studies free-running tidal rhythms have been detected under constant conditions. The most extensive and profound analysis was given by Enright (1963a) with the amphipod *Synchelidium* and by Klapow (1972) with the isopod *Excirolana*. In both cases it was supposed that the rhythms were based on a circadian oscillator which was entrained by tidal factors such as turbulence instead of the daily light–dark cycle. Until now clear evidence for a circatidal oscillator is lacking. During the last decade most biorhythm ecologists concentrated on self-sustained oscillations and perhaps ignored other mechanisms. The arctic *Clunio* is not the only case of an hourglass timer in intertidal organisms. Recently Lehmann (personal communication) found hourglass programming in the filter feeding activity of the barnacle *Balanus improvisus*. Furthermore, in African populations of the fiddler crab, the tidal timing mechanism of locomotory activity is also not based on a self-sustained oscillator (Lehmann *et al.*, 1974). Because these examples are outside the scope of this chapter they will be discussed elsewhere.

Summary

Intertidal organisms are confronted with remarkable fluctuations of temperature, light, submergence, turbulence, hydrostatic pressure and other factors. These fluctuations depend upon the beach level occupied, on the geographic location, and, last but not least, on the actual weather. In spite of such complexity and variability, advantageous intertidal conditions reoccur at regular, precise intervals. Presumably an accurate synchronization of development and reproduction with favorable situations by means of timing mechanisms confers a high selective advantage. In summary, it can be stated for *Clunio* that: (1) the timing mechanisms allow synchronization with environmental cycles; (2) the timing mechanisms can adapt to reliable time cues; (3) the combination of two timing mechanisms during development results in a very precise temporal programming.

An important question remains unanswered: What are the gene controlled adaptations of the timing mechanisms? Finding an answer to this question will be difficult because of the multiple factors involved. Receptor sensitivity, the entraining system, the basic clock itself, and coupling processes must all be considered, as has been shown in classical experiments with *Drosophila*, cockroaches, and silkmoths (Pittendrigh, 1967; Brady, 1969; Truman, 1971). Studies with intertidal organisms, including *Clunio*, may offer deeper insight into the adaptive aspects of timing mechanisms and its gene-controlled parameters.

Acknowledgment

Supported by a grant from the Deutsche Forschungsgemeinschaft.

References

Brady, J. (1969). How are insect circadian rhythms controlled? *Nature London* **223**, 781–784.

Bünning, E. (1967). "The Physiological Clock." Springer, New York.

Bünning, E., and Müller, D. (1961). Wie messen Organismen lunare Zyklen? *Z. Naturforsch.* **16b**, 391–395.

Caspers, H. (1951). Rhythmische Erscheinungen in der Fortpflanzung von *Clunio marinus* (Dipt. Chiron.) und das Problem der lunaren Periodizität bei Organismen. *Arch. Hydrobiol.* (Suppl.) **18**, 415–594.

Enright, J. T. (1963a). The tidal rhythms of activity of a sandbeach amphipod. *Z. Vergl. Physiol.* **46**, 276–313.

Enright, J. T. (1963b). Endogenous tidal and lunar rhythms. *Int. Congr. Zool.* **16** (4), 355–359.

Gibson, R. N. (1970). The tidal rhythm of activity of *Coryphoblennius galerita* (L.) (Teleostei, Blenniidae). *Anim. Behav.* **18**, 539–543.

Hauenschild, C. (1956). Neue experimentelle Untersuchungen zum Problem der Lunarperiodizität. *Naturwissenschaften* **43**, 361–363.

Hauenschild, C. (1960). Lunar periodicity. *Cold Springs Harbor Symp. Quant. Biol.* **25**, 491–497.

Hauenschild, C., Fischer, A., and Hoffmann, D. K. (1968). Untersuchungen am pazifischen Palolowurm *Eunice viridis* (Polychaeta) in Samoa. *Helg. Wiss. Meeresunters* **18**, 254–295.

Klapow, L. A. (1972). Natural and artificial rephasing of a tidal rhythm. *J. Comp. Physiol.* **79**, 233–258.

Lehmann, U., Neumann, D., and Kaiser, H. (1974). Gezeitenrhythmische und spontane Aktivitätsmuster von Winkerkrabben—ein neuer Ansatz zur quantitativen Analyse von Lokomotionsrhythmen *J. Comp. Physiol.* **91**, 187–221.

Naylor, E. (1958). Tidal and diurnal rhythms of locomotory activity in *Carcinus maenas* (L.). *J. Exp. Biol.* **35**, 602–610.

Neumann, D. (1966). Die lunare und tägliche Schlupfperiodik der Mücke *Clunio*—Steuerung und Abstimmung auf die Gezeitenperiodik. *Z. Vergl. Physiol.* **53**, 1–61.

Neumann, D. (1967). Genetic adaptation in the emergence time of *Clunio* populations to different tidal conditions. *Helg. Wiss. Meeresunters.* **15**, 163–171.

Neumann, D. (1968). Die Steuerung einer semilunaren Sclüpfperiodik mit Hilfe eines künstlichen Gezeitenzyklus. *Z. Vergl. Physiol.* **60**, 63–78.

Neumann, D. (1969). Die Kombination verschiedener endogener Rhythmen bei der zeitlichen Programmierung von Entwicklung und Verhalten. *Oecologia* **3**, 166–183.

Neumann, D., and Honegger, H. W. (1969). Adaptations of the intertidal midge *Clunio* to arctic conditions. *Oecologia* **3**, 1–13.

Pflüger, W. (1973). Die Sanduhrsteuerung der gezeitensynchronen Schlüpfrhythmik der Mucke *Clunio marinus* im arktischen Mitsommer. *Oecologia* **11**, 113–150.

Pflüger, W., and Neumann, D. (1971). Die Steuerung einer gezeitenparallelen Schlüpfrhythmik nach dem Sanduhr-Prinzip. *Oecologia* **7**, 262–266.

Pittendrigh, C. S. (1966). The circadian oscillation in *Drosophila pseudoobscura* pupae: a model for the photoperiodic clock. *Z. Pflanz. Physiol.* **54**, 275–307.

Pittendrigh, C. S. (1967). Circadian systems. 1. The driving oscillation and its assay in *Drosophila pseudoobscura*. *Proc. Nat. Acad. Sci* **58**, 1762–1767.

Pittendrigh, C. S. (1972). Circadian surfaces and the diversity of possible roles of circadian organization in photoperiodic induction. *Proc. Nat. Acad. Sci* **69**, 2734–2737.

Remmert, H. (1965). Über den Tagesrhythmus arktischer Tiere. *Z. Morp. Ökol. Tiere* **55**, 142–160.

Truman, J. W. (1971). Circadian rhythms and physiology with special reference to neuroendocrine processes in insects. *Proc. Int. Symp. Circadian Rhythmicity* Wageningen, 111–135.

Vielhaben, V. (1963). Zur Deutung des semilunaren Fortpflanzungszyklus von *Dictyota dichotoma*. *Z. Bot* **51**, 156–173.

Walker, B. W. (1949). Periodicity of spawning of the grunion, *Leuresthes tenuis*, an antherine fish. Ph.D. thesis, Univ. of California at Los Angeles, California.

Zann, L. P. (1973). Interactions of the circadian and circatidal rhythms of the littoral gastropod *Melanerita atramentosa* Reeve. *J. Exp. Mar. Biol. Ecol.* **11**, 249–261.

The Circadian Tape Recorder and its Entrainment

J. T. Enright

Scripps Institution of Oceanography
University of California
La Jolla, California

Introduction

Rhythmicity is such a widespread and essential aspect of the functioning of living systems that most biologists have tended to take its existence and generality for granted without further consideration. High-frequency rhythms are evident in the firing of spontaneously active neurons, in the tonic discharge of sensory systems, and in the cardiac and respiratory systems. Somewhat longer periods are evident in the rhythm of brainwave records, particularly during sleep; and the spectrum of rhythmicity extends to tidal and daily biological cycles, including those which underlie the wake – sleep cycle; fortnightly and monthly rhythms, as seen in the reproduction and activity of intertidal organisms and in the human menstrual cycle; and annual rhythms as observed in growth and reproductive processes of a large array of arctic and temperate zone plants and animals.

While any regular rhythmic system could, in principle, be used for time measurement, all the so-called biological clocks which underlie biological time measurement represent rhythms of a special sort, sharing at least two essential properties. (1) Timing rhythms have natural (i.e., spontaneous or free-running) periods which are close to those of certain natural environmental cycles: the tidal and the daily cycles; the semilunar and lunar cycles; and the yearly cycle; and (2) these biological clocks represent rhythms which can be entrained by (i. e., synchronized with) the natural environmental cycle which they approximate in period.

Entrainment is the essential key to biological time measurement, the *sine qua non* of its adaptive value. The teleonomic, evolutionary "purpose" of these special rhythms is to permit organisms to synchronize their life processes, their physiology, and behavior with the environment, just as our electric and mechanical clocks permit us to synchronize our activities with our physical and social environment. A free-running circadian rhythm with a period of, say, 23½ hours, would have no ecological usefulness in the field; it would lead the animal to wake up 30 min earlier each successive day, which would, in fact, ordinarily be badly maladaptive. A free-running rhythm of this sort might well be able to produce internal coordination of physiological processes within the individual; but for this function alone the period of the rhythm might equally well be 10 hr, or 40 hr, corresponding to nothing of environmental consequence. Only when a circadian rhythm has been synchronized with and by the environment can its true adaptive significance, as a mechanism for time measurement, be realized.

Entrainment as a General Process

How is this environmental synchronization accomplished? The method commonly used by physiologists to answer this question has been to observe the free-running rhythm of the organism under constant conditions, and then to give a single, appropriate stimulus, such as a light pulse, in order to determine the extent to which this stimulus shifts the phase of (i. e., resets) the system. Probably the simplest kind of synchronization process which can be envisioned is illustrated in Figure 1A: the stimulus might immediately produce "complete reset" of the rhythm to a new timing determined by the phase in the cycle at which the stimulus is given. One can easily imagine such a process as operative in an electronic oscillator based upon charging and discharging of a capacitor; and comparable results have been obtained experimentally in certain neurological preparations (Perkel *et al.*, 1964).

A common method for summarizing data from an array of experiments of this sort is called a "phase-response curve," such as shown in Figure 1B based on the idealized system of Figure 1A. Since the decision about whether a given phase shift in a system of this sort represents an advance or a delay is rather arbitrary, two separate response-curve lines can be drawn for the hypothetical data; and as shown in Figure 1C, depending upon the convention adopted (for example, assuming that a phase shift is never more than 180°) additional variations in the method of presenting the same basic data are available.

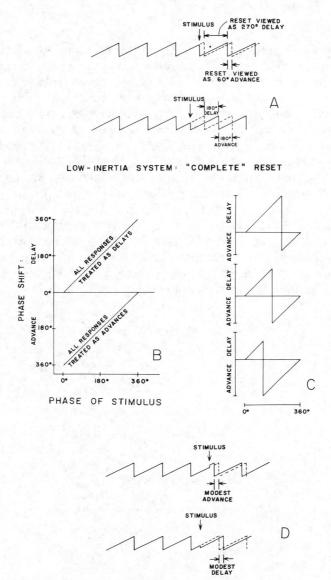

Figure 1 Theoretical possibilities for rephasing an oscillating system. A, Stimulus causes an immediate and complete reset of the rhythm (expected oscillations without stimulus indicated by dashed line). B, Phase-response curves for a system which shows complete reset, as in (A); rephasing can be regarded as either advance or delay, depending upon interpretation of cycle(s) in which stimulus is given. C, Alternative presentations of the results shown in (A) and (B). D, Stimulus causes only partial reset of the rhythm, with amount and direction of reset dependent upon phase of stimulation.

The practical ecological problem with synchronization of this elementary sort is that it would characterize a system which is extremely sensitive to perturbation. The biological system would have a very low inertia in the time domain, and a single mistimed stimulus, such as might be provided by a lightning storm or bright moonlight, would lead to reset of the biological clock to an inappropriate phase. A day-active burrowing ground squirrel, for example, might find his biological clock completely reset each time he emerges from his burrow. Figure 1D shows a slightly more complex form of resetting which involves reduced sensitivity to perturbation: the stimulus produces only a partial reset, a phase-shift which compensates only in part for the out-of-time stimulus. Experimental data indicate that this is the more usual situation in the responsiveness of circadian rhythms to stimuli. Figure 2 summarizes experimentally obtained phase-response curves for light stimuli administered to several circadian systems. None of these curves indicates "complete reset" by the stimulus throughout the entire cycle; the data for nocturnal

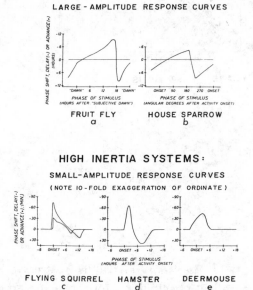

Figure 2 Measured phase-response curves for several circadian systems. a, *Drosophila pseudoobscura,* data for 4-hr stimuli from Pittendrigh, 1960. b, *Passer domesticus,* data from Eskin, 1971. c, *Glaucomys volans,* data from DeCoursey, 1961. d, *Mesocricetus auratus,* data from DeCoursey, 1964. e, *Peromyscus leucopus,* data from Rawson, 1960. Note that none of these curves involves complete reset of the rhythm at all phases of the cycle; thus, the systems are comparable with Figure 1 D, and not Figure 1 A.

mammals indicate, in fact, a quite low sensitivity to resetting stimuli. In other words, these latter biological rhythms have a high temporal inertia: a single stimulus produces only modest reset of the timing processess; and major rephasing of the biological clock, which represents the true process of entrainment, requires stimuli repeatedly experienced over many cycles.

This, then, is the process of entrainment as commonly studied by the physiologist. The stimuli involved need not be light; changes of temperature are quite effective as entraining stimuli for poikilotherms (Hoffmann, 1968); cycles of conspecific song (Gwinner, 1966; Menaker and Eskin, 1966), as well as of a loud buzzer (Lohmann and Enright, 1967) can entrain the activity rhythms of birds; cycles of barometric pressure have entrained the activity cycles of pocket mice (Hayden and Lindberg, 1969); and mechanical stimuli can produce entrainment of the activity rhythms of certain beach crustaceans (Enright, 1965; Klapow, 1972) as was well as birds (Figure 3). This latter case is clearly only a laboratory curiosity, since comparable stimulus cycles would be unlikely in a natural environment, but the result indicates that sensory stimuli of a wide variety can potentially act as entraining agents for circadian rhythms.

What is the physiological mechanism involved in this process of resetting and entraining biological timing systems? At this point, no detailed general answer can be given. The question is under study in several laboratories, and perhaps it is not surprising that we do not yet fully understand the mechanisms. Only very recently have we learned that even our casual assumptions about the sensory systems involved in entrainment can be badly mistaken. Menaker and one of his students (Menaker, 1968; Underwood and Menaker, 1970) have demonstrated that the action of light upon the circadian rhythms of both birds and reptiles is apparently not mediated throught the ordinary visual system, but instead is based upon extraretinal light receptors, located in the brain.

While the physiologist may be frustrated by how little is known about the details of the entrainment process, this volume is organized around the theme of the adaptive significance of biological timing, and therefore for the moment, we need not concern ourselves further with such questions.

A 24-Hour Tape Recorder?

In the process of studying circadian rhythms in the laboratory, it appears to me that physiologists have paid too little attention to a particularly interesting and potentially important feature of their data: the fact

Figure 3 Perch-hopping record of an isolated house finch, subject to treatment by cage-shaking: double-plotted data, with number of 22 hr, 40 min cycles or "days" shown on left margin. Light intensity of about 0.5 lx; temperature of 20°C. During treatment, the cage was slowly raised by about 1 cm, and then suddenly dropped onto rubber cushions, at a rate of three cage oscillations per minute. Treatment was applied for 6 hr, in cycles with a period 22 hr, 40 min, with one phase shift, between "days" 40 and 74, and between "days" 84 and 125; treatment was continuous on "days" 145 to 161. Times of cyclic treatment have been enclosed by rectangles on only one of the two records, so that activity onsets during treatment can also be inspected without the bias introduced by vertical lines superimposed on the record. During continous treatment, the free-running period was shortened by about 10 min, relative to pre- and post-treatment values. While entrainment by treatment was somewhat labile from "days" 50 to 74 and 90 to 125, an examination of activity onsets in the unenclosed portions of the record leaves little doubt that treatment affected the activity rhythm to produce synchronization. In the second comparable experiment performed with another bird, the finch's activity rhythm initially had a free-running period of 23 hr 2 min, for 22 cycles. Following eight cycles, during which the onset of activity gradually approached onset of shaking, the rhythm showed stable entrainment, (T = 22 hr, 40 min), with activity onset exactly coincident with onset of shaking, for 16 cycles. During the subsequent free run, the period gradually lengthened, over seven transient cycles, before stabilizing on a value of 22 hr, 59 min, for 34 cycles.

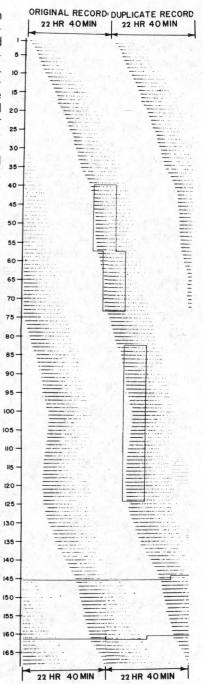

that a circadian rhythm of locomotor activity often involves the cycle-after-cycle repetition of a rather complex "pattern" of behavior. When dealing with the process of entrainment, most workers have tended to focus attention upon some single phase-reference point in the cycle, such as onset or midpoint of locomotor activity, to the neglect of the entire repetitive pattern.

I first became interested in this phenomenon in conjunction with laboratory data on tidal rhythms, in which there is circadian repetition of an asymmetric bimodal pattern of activity, with intense swimming by the crustaceans at times of the higher of the two daily high tides, and a burst of lesser activity correlated with times of the lower high tide (Enright, 1963; Klapow, 1972). This pattern which parallels the tides is reflected both in the behavior of populations of animals (Klapow, 1972) and in single individuals (Enright, 1972.) The fact that the pattern observed reflects prior field conditions has suggested to me the analogy of a 24-hr closed-loop tape recorder.

Comparable repetition of activity patterns in the laboratory is not, however, just characteristic of animals which are ordinarily synchronized by the tides. Examples can be found in the activity records of many species of mammals and birds when studied under both free-running conditions and under entrainment by a light–dark cycle in the laboratory. The repetitive patterns range from weak bimodality [DeCoursey, 1961 (Figure 9); Aschoff and Wever, 1962 (Figure 1), 1963, (Figure 1)] through clear three-peaked patterns [Pittendrigh, 1967 (Figure 2); Hoffmann, 1969 (Figure 3), 1970 (Figure 4)] on to multimodal repetition [DeCoursey, 1961, (Figure 3); Pittendrigh, 1960, (Figure 12)]. Sometimes an observed pattern of activity will persist for many weeks; in other cases, there may be gradual changes in pattern, over intervals of a few days or weeks [Aschoff, 1966 (Figure 2); Enright, 1966 (Figure 3)].

Figure 4 represents a striking example of the kind of detailed pattern which may be repeated, and the ways in which patterns may change under constant conditions. For the first 27 days, the finch began its daily cycle with a 3- 4-hr burst of intense activity, followed by scattered activity for 8 – 9 hr, and then a 5- to 10- min burst of very intense activity just before going to sleep on the perch (note pen position during inactivity). Beginning on about day 12, the bird began to show a 2- to 3-hr rest interval—while remaining *off* the perch—just before the final 10-min burst; this feature persisted until at least day 27, when the entire morning burst of activity was nearly completely "erased from the tape"—perhaps precipitated by the feeding disturbance on day 27. The brief end-of-the-day burst of activity, before retirement on the perch, persisted more or less unchanged throughout the recording. The pre-retirement rest interval

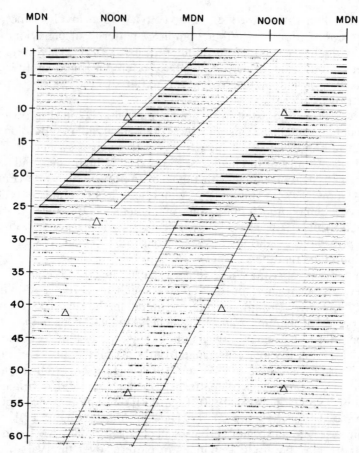

Figure 4 Perch-hopping record of an isolated house finch under constant dim light (approximately 0.5 lx) and constant temperature
(20°C); double-plotted data, with number 24-hr days indicated on left
margin. Five-min feeding disturbances indicated by triangles. *No*
change in constant conditions (light, temperature, etc.) occurred on
day 27; the change in activity pattern and period of the rhythm was
perhaps induced by the feeding disturbance. See text for detailed
discussion of activity pattern.

became clear again by about day 30, only to disappear spontaneously by
about day 39. A careful examination of records such as this indicates
remarkably detailed circadian repetition of daily activity patterns. One
way of describing results of this sort would be to say that the animal
"gets into daily habits," just as do you and I. Another way of phrasing it
is to say that the animal has a strong tendency to repeat the timing pattern

of activity from preceding days, like a circa 24-hr closed loop on a tape recorder, even under conditions of no external reinforcement of the pattern.

What is the mechanism for such repetition? Does it mean that the circadian system underlying locomotor activity represents a multioscillator system? This is an important question for the physiologist, and the answer today is in most cases by no means clear: perhaps there are many "circadian clocks," each associated with a separate aspect of the pattern; perhaps there is only one basic circadian timing system, with the possibility of many separate reference points throughout the cycle, analogous, indeed, with a closed-loop tape recorder. For present purposes, the question of physiological mechanism is less important than the recognition that repetitive patterns of this sort occur.

What is the meaning of this phenomenon for the ecologist? What is its adaptive significance under field conditions? My answer would be that under the greater environmental complexity of the natural environment, one should expect the animal to be much more a "victim of its habits" than in the laboratory; that one should expect an animal more or less to repeat, day after day, its general pattern of behavior on a time-dependent basis. If a particular animal was observed yesterday to be feeding at a given location, at a given time of the day, one should expect the same animal at the same locaction at about the same time today. If a given bird sang yesterday to announce his territory from a given tree at a given time, or took a noonday rest in a particular bush, he should, with high probability, be expected to be there today. And such a repetitive pattern is, *a priori*, a good strategy for today: if the animal is still alive and healthy this morning, this means that what he did yesterday was more or less the "right" thing to do. Therefore, his best "guess" for survival is to repeat approximately what he did yesterday, on a time-dependent basis. Not too rigidly, however; he should be prepared to take advantage of a new opportunity when it is offered, and to incorporate the attendant behavior into his strategy—his tape loop—for tomorrow. But yesterday's strategy "worked," and it is far more reasonable for the animal to repeat yesterday's daily pattern of behavior than to make a random choice of what to do, and when to do it.

In studying circadian rhythms in the laboratory in a topographically and temporally simplified environment, we give the animal very little chance to show this kind of complexity in his circadian pattern; the amazing thing to me is that we see as much repeating pattern as we do under constant conditions of only self-generated reinforcement.

Does such daily repetition of temporal and spatial patterning of behavior really take place in the field, under natural conditions? One clear line of evidence that it does is found in the time-training of bees, in which the same individual can be induced to come to a given feeder at one time of day, and to another feeder at a second time of day. Comparable experiments have been conducted with birds (Stein, 1951), and similar behavior has been observed of bees in a more natural ecological situation (Janzen, 1970). Nearly all other evidence for such regular daily programming of behavior is anecdotal. I could describe many isolated cases, unsupported by adequate documentation: situations in which a given animal—a house pet, a bird in the field, or the like—has "gotten in the habit" of doing something at the same time each day, a habit which persists for at least several days; and most readers will probably know of similar instances from their own experiences. Such anecdotes do not, however, provide proper foundation for evaluation of the present hypothesis. In order to determine how general such timing of behavior may be under field conditions, a careful and systematic investigation will be necessary by experienced naturalists. On the basis of the laboratory data, it is evident that we should be looking for patterns of behavior which are characteristic of a particular individual, rather than of an entire species. And, as every ecologist will recognize, one should not expect time-dependent "habits" to be completely independent of prevailing environmental conditions. An animal's behavior in the field is a complex, nonadditive resultant of the endogenous "readiness" to behave in a given way and of exogenous stimuli which modify these internally generated tendencies. Time-trained bees, for example, will remain in the hive for up to several days during inclement weather, only to return to the feeder at the appropriate time of day when clear weather returns. Furthermore, because of secular trends in environmental factors and because behavior which is well rewarded one day may thus become gradually less successful, one should not expect an animal under field conditions to show time-dependent habits which persist for as long as we observe under constant laboratory conditions. Temporal patterning of behavior under constant laboratory conditions can persist unmodified for long intervals because the environment provides little if anything in the way of reward, or of punishment in the form of lack of success: essentially any pattern the animal settles upon is as "good" as any other. In a natural environment, in contrast, we should expect time-correlated habits to be frequently "erased from the tape loop," to be replaced by the recording of some new element in the pattern.

Can one refer to this process as circadian entrainment? Probably not, at least as the term "entrainment" is usually used. Maybe the process is real entrainment of separate circadian oscillators; and maybe it is analogous with recording something on a circadian "tape loop." For the ecological application of circadian rhythmicity, the formation of such patterns is in itself of broad significance, regardless of mechanism. Is the process really "learning" in the usual sense? The behavioral events may in some cases seem to be comparable with learned habits, associated with an obvious reward, a process like conditioning. In other cases, the mere act of behavior itself (e.g., territoral singing at a given time) may be self-rewarding. I should emphasize, however, that the basic circadian oscillation system is inborn: genetically fixed in period, and not learned. In other words, the length of the circadian tape loop is not determined by experience; hence, if we wish to make analogies with more usual learning processes, we must confine our attention to the messages on the inborn tape loop, which can be recorded or erased, as dictated by experience.

It is my contention that these repeated circadian patterns of behavior may represent the real ecological meaning, the primary adaptive significance of biological clocks for higher animals: a time-dependent environmental entrainment of "habits," so that the animal can exploit the strategy of getting into a "behavioral rut." For an animal trying to deal with a hostile and erratic environment, "getting into a rut" in this way—tending to pattern each day's routine after yesterday's—has a high *a priori* probability of being a good strategy: perhaps not optimal strategy, but at least far better as a point of departure than a random choice.

Acknowledgment

Preparation of this manuscript was supported by Grant GB-36750 of the National Science Foundation.

References

Aschoff, J. (1966). Circadian activity rhythms of chaffinches *(Fringilla coelebs)* under constant conditions. *Jap. J. Physiol.* **16**, 363–370.

Aschoff, J., and Wever, R. (1962). Über Phasenbeziehungen zwischen biologisher Tagesperiodik und Zeitgeberperiodik. *Z. Vergl. Physiol.* **46**, 115–128.

Aschoff, J., and Wever, R. (1963). Resynchronization der Tagesperiodik von Vögeln nach Phasensprung des Zeitgebers. *Z. Vergl. Physiol.* **46**, 321–335.

Aschoff, J., and Wever, R. (1965). Circadian rhythms of finches in light-dark cycles with interposed twilights. *Comp. Biochem. Physiol.* **16**, 507–514.

DeCoursey, P. J. (1961). Effect of light on the circadian activity rhythm of the flying squirrel, *Glacomys volans. Z. Vergl. Physiol.* **44**, 331–354.

DeCoursey, P. J. (1964). Functions of a light response rhythm in hamsters. *J. Cell. Comp. Physiol.* **63**, 189–197.

Enright, J. T. (1963). The tidal rhythm of activity of a sand-beach amphipod. *Z. Vergl. Physiol.* **46**, 276–313.

Enright, J. T. (1965). Entrainment of a tidal rhythm. *Science* **147**, 864–867.

Enright, J. T. (1966). Influences of seasonal factors on the activity onset of the House Finch. *Ecology* **47**, 662–666.

Enright, J. T. (1972). A virtuoso isopod: circa-lunar rhythms and their tidal fine-structure. *J. Comp. Physiol.* **77**, 141–162.

Eskin, A. (1971). Some properties of the system controlling the circadian activity rhythms of sparrows. *In* "Biochronometry," (M. Menaker, ed.), pp. 55–80. Nat. Acad. Sci., Washington, D.C.

Gwinner, E. (1966). Entrainment of a circadian rhythm in birds by species-specific song cycles (Aves, Fringillidae: *Carduelis spinus*, *Serinus serinus*). *Experientia* **22**, 765.

Hayden, P., and Lindberg, R. G. (1969). Circadian rhythm in mammalian body temperature entrained by cyclic pressure changes. *Science* **164**, 1288–1289.

Hoffmann, K. (1968). Synchronization der circadianen Aktivitätsperiodik von Eidechsen durch Temperaturcyclen verschiedener Amplitude. *Z. Vergl. Physiol.* **58**, 225–228.

Hoffmann, K. (1969). Circadiane Periodik bei Tupajas in konstanten Bedingungen. *Verh. deutsch. Zool. Ges. 1969*, 171–177.

Hoffmann, K. 1970. Zur Synchronization biologischer Rhythmen. *Verh. d Deutsch. Zool. Ges. 1970*, 266–273.

Janzen, D. H. (1970). "Traplining by Tropical Bees, and Plant Spatial and Temporal Proximity." Univ. of Chicago Press, Chicago, Illinois.

Klapow, L. A. (1972). Natural and artificial rephasing of a tidal rhythm. *J. Comp. Physiol.* **79**, 233–258.

Lohmann, M., and Enright, J. T. (1967). The influence of mechanical noise on the activity rhythms of finches. *Comp. Biochem. Physiol.* **22**, 289–296.

Menaker, M. (1968). Extraretinal light perception in the sparrow. I. Entrainment of the biological clock. *Proc. Nat. Acad. Sci.* **59**, 414–421.

Menaker, M., and Eskin, A. (1966). Entrainment of circadian rhythms by sound in *Passer domesticus*. *Science* **154**, 1579–1581.

Perkel, D. H., Schulman, J. H., Bullock, T. H., Moore, G. P., and Segundo, J. P. (1964). Pacemaker neurons: effects of regularly spaced synaptic input. *Science* **145**, 61–63.

Pittendrigh, C. S. (1960). Circadian rhythms and the circadian organization of living systems. *Cold Springs Harbor Symp. Quant. Biol.* **25**, 159–184.

Pittendrigh, C. S. (1967). Circadian rhythms, space research and manned space flight. *In* "Life Sciences and Space Research," pp. 122–134. North-Holland, Amsterdam.

Rawson, K. S. (1960). Effects of tissue temperature on mammalian activity rhythms. *Cold Springs Harbor Symp. Quant. Biol.* **25**, 105–113.

Stein, H. (1951). Untersuchungen über den Zeitsinn bei Vögeln. *Z. Vergl. Physiol.* **33**, 387–403.

Underwood, H., and Menaker, M. (1970). Extra-retinal light perception: entrainment of the biological clock controlling lizard locomotor activity. *Science* **170**, 190–193.

Plant Photoperiodism and Circadian Rhythms: A Hypothesis Concerning "Dawn" and "Dusk" Master Clocks

K. C. Hamner and T. Hoshizaki

Department of Biology
University of California
Los Angeles, California

Photoperiodism is the term introduced by Garner and Allard (1920) to designate the responses of living organisms to changes in the environmental variable, the relative length of day to night, usually referred to simply as day length or length of day. A large percentage of the living organisms on the earth live in the temperate zones where seasonal changes associated with day length changes are very marked. While many of these changes are fairly predictable during the course of the year, there is a great deal of variation from year to year in the individual variables at a given location except for variable day length. Changes in this environmental variable are entirely predictable from day to day, week to week, and year to year. As might be expected living organisms have become adapted to monitor variations in day length and thereby to anticipate forthcoming seasonal changes.

Photoperiodism in plants involves many physiological changes. Perhaps, the most spectacular response is the induction of flowering. It is obviously advantageous to a plant to produce its flowers and seeds at the time of year most favorable for survival of the species, and in many plants the initiation of the flowering process is triggered when the appropriate day length is reached. The so-called long-day plants are induced to flower when the days become long enough in the summer while short-day plants are induced to flower by the decreasing day length of the late

477

summer and fall. While there are a large group of plants (the indeterminate plants) which are not limited in their flowering by the length of day and while there are many other photoperiodic responses in plants, most of the work on photoperiodism has dealt with the flowering responses of the two groups of photoperiodically sensitive plants, the long-day plants and the short-day plants. Throughout the course of organic evolution organisms have been exposed to cyclic changes in day length year after year. It might not be surprising, therefore, if organisms had explored every possible method of measuring day length and utilized this information in their physiological behavior. Furthermore, any given species may contain the basic genetic information for the utilization of all the methods of measurement.

In discussing length of day an as environmental variable, one immediately runs into difficulties of terminology. Day is sometimes referred to as a 24-hr period representing one revolution of the earth with respect to the sun (i.e., a solar day). On the other hand, when we are discussing day length, we usually refer to the day as that portion of the 24-hr period from sunrise to sunet. In connection with photoperiodism the illuminated portion of the 24-hr cycle is referred to as the photoperiod. Since a solar day consists of a photoperiod and a dark period and since the solar day is constant, it is obvious that any change in the day length will produce a change in two variables, the photoperiod and the dark period, which vary inversely one to the other. Therefore, an organism can measure day length by measuring either the length of the photoperiod or the length of the dark period, or it might determine day length by the ratio of these two. Since photoperiods increase day by day throughout half of the year and then decrease day by day through the second half of the year, it also seems possible that the rate of change in day length and the direction of such change may be factors in determining or timing physiological responses.

It is generally accepted that all living organisms (with the possible exception of viruses and bacteria) possess a mechanism whereby they can meter the passage of time, tell the time of day, or measure the length of day with surprising accuracy. This mechanism is usually referred to as the biological clock (or clocks). This clock (or clocks) is (or are) useful to organisms in many ways. It enables them to anticipate the most suitable time of day for certain activities or processes; it provides information concerning the movement of the sun and stars in direction finding, and many other values in addition to measurement of length of day. Many recent investigators have concluded that this clock (or clocks) involves some kind of an oscillator mechanism. This subject has been reviewed extensively in recent years (Brown et al., 1970; Cold Spring Harbor Symposium, 1960; Danilevsky et al., 1970; Hamner and

Takimoto, 1964) Endogenous circadian rhythms have been clearly implicated. The purpose of this chapter is to present a somewhat new viewpoint on the basic processes.

Hypothesis Concerning "Dawn" and "Dusk" Master Clocks

The present hypothesis proposes that there are four distinct methods of time measurement involved in biological response: (1) an oscillatory type of clock involving an endogenous circadian rhythm which is rephased and entrained by the "light-on" signal; (2) an oscillatory type of clock involving an endogenous circadian rhythm which is rephased and entrained by the "light-off" signal; (3) an oscillatory type of clock involving an endogenous circadian rhythm which represents the summation or composite of the above two; and (4) an hourglass type of clock in which time measurement involves a process which proceeds in a given direction and time is measured by the disappearance of substrate (or substrates) or the accumulation of a product (or products). In the following discussion we will refer to these various clocks respectively as: (1) the dawn clock, (2) the dusk clock, (3) the composite oscillator or the composite rhythm, and (4) the hourglass clock. Clocks (1) and (2), the "dawn" and "dusk" clocks, are considered master clocks since they control clock (3). They are essentially independent one from the other, and any particular overt response may depend entirely upon one or entirely upon the other as well as depending upon the action of both together. Furthermore, it is proposed that in multicellular organisms the basic genetic information for response to both clocks may be present in all of the cells, but during the process of differentiation, certain cells may retain the ability to respond only to one of the clocks while other cells may retain ability to respond only to the other, while still other cells of the organism may respond to both at the same time. It seem possible also that the light quality, intensity, and quantity most effective in producing the light-on signal may differ from that for the light-off signal. Each of these two master clocks may have different temperature responses. In any event, it seems that the above hypothesis presents a fresh approach to the problem of the biological clock and in the present discussion we will examine in a cursory fashion some of the available data to see whether or not there is sufficient indications of support to the above hypothesis to justify its serious consideration. If such is the case, it is hoped that various experimenters will reexamine their own data to see whether or not the above hypothesis is in any way applicable and perhaps devise new experiments to test it or modify it if necessary.

Evidence from *Pharbitis nil*

In our laboratory we first proposed the possibility that these four clocks existed in 1964 from the work by Takimoto and Hamner (1964) with Japanese morning glory *Pharbitis nil. Pharbitis* is a short-day plant and remains vegetative when growing under long-day conditions, but it will be induced to flower as a result of exposure to a single short day. An effective short day must have a dark period longer than a certain critical length, and the plant will not flower regardless of the conditions unless a dark period beyond the critical length is used. Furthermore, the seeds of this plant may be planted under continuous light and maintained under continuous light for 96 hr at which time the plant is ready for experimentation. This work has recently been reviewed by Hamner and Hoshizaki (1973), and a quotation from this review seems pertinent.

> At dark periods longer than the critical length, the number of flowers is proportional to the length of that segment of the dark period beyond the critical length. The quantity of flowers produced, therefore, is controlled by a mechanism on the hourglass principle. This mechanism is very sensitive to temperature, as is shown in Figure 1.
>
> The critical length of the dark period is determined, however, not by a mechanism on the hourglass principle but by a circadian rhythm of sensitivity to light. This is illustrated in Figure 2. When the plant is exposed to a single, long, dark period and the dark period is interrupted at various times with brief exposures to light, it is found (Takimoto and Hamner, 1964) that such exposures inhibit flowering to different degrees, depending upon the time

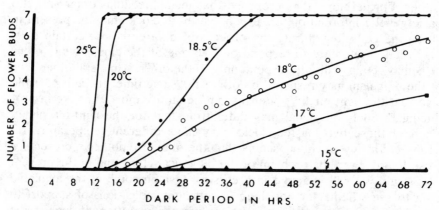

Figure 1 Flowering response of *Pharbitis nil* exposed to a single dark period of various duration at different temperatures. The plants were exposed to continuous illumination before the dark treatments. After Takimoto and Hamner (1964).

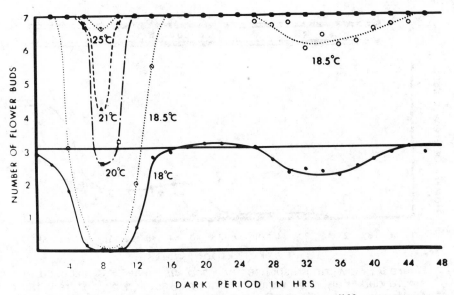

Figure 2 Flowering responses of *Pharbitis nil* at different temperatures when exposed to 5 min of red light at different times in a 48-hr dark period. The plants were exposed to continuous illumination before the dark treatments. After Takimoto and Hamner (1964).

during the dark period at which the exposure is made. This sensitivity to brief light interruptions exhibits a circadian rhythm whose periodicity is not affected by temperature (i.e., it is temperature compensated). Since the plants were previously exposed to continuous light, it is apparent from Figure 2 that this circadian rhythm of sensitivity to light is initiated by the onset of darkness, and so we call it the "light-off" rhythm.

The light-on rhythm may be demonstrated by introducing a photoperiodic treatment prior to exposure to the long experimental dark period. If the plant is exposed to an 8-hr noninductive dark period prior to the longer experimental dark period (which causes floral induction), and this is followed by either a 12-hr light period or an 8-hr light period, the results shown in Figure 3 are obtained. These results show that the increase in flowering with the increasing length of the dark period is stepwise, indicating not only the effects of the hourglass mechanism but also the working presence of a circadian rhythm. The two curves shown in Figure 3 become superimposed if they are plotted in relation to the beginning of the preconditioning light period. Thus, the rhythmic response is relative to the time the light was turned on.

Through a series of experiments too complex to be outlined here but which involve a pretreatment with a light-on signal and scanning a long dark period with brief light exposures, it has been shown . . . that the overt rhythm of sensitivity to light which is involved in the reaction of this plant to

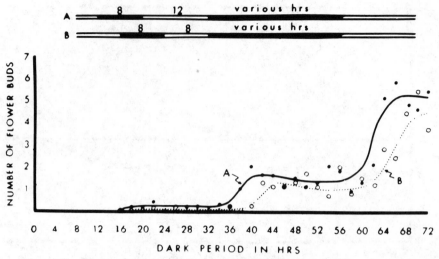

Figure 3 Flowering responses of *Pharbitis nil* at 18°C, exposed to a single dark period of various duration preceded by different light conditions. Group A and B were exposed to an 8-hr dark period followed by 12- and 8-hr light periods, respectively, preceding the main dark period. After Takimoto and Hamner (1964).

light interruptions during a long dark period is a summation of the above two circadian rhythms, the light-on and the light-off rhythms. Disregarding the hourglass mechanism, one may say therefore that manifestations of the biological clock may be related to three distinct mechanisms: (1) an internal circadian rhythm initiated by turning the light on, (2) an internal circadian rhythm initiated by turning the light off, and (3) an internal circadian rhythm resulting from the summation of the first two.

It might be argued that we are dealing here with a single rhythm which is phase shifted by both the light-on and the light-off signals. However such does not seem to be the case, at least in *Pharbitis nil*. A comparison of Figures 1, 2, and 3 indicates that the light-on rhythm is qualitatively different from the light-off rhythm. When the plants are exposed only to the light-off signal by giving them continuous light from germination until the experimental period and then simply exposing them to dark periods of various lengths there is no evidence of a rhythm in the flowering response (Figure 1). However such a treatment does initiate an internal rhythm as is shown in Figure 2 when a long dark period is scanned with a brief exposure to light. Thus, this light-off rhythm does not express itself in a length of dark experiment. On the other hand, if a light-on signal is introduced prior to the experimental dark period, exposing the plants to various lengths of dark periods does result in a step-wise increase in flowering (Figure 3) showing the presence of a circadian rhythm qualitatively different from that caused by the "light-off" signal.

Evidence from Leaf and Petal Movement Rhythms*

In 1967 Engelmann and Honegger in their studies of petal movements of *Kalanchoe blossfeldiana,* found that the light-on signal and the light-off signal each start rhythmic processes independent of each other and that the final position of maximum opening of the petals is determined by a composite of the two. They further found that what might be called the free-running periodicity of each rhythm was different, and they found no evidence of coupling of one rhythm with the other, so that the phase relationships between the two rhythms was constantly changing under constant conditions over a period of days.

Holdsworth in 1959, investigating the effects of day lengths on the movements of pulvinate leaves, presented evidence which we think also shows clearly the presence of a light-on and a light-off rhythm being involved in these leaf movements. A graph (Figure 4) has been replotted from one of Holdsworth's figures to illustrate the hypothetical participation of the "light-on" and "light-off" rhythms in *Bauhinia.* The data are from plants exposed to five different light-dark treatments. The light treatment began at 6 A.M. and some plants received light until midnight, others only until 9 P.M., 6 P.M., 3 P.M., or noon. Following the light treatment, all plants received a dark period until 6 A.M. of the following day. Thus the dark period varied from 6 to 18 hr in the different treatments. At 6 A.M. all plants were subjected to continuous light. The resulting leaf movements were interpreted by making two assumptions. Firstly, the light-on signal initiated a light-on rhythm and the beginning of this rhythm is indicated by the opening of the leaf and also by a closure 12 hr later. In Figure 4 the time of opening (curve moving upward) and closing (curve moving downward) of the leaves by the light-on rhythm is indicated respectively by the solid parallel vertical lines 12 hr apart. Secondly, the light-off signal initiates a light-off rhythm and the rhythm is indicated by a closure of the leaf immediately after the beginning of the dark period and also 24 hr later. The closure time of the leaves by the light-off rhythm is marked by the broken parallel lines 24 hr apart in Figure 4. It appears that leaf closure in *Bauhinia* under continuous light can be related to a signal for closure either from the light-on or the light-off rhythm and by whichever one occurs first. If the previous dark period was shorter than 12 hr, the leaf closure occurred about 12 hr after the continuous light period began (see upper three curves of Figure 4). On the other hand, if the previous dark period was longer than 12 hr, the leaf closure occurred 24 hr after the beginning of the previous (last) dark

---

*The discussion in this section is taken almost verbatim from a paper by Hoshizaki *et al.* (1974).

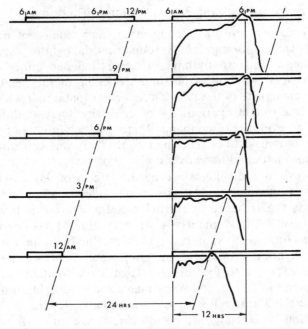

Figure 4 Interpretation of *Bauhinia monandra* leaf movement data using the participation of two rhythm hypothesis. The leaf movements of *Bauhinia* were analyzed from the original data of Holdsworth's and one set was separated into individual plots. The plants were exposed to five different light–dark treatments. The light treatment is shown as horizontal open bars and a dark period is shown as a horizontal bar. The light-on rhythm is interpreted to be the opening of the leaf at the beginning of the light period (curve moving upward) and a closure 12 hr later (curve moving downward). The vertical parallel lines 12 hr apart designate this period of the light-on rhythm (6 A.M. to 6 P.M.). The "light-off" rhythm is interpreted to be the closure of the leaf at the end of the light period and also 24 hr later (parallel broken lines 24 hr apart). Thus leaf closure in light occurs approximately 12 hr after the beginning of the light period, or approximately 24 hr after the end of the previous light period, whichever occurs first. From Hoshizaki *et al.* (1974).

period (see lower two curves of Figure 4). Thus in the case of *Bauhinia* where the proper light-dark treatments were given, the application of the two-rhythm concept for the analysis of leaf movement gave a surprisingly good fit.

Hoshizaki *et al.* (1974) have investigated leaf movements in *Xanthium strumarium* under different photoperiodic conditions. It had been previously shown that this plant exhibited two distinct leaf movement rhythms with one occurring in continuous light and presumably related to an endogenous rhythm initiated by the light-on signal and the other occurring in continuous dark and presumably related to an endogenous rhythm initiated by the light-off signal. The light-on rhythm is characterized by a sudden and rapid downward movement of the leaf occurring about 16 hr after the light-on signal. The light-off rhythm is characterized by an immediate and sudden upward movement following the light-off signal. Under certain photoperiodic treatments, the two movements seem to be in conflict.

The characteristic light-on downward movement was predominant in the LD 14:10 and LD 16:8 treatments while the light-off upward movement was predominant in LD 8:16 and LD 10:14 treatments. In the LD 12:12 treatment, one movement was predominant in about half of the cases and vice versa. Thus leaf movements of *Xanthium strumarium* plants given these light-dark treatments were found to fit hypothetical curves based on the participation of both a light-on and a light-off rhythm.

Evidence from Animals

Dr. Klaus Hoffmann (1971) has presented what we consider strong evidence of two independent circadian rhythms being involved in animal activity. He has kindly furnished us with one of his figures which is reproduced in our Figure 5. A tree shrew *Tupaia belangeri* was allowed to free-run at 9.5 lx light intensity. It exhibited a clear-cut circadian rhythm of activity. When, however, the light intensity was decreased to 1.1 lx, the rhythm split into two components. To quote Dr. Hoffmann, "the actograms do not suggest the separation of two peaks of a bimodal activity pattern, but rather the separation of two oscillators that have been in phase, and then shift toward a new phase relationship." This seems to be an example of the operation of both the dawn and the dusk clocks in this activity rhythm. It appears that both clocks have some control over the onset as well as the cessation of activity, but that one clock has more control over onset than the other, and vice versa, the other has more control over cessation of activity. We have no way of knowing at present which clock is which, but it appears that one of the clocks has a free-running periodicity that is affected by light intensity. One wonders whether or not such a possibility might influence the interpretation of Aschoff's Rule (Aschoff, 1960).

It is of interest to compare the results obtained by Hoffmann with animals (see above) with the results obtained with plants by Mayer and Sadleder (1972). Leaf movements in the plant *Phaseolus coccineus* depend upon activity in both the primary and secondary pulvini. The free-

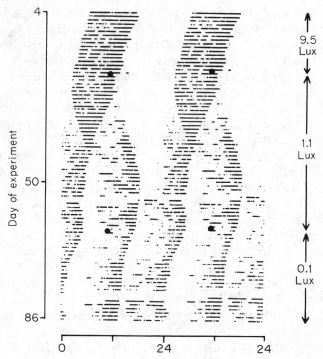

Figure 5 Splitting of the circadian rhythm of locomotor activity into two components after abrupt reduction of the otherwise constant illumination in a tree shrew *Tupaia belangeri*. Running wheel activity was registered by an event recorder. Activity is indicated by the vertical pen markings on the line, which can fuse to give a band of solid activity; successive days are plotted one below the other. To facilitate visual following of the different components of the rhythm the total record, or a part of it, has been reproduced on the right, displaced upward 1 day. The black dots indicate the times at which light intensity was changed. At the left the number of days under experimental conditions is given, at the right the intensity of constant illumination is indicated. From Hoffman (1971) with author's permission.

running periods of both sets of pulvini were measured in continuous darkness (DD) and in continuous light (LL) of different intensities. The free-running periods of the two pulvini did not differ either in constant darkness or in constant high intensity light. However, at low light intensities, the periods of the two did differ. Our interpretation of these results would be that the two sets of pulvini are operating on different clocks, perhaps one set on the dawn clock and the other on the dusk clock, and that the free-running period of one of the clocks is affected by light intensity. Surprisingly, the situation closely parallels Hoffmann's work with animals. The two clocks in both organisms seem to be in synchrony; i.e., have the same free-running period in constant darkness or in high intensity light, but in low intensity light one of the clocks changes its free-running period. This interpretation also implies that in *Phaseolus* all of the cells of the plant have the basic information for a response to either clock and in the process of differentiation one set of pulvini cells differentiated to respond to one clock and the other set of pulvini cells differentiated to respond to the other clock.

Evidence from Arthropods

The present authors are not qualified to discuss the literature on biological rhythms in terrestrial arthropods. However, an excellent and comprehensive review has recently been prepared by Danilevsky *et al.* (1970). Throughout their review they refer to the separate effects of the light-on signal and the light-off signal. In fact, in the latter part of their review they give considerable space to a hypothesis developed in 1966 by Tyshchenko in which he interprets photoperiodic response on the basis of a model involving two oscillators (A and B). To quote from Danilevsky *et al.* (1970):

> The phase of the A oscillator is assumed to switch on at "dawn" and the phase of the B oscillator, in darkness. Rhythmic processes which are controlled by the oscillators are thus synchronized in the first case only with light rhythm; in the second case, only with darkness rhythm.

Tyshchenko has developed a theory explaining photoperiodism on the basis of interaction between these two independent circadian rhythms. Our interpretation of the photoperiodic response differs from Tyschchenko's and we will not have time to critically evaluate his theory in comparison with ours. We may say that our hypothesis was developed entirely independently from Tyshchenko's since we were not aware of his hypothesis until a short time ago. It is surprising how parallel the two hypotheses have become.

An Interpretation of Photoperiodism Based on the Hypothesis of Dawn and Dusk Clocks

We propose that both of the master clocks, the dawn and the dusk clocks, oscillate through two distinct equal phases, a *photophase* and a *scotophase** making a complete oscillation in approximately twenty-four hours. At the light-on signal, the dawn clock enters the photophase of its oscillation and this oscillation proceeds to completion unless another light-on signal is received. The dusk clock, upon receiving the light-off signal enters the scotophase of its oscillation, and this proceeds to completion unless another light-off signal is received. The two clocks are essentially independent of each other. However, when both clocks are involved in the same overt response on the part of the organism, then that overt response depends upon a simple summation of the status of the two clocks. In other words, a new composite rhythm or oscillation is obtained which goes through photophase and scotophase stages as do the master clocks. When the organism is exposed to a day length of 12 hr, i.e., an LD 12:12 treatment, the two master clocks are completely in phase and such treatment has no photoperiodic effect, i.e., photoperiodically it is completely inactive. We propose that in plant photoperiodism the response depends primarily on the composite clock in the following fashion: in both long-day and short-day plants high intensity illumination during the photophase of the oscillation is *promotive* to flowering (and in most cases essential); on the other hand, illumination during the scotophase is *inhibitory* to flowering in short-day plants and *promotive* to flowering in the long-day plants.

Another distinction between the long-day plants and the short-day plants lies in the fact that flowering in the long-day plants depends entirely upon the promotive effect of favorable day lengths and in the short-day plants flowering depends on the inhibitory effects of unfavorable day lengths. Thus, in long-day plants when a particular photoperiodic cycle produces sufficient promotive effect to cross a threshhold value, a more-or-less permanent change is brought about in the cells of the leaves and the plant may be considered as partially photoperiodically induced. This change is relatively stable, persisting through a considerable number of unfavorable cycles, and may be supplemented in an additive manner by any subsequent promotive cycles while in this state. After a sufficient number of hours of exposure to promotion or promotive effects above the threshold value, the cells of the leaf are sufficiently changed so

---

*The use of the terms photophase and scotophase may be of value in connection with discussions other than those dealing with photoperiodism. For instance, in the free-running condition the two terms might at times be substituted for the terms "subjective day" and "subjective night." If for example, future investigations indicate that two independent oscillators of the type described above are involved in many circadian rhythms, it may prove useful to use these two terms in discussing problems of synchronization of the oscillators. It is realized that these two terms are but slight modifications of the original terms proposed by Bunning (1936), namely "photophil" and "scotophil."

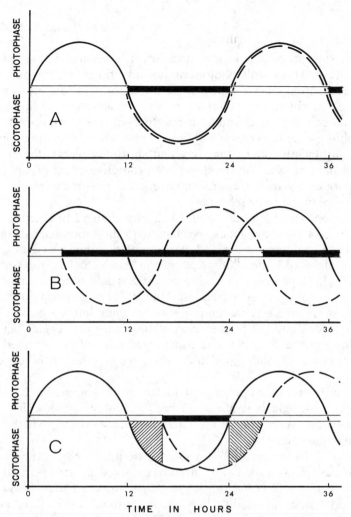

Figure 6 An interpretation of photoperiodism effects with the hypothesis of "dawn" and "dusk" clocks. During a 36-hr period, the light periods are represented by an open horizontal bar and the dark periods by a horizontal bar. The "dawn" oscillator is shown as a solid curve, the "dusk" oscillator by a broken line. Each curve is considered to be in photophase when above the median and in scotophase when below. A, at day lengths of 12 hr, the photophase and the scottophase of both the "dawn" and the "dusk" clocks are in phase. B, at day lengths shorter than 12 hr (i.e., short day) light is not received during the scotophase of either clocks. C, at day lengths longer than 12 hr (i.e., long day), the photoperiod extends into the scotophase of the "dawn" clock (shaded area of left) and the photoperiod of the next cycle begins before the scotophase of the "dusk" clock is complete (shaded area on right).

that they start producing florigen (the flower hormone), and the plant has undergone what we call photoperiodic induction. On the other hand, with the short-day plants, unfavorable photoperiodic conditions produce in the leaf a condition inhibitory to the manufacture of florigen and, while this condition is unstable, it may persist over a number of subsequent photoperiodic cycles which would be favorable for flowering. The critical day lengths of the long-day and short-day plants, therefore, depend, in the first case, on the degree of promotive effect of a photoperiodic treatment, and, in the second case, on the degree of inhibition of a particular photoperiodic treatment.

It is proposed that at day lengths shorter than 12 hr (Figure 6B) the photophase of the dawn clock overlaps with the scotophase of the dusk clock at the beginning of the dark period and the photophase of the dusk clock overlaps with the scotophase of the dawn clock at the end of the dark period. Thus, under short-day conditions light is not received during the scotophase of either oscillation. Under day length conditions longer than 12 hr (Figure 6C) the photoperiod extends into the scotophase of the dawn clock and the photoperiod of the next cycle begins before the scotophase of the dusk clock is complete. Thus light is received during the scotophase of both oscillators when the day length is longer than 12 hr.

In our hypothesis one critical factor in photoperiodic response is whether or not light is received during the scotophase of either oscillation. The only natural conditions where this occurs is shown in the shaded areas of Figure 6C.

So far, we have said nothing about the hourglass clock. It is proposed that the hourglass clock is not directly involved in the essential timing mechanism of photoperiodism. Rather, it is proposed that the hourglass clock participates to modify the response, much as in the case with *Pharbitis*, as shown in Figures 1–3. Recently, some investigators have been inclined to the hypothesis that the photoperiodic response in some organisms is based entirely upon a hourglass type of clock. We feel there is reason to believe that these particular cases involve a response solely to the dusk clock and that the response to the dusk clock is modified by factors operating on the hourglass principle. Reasons for these conclusions are given below.

There are many reports in the literature which might be discussed in support of the above hypothesis. However we will discuss only a few special cases which seem particularly pertinent. We have also raised questions concerning certain other interpretations and approaches partly for the sake of provoking discussion.

Special Cases

Biloxi Soybean

Evidence in support of and to illustrate the above interpretation is found in the work of Sirohi and Hamner (1962) with Biloxi soybean, a short-day plant. All plants were exposed to seven cycles of a standard short day (8 hr of light and 16 hr of darkness). The standard short days were separated from each other by 24-hr experimental period. If this experimental period was complete darkness, there was no effect on the overall response. In other words, the number of flowers produced was exactly the same as the numbers produced by 7 standard short days in succession. If the intervening experimental period consisted of 12 hr of light and 12 hr of darkness, it was also without photoperiodic effect, and the number of flowers produced was exactly the same as if the intervening period had been complete darkness. However, if the intervening experimental period consisted of high intensity photoperiods, shorter than 12 hr, flowering was stimulated, and if the photoperiod was longer than 12 hr, flowering was strongly inhibited. It should be remembered that a day length of 12 hr is below the critical day length of Biloxi soybean, and plants exposed continuously to a LD 12:12 cycle will flower. Thus, a photoperiodic treatment of Biloxi soybean, which is innocuous when presented as an intervening cycle, permits the plant to flower when given as successive treatments indicating that Biloxi soybean is a short-day plant because long days inhibit flowering.

Circadian Surfaces

Recently Pittendrigh (1973) has presented what he calls a circadian surface based upon Beck's data (Beck, 1962) for the moth *Ostrinia nubilalis* (Figure 7, left). The contour lines in Figure 7 (left) representing equivalent amounts of induction (from 60 to 100% diapause) define a surface which peaks (100% diapause) when the dark period is 12 hr in length and the light period is from 10 to 12 hr. It is obvious that this surface is contoured in relation to line c of the diagram, in other words with a dark period of 12 hr in duration. We believe such a surface might be obtained if the organism were responding primarily or entirely to the dusk clock. We have presented a graph of the available data we have for Biloxi soybean (Figure 7, right) for comparison with Pittendrigh's graph. It is unfortunate that, with all of the work that we have done with Biloxi soybean, we could not present a more complete figure. However, we believe that there is sufficient data to indicate that this cicadian surface is contoured around a line represented by a on the graph: in other words

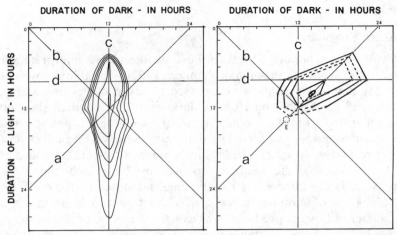

Figure 7 Two circadian surfaces. The left hand panel is based on a figure from Pittendrigh (1973) which was based on Beck's data of 1962. Reproduced with permission from Prof. C. S. Pittendrigh. The amount of induced effect (diapause) in the moth *Ostrinis nubilalis* is plotted on coordinates indicating the duration of both light and dark. Any given level of induction can be effected by an infinite number of light–dark cycles which form a closed loop—an *isoinduction contour* —on the light-versus-dark coordinates. Six isoinduction contours define the light cycles that induce 60, 80, 90, 95, and 100% diapause.

In the righthand panel the circadian surfaces for the floral induction of Biloxi soybean *Glycine max* is given with data obtained from various investigations in our laboratory. Five isoinduction contours define the light–dark treatments that induce 5, 10, 20, 30, and 40 nodes to flower in 10 plants of soybeans receiving seven cycles of treatments. Solid contour lines connect points derived from actual experimental data. Broken contour lines are extrapolated contours. The area designating the critical dark period of Biloxi soybean given 24-hr cycles (0 nodes flowering) is the broken circle above E.

Line a defines a locus of treatments whose sum of light and dark durations is 24 hr. Line b defines a locus of treatments whose light and dark durations are equal. Line c defines a locus of treatments whose dark treatment is 12 hr long with light of various durations. Line d defines a locus of treatments whose light treatments is 8 hr long with dark of various durations. The numbers along the sides of the figures represent the duration in hours of light or dark.

around a 24-hr cycle. We believe that this indicates Biloxi soybean is responding both to the dawn and to the dusk clocks.

Response Solely to the Dusk Clock

In *Pharbitis*, Takimoto and Hamner (1964) have found a remarkable sensitivity to a light interruption about 8 hr after the onset of darkness (see Figure 2). A similar sensitivity to light interruptions 8 hr after the onset of darkness has been found in Biloxi soybean (Nanda and Hamner, 1962) and in *Xanthium* (Reid *et al.,* 1967). In *Pharbitis* as is shown in Figure 2 this sensitivity is clearly related to the endogenous rhythm associated with the light-off signal, i.e., in relation to the dusk clock. We assume that the responses of *Xanthium* and Biloxi soybean are similar to those of *Pharbitis* although we have not been able to devise an experiment to prove this. Lees (1965) has found a somewhat similar situation in insects, and as a result has developed a theory of insect photoperiodism based upon a clock operating on the hourglass principle. One wonders whether or not the time measurement in his case is temperature compensated as it is in *Pharbitis*. In any event, we do not believe that it is necessary to introduce the hourglass hypothesis as responsible for the essential timing in photoperiodism since evidence for the presence of both the dawn and the dusk clocks in insects is indicated and since we feel most of his results could be explained on the basis of a response to the dusk clock.

Skeletal Photoperiods

A considerable amount of investigative work has been done using what have been called skeletal photoperiods. In such experiments the organisms are exposed during the experimental period to two short photoperiods in each 24-hr cycle and the interval between the two photoperoids is varied in the different treatments. Furthermore the two photoperiods have been of equal duration and light intensity or one has been longer than the other. In another type of experiment, the experimental period has been signaled by the transfer of the organism from light to darkness. In the continuous darkness subsequent to a transfer from light to dark an overt circadian rhythm of response is observed. However, if the dark period is interrupted at different times with a short period of light the light interruption may cause an advance in time or a delay in the overt response. Whether an advance or a delay occurs depends upon when the light interruption occurs. At some point in the dark period there is usually a sudden reversal of response from advance to delay or vice versa. It is tempting to try to explain these results on the basis of the two clocks postulated above. Thus, for example, if two photoperiods of equal duration and intensity occur within a 12-hr period (a typical skeletal photoperiod experiment) the "dawn" and the "dusk" clocks may be partially synchronized in a fashion to make that 12-hr period the photophase of the overall response curve. Furthermore, when the light-on signal of each photoperiod is exactly 12 hr apart, one might reach the critical stage where there is a sudden shift and that part of the cycle which had formerly been a photophase might suddenly become a scoto-phase. It is difficult to postulate exact curves and draw graphs to represent the various possibilities since we know so little about the entrainment properties of each of the clocks and so little about the *zeitgebers*. For example, the effectiveness of the light-on signal may be related to light intensity or light quality and may even be related to the amount of light received after the signal is given. Similarly the effectiveness of the light-off signal might depend upon the previous light duration and/or intensity and even upon light quality. It was found (Takimoto and Hamner, 1964), for example, that *Pharbitis nil* plants which have received only the light-off signal (grown for 4 days in continuous light and transferred to darkness) exhibit a rhythmic sensitivity to light perturbations. Maximum sensitivity to such perturbations occurs 8 hr after the beginning of the dark period. If the perturbation is very brief (i.e., 3 min, which has a inhibitory effect on flowering), the perturbation has no effect upon the endogenous rhythm. On the other hand, it was shown that a light perturbation given 8 hr after the beginning of the dark period must be about 2 hr in length to overcome the rhythm produced by the initial light-off signal and must be about 4 hr in length to produce its own light-off signal. Various experimenters use perturbations varying from 1 sec to 6 hr or more and since each perturbation provides its own light-on and light-off signal, interpretations in terms of the above hypothesis of the dawn and dusk clocks and the composite clock are indeed complicated.

Temperature Effects

It has often been said that the relative length of day to night, i.e., day length, is the most noise-free signal whereby the organism may obtain information concerning the calendar day. It should be remembered that the annual cycle of temperature changes could also provide information concerning the calendar day. It is recognized however that this signal is certainly not noise free. It seems to the authors that certain organisms such as insects might find it advantageous to use the temperature signal in combination with or perhaps in place of the day length signal as the primary guideline to seasonal behavior. Many insects have several life cycles in a given year and it may be advantageous to a particular species to, in a sense, take advantage of the relatively warm fall or an early spring. In any event it might be expected that response to day length in many insects would be considerably modified by temperature.

One example of how temperature can affect the life cycle of plants is found with biennial plants. These plants grow vegetatively during the first summer after planting. The following winter they are exposed to low temperatures and then in the subsequent summer many of them behave as long-day plants. It has been shown that there is a specific cold requirement in order for these plants to become sensitive to photoperiod and to flower as a result of photoperiodic exposure.

We have had great difficulties in our attempts to incorporate the effects of temperature into some overall concept of photoperiodism using our own data and those recorded in the literature. Throughout the above discussion, therefore, we have largely disregarded the effects of what might be called abnormal temperature changes or levels. Probably the next area of investigation might be temperature effects on the dawn and dusk clocks. Such studies might promise some further clues as to the nature of these clocks.

Summary

Thus we have seen that the hypothesis of the dawn and dusk clocks controlling the biological rhythms of organisms fits well with the data just discussed. It might be justified now as mentioned earlier to reexamine carefully the more pertinent data previously obtained and to modify experimental procedures to test the two clocks hypothesis. Of course more experimentation is necessary to sharply define the various parameters of the dawn and dusk clocks. Although much can be surmised about these clocks from the extensive and intensive studies in *Pharbitis nil* (Imamura, 1967) it would be satisfying to find similar evidence of the various light intensity, quality, and duration effects and temperature effects in other plants. Of great value, of course, would be to determine whether or not the various parameters of the dawn and dusk clocks in animals are similar to those found in plants.

The authors are well aware of the many inadequacies in the hypothesis presented above. Since activities in our laboratory in this field will be terminated in the not too distant future, we felt justified in presenting our best assessment of the situation as we see it at the moment. In some of our statements we have been deliberately provocative. Perhaps our statements will stimulate thought and activity on the part of others. Perhaps that is what meetings such as this are all about.

Acknowledgment

This work was supported in part by a National Science Foundation Grant GB-30608. We gratefully acknowledge the technical assistance of Jack Rader.

References

Aschoff, J. (1960). Exogenous and endogenous components in circadian rhythms. *Cold Spring Harbor Symp. Quant. Bio.* **25**, 11–28.

Beck, S. D. (1962). Photoperiodic induction of diapause in an insect. *Biol. Bull.* **122**, 1–12.

Brown, F. A., Hastings, J. W., and Palmer, J. D. (1970). "The Biological Clock: Two Views." Academic Press, New York.

Bünning, E. (1936). Die endonome Tagesrhythmik als Grundlage der photoperiodischen Reaktion. *Ber. Deut. Bot. Ges.* **54**, 590.

Cold Spring Harbor Symposia on Quantitative Biology 25 (1960). "Biological Clocks." Long Island Biol. Ass., Cold Spring Harbor, Long Island, New York.

Danilevsky, A. S., Goryshin, N. I., and Tyshchenko, V. P. (1970). Biological rhythms in terrestrial arthropods. *Annu. Rev. Entomol.* **15**, 201–244.

Englemann, W., and Honnegger, H. (1967). Veruche zur Phasenverschiebung endogener Rhythmne: Blutenblattbewegung von *Kalanchoe blossfeldiana*. *Z. Natur.* **22**, 200–204.

Garner, W. W., and Allard, H. A. (1920). Effect of the relative length of day and night and other factors of the environment on growth and reproduction in plants. *Agr. Res.* **18**, 553–606.

Hamner, K. C., and Hoshizaki, T. (1973). Multiplicity of biological clocks. *In* "Chronobiology." (L. E. Scheving *et al.*, eds.) pp. 671–674. *Int. Soc. Study Biol. Rhythms*, Little Rock, Arkansas. Igaku Shoin, Tokyo.

Hamner, K. C., and Takimoto, A. (1964). Circadian rhythms and plant photoperiodism. *Amer. Natur.* **98**, 295–322.

Hoffmann, K. (1971). Splitting of the circadian rhythm as a function of light intensity. "Biochronometry." (M. Menaker, ed.), pp. 134–154. Nat. Acad. Sci. Washington, D.C.

Holdsworth, M. (1959). The effects of daylength on the movements of pulvinate leaves. *New Phytol.* **58**, 29–45.

Hoshizaki, T., Brest, D. E., and Hamner, K. C. (1974). The participation of two rhythms in the leaf movements of Xanthium plants given various light-dark cycles. *Plant Physiol.* **53**, 176–179.

Imamura, S. (1967). Physiology of flowering in *Pharbitis nil.* Jap. Soc. Plant Physiol., Tokyo, Japan.

Lees, A. D. (1965). Is there a circadian component in the *Megoura* photoperiodic clock? *"Circadian Clocks," Proc. Feldafing Summer School*, (J. Aschoff, ed.) pp. 351–356. North Holland, Amsterdam.

Mayer, W., and Sadleder, D. (1972). Unterschiedliche Lichtintensitatabhängigkeit der Spontanperioden als Ursache interner Desynchronisation circadianer Rhythmen bei *Phaseolus coccineus. Planta* **108**, 173–178.

Nanda, K. K., and Hamner, K. C. (1962). Investigations on the effect of light break on the nature of endogenous rhythms in the flowering response of Biloxi soybean (*Glycine max* L. Merr.). *Planta* **58**, 164–174.

Pittendrigh, C. S. (1973). Circadian oscillations in cells and the circadian organization of multicellular systems. *"The Neurosciences,"* Third Study Program, (F. O. Schmitt, ed.). MIT Press, Cambridge, Massachusetts.

Reid, H. B., Moore, P. H., and Hamner, K. C. (1967). Control of flowering of *Xanthium pennsylvanicum* by red and far-red light. *Plant Physiol.* **42**, 532 – 540.

Sirohi, G. S., and Hamner, K. C. (1962). Floral inhibition in relation to photoperiodism in Biloxi soybean. *Plant Physiol.* **37**, 785 – 790.

Takimoto, A., and Hamner, K. C. (1964). Effect of temperature and preconditioning on photoperiodic response of *Pharbitis nil. Plant Physiol.* **39**, 1024 – 1030.

Tyshchenko, V. P. (1966). Two-oscillatory model of the physiological mechanism of insect photoperiodic reaction. *Zh. Obshch. Biol.* **27**, 209 – 222 (in Russian).

Part VI

Synergisms, Models, and What Next

Multiple Factor Effects on Plants

Frank B. Salisbury

Plant Science Department
Utah State University,
Logan, Utah

It seems appropriate to begin this discussion with a brief excerpt from the history of this symposium. Someone on the planning committee (I'm haunted by the thought that it might have been me) suggested that recent work on multiple factor effects appeared interesting. New statistical tools were mentioned. "Let's get some specialist to tell us all about it," someone said. Names were suggested. Rather recently I was informed that the individual we wanted couldn't give this talk. Could I give it? Having forgotten what we originally had in mind but being interested in the topic, I accepted! Since then I have been remembering what we had in mind, realizing that I'm not that specialist and that I know virtually nothing about the topic — and worrying about what I might say! Actually, work on the talk has been fun. It seems that there might be three general aspects to the problem:

1. *Sorting out the interactions.* Breathes there a biologist with soul so dead that he isn't constantly contending with these interactions? Statistical tools have been developed to sort them out, but so far as I have been able to learn, the tools are not new in principle. They involve primarily Fisher's analysis of variance, which is a highly sophisticated application of the principle of regression analysis — a tool itself highly valuable in situations where data must be taken as they

come rather than obtained from an experiment that was carefully designed in advance. This approach is often used in agriculture and in physiological ecology.

2. *Understanding the interactions.* What are the mechanisms of interaction? To obtain answers, graphs are plotted, models are formulated, and kinetic concepts are applied. I think of this as largely a physiological approach, although it could well have important applications in ecology.

3. *Incorporating the results of the first two studies into our thinking about specific problems.* What do the results of our analysis mean to the problem that originally motivated the research? Of course this can be the primary question in physiological ecology, but it is also important in physiology, agriculture, or biology in general.

Mineral Nutrition: A Simple Model

One of the first and still one of the most important principles of factor interaction was the law of the minimum, formulated by Justus von Liebig in 1840 (see Liebig, 1885). This law seemed to imply that only one environmental factor might be limiting the growth of a plant at any given time. The application in agriculture was obvious: find the limiting factor and remedy it to increase yield. Food surpluses of a few years back attest to the success of this approach (combined, of course, with others). We should not let this success in agriculture, or the difficulties (some discussed below) encountered with this law distract us from realizing its fundamental importance in such disciplines as physiological ecology.

Liebig formulated the principle as it applied to the mineral nutrition of plants, and it seemed to me that this might be an appropriate topic around which I could build my discussion. In a rather cursory search of the literature (extending at a very superficial level over many years), I have been unable to find the kind of "clean" data that might lend themselves to a discussion such as this (although I feel certain such data must exist). Most of the data that I have encountered were obtained from agricultural field trials. (Numerous examples are summarized by Clements, 1964.) A few weeks after accepting the assignment to give this talk, I decided the only way out was to perform the experiment myself. Luckily, this proved to be simple enough so that I could make three runs, beginning the first one on April 12, 1973.

Four-inch, square plastic pots were filled with medium-sized vermiculite, and four tomato (cherry) seedlings were transplanted from soil (first experiment), from vermiculite (second experiment), or from pearlite (third experiment) into each of these pots. Three pots (12 plants) were used for each treatment. The pots were placed on galvanized hardware cloth held above a wooden greenhouse bench by dowels or slats (so that solutions could not run from one pot to another). The pots were watered on Mondays, Wednesdays, and Fridays with nutrient solutions and on the other days with distilled water.

The complete solution was prepared according to the recipe in Machlis and Torrey (p. 44, 1956). This recipe was modified slightly in minor nutrients and iron as dictated by the salts available to me. Molarities of the control solution are shown in Table 1. In the first experiment, nitrogen was varied from 0 to 100% of the control, and phosphorus was applied at 25, 50, and 100%. Phosphate or nitrate were replaced by chloride ($CaCl_2$ or KCl) in deficient solutions. As it turned out, the lowest phosphate (25%) was already saturating (it is the level recommended in Shrive's solution), and hence there was virtually no response to phosphate level in this experiment. In the second experiment, more nitrogen levels were added, and phosphorus was applied at 15 and 100%. In the third experiment, phosphorus was varied from 0 to 100% at 15, 30, and 100% nitrogen.

After 2–2½ weeks, two plants were harvested from each pot and their fresh and dry weights were determined. (In the second experiment, many pots contained only two or three plants, so only the one extra plant could be harvested early, meaning that each treatment was represented by only two or three plants.) The second and final harvest was when the plants were about 1 month old. Flower buds were just beginning to appear on a few plants at that time, but roots were so extensive that it was impossible to remove all the vermiculite.

Table 1 Molarities of Nutrient Elements in Complete Solution[a]

NO_3^-	0.015	Fe-chelate	0.0001
K^+	0.006	H_3BO_3	0.00005
Ca^{2+}	0.005	$MnCl_2 \cdot 4H_2O$	0.00001
Mg^{2+}	0.002	$ZnSO_4 \cdot H_2O$	0.0000008
SO^{2-}	0.002	$CuSO_4 \cdot 4H_2O$	0.0000004
$H_2PO_4^-$	0.001	MoO_3	0.0000001

[a]From Machlis and Torrey, 1956. For the sake of convenience, solutions were mixed in completely filled gallon jugs, about 3.94 liters, rather than 4.00 liters. Hence true values are more closely approximated by multiplying the figures in the table by 1.018. Values for minor elements are only approximate. When NO_3^- or $H_2PO_4^-$ were decreased in the solutions, they were replaced by Cl^- (as $CaCl_2$ and/or KCl).

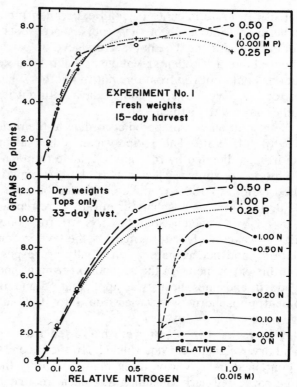

Figure 1 Results of Experiment 1. All phosphate levels are essentially saturating, as indicated by the insert at lower right. The data in the insert are the same as those in the curves to its left, but are plotted as a function of phosphorus instead of nitrogen.

Experimental Results

The 15-Day Harvest of Experiment 1 (April 27th)

It was evident at the first harvest that all phosphorus levels were saturating (Figure 1). Nevertheless, the experiment gives some indication of the range of variability. Note also that nitrogen saturation occurs at about 25% (0.004 M) of the control.

The 33-Day Harvest of Experiment 1 (May 15th)

Note that by the time the plants are older, nitrogen saturation occurs at about 50% of the control, indicating that nitrogen requirements change as a function of age (Figure 1). This is an interesting interaction in itself. Phosphorus is still saturating at 25% (0.00025 M) of the control. All of this was disappointing to me, because I wanted to see Liebig's law of the minimum illustrated. I was able to do so by plotting the results as a function of phosphorus concentration at the various nitrogen levels — although to see Liebig's law in operation, I had to fill in a lot of dashed lines where there were no data points!

The 14-Day Harvest of Experiment 2 (May 17th)

Although there are only two or three plants per treatment, the second experiment beautifully illustrates the law of the minimum (Figure 2). Indeed, the curves closely resemble those of Blackman (1905). Saturation occurs at 20% nitrogen for 15% phosphorus and at 40% nitrogen for 100% phosphorus. There also seems to be an indication of a high nitrate inhibition, although this is somewhat less clear for the dry weights than for the fresh weights. This is not due to high salts, because the total salt

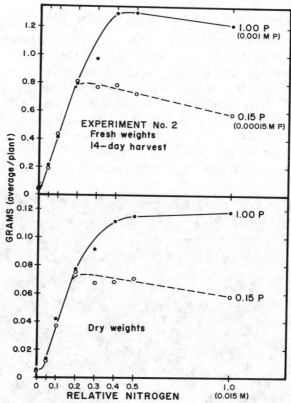

Figure 2 The 14-day harvest of Experiment 2, showing both fresh and dry weights. Note that curves are essentially similar.

molarity was held constant at about 0.0261 M. (Fresh weights in the early experiments are probably less reliable than dry weights, because plants tended to dry out during the weighing process—a problem that was avoided in later weighings by wrapping the plants in moist toweling.)

The 29-Day Harvest of Experiment 2 (June 1st)

Again the nitrogen saturation concentration seems to be higher with the older plants: 20–50% at 15% phosphorus and 50% or higher at 100% phosphorus (Figures 3 and 4). Note that the curves are not exactly superimposed at 5–20% nitrogen. They are close, however, from 0 to 20%, and repetitions of the experiment plus statistical analysis would be required to see whether they are statistically different in this range. (Figure 4 shows only fresh weights of tops, because the roots included considerable vermiculite.)

The 18-Day Harvest of Experiment 3 (June 4th)

Although there is some scatter in the data (Figure 5), the curves nevertheless illustrate Liebig's law when yield is plotted as a function of phosphorus level at three nitrogen levels. Again it would require repeats of the experiment plus statistics to determine whether nitrogen is limiting at 0–20% phosphorus. The curves as drawn indicate that this is the case. Incidentally, there is no sign of inhibition by high phosphate at high nitrogen levels as appeared to be the case in Figure 1.

The results of Figure 1 could be due to chance, but changes did occur in the greenhouse growing conditions as spring progressed. In the

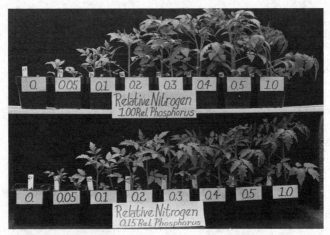

Figure 3 Photographs of the plants of Experiment 2 taken just before harvesting on June 1 (29 days after planting).

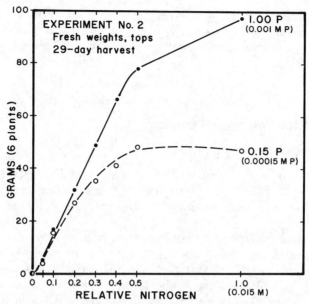

Figure 4 Fresh weights of the plants of Experiment 2, harvested 29 days after planting. Examples are shown in Figure 3.

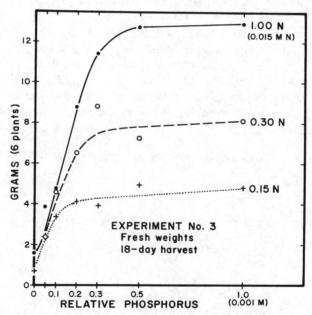

Figure 5 Fresh weights of representative plants from Experiment 3, harvested after 18 days.

early experiments, plants in a given treatment showed little statistical variability, but in the last experiment, plants closest to the cooling pads (which did not operate earlier) were noticeably smaller than plants farther along the bench—illustrating again the numerous complex interactions.

Analysis of Multiple Factor Effects

Sorting out the Interactions

After obtaining experimental data such as those discussed above, our assignment is to make sense of the interactions. The first step is to plot the data as we have been doing. Often this provides immediate insights, as we have seen.

A second approach is statistics. A regression analysis is often valuable when field data are used and one has little or no control over experimental design. Clements (1964) argues strongly and convincingly for this approach in agricultural field studies. One may come closer to understanding the truth by taking things as they occur in the field (in physiological ecology as well as agriculture) than might be achieved in an experimental situation where several factors, though controlled, may differ markedly from those present in the field situation that gave rise to the problem.

In experiments such as those of Figures 1–5, analysis of variance is more appropriate than regression analysis. Table 2 shows the results of an analysis of variance of the plotted data in Figure 4 (fresh weights of tops in the 29-day harvest of experiment 2). Variability within replications is extremely low, as is experimental and sampling error. (Actually, there was slightly more variability between two plants in a pot than between different pots in the same treatment—indicating perhaps that one

Table 2 Analysis of Variance, Experiment No. 2, June 1 (29-Day) Harvest (Tops Only)

Source of variation	Degree of freedom	Sum of squares	Mean square	F
Reps	2	1.0121	0.5060	<1
P	1	165.4459	165.4459	112.068**
N	7	1695.2000	242.1714	164.039**
P × N	7	189.9490	27.1356	18.381**
Exp. error	30	44.2883	1.4763	—
Sampling	48	198.9706	4.1452	—
TOTAL	95	2294.8659		

plant might tend to "dominate" the other.) Yield is strongly influenced by phosphorus and by nitrogen level, and there is a significant interaction between phosphorus and nitrogen.

The analysis of variance is a powerful tool in the study of interactions. Indeed, as Lockhart (1965) points out, the results of such an analysis are quite independent of the interaction mechanism.

Understanding the Interactions

When plots of the data plus statistical analysis indicate interaction or no interaction, then it is often of interest to attempt an understanding of the mechanism of interaction. In physiological studies, this understanding would probably be at the molecular level; various other levels are conceivable in ecological or agricultural studies. Several workers have attempted to derive principles upon which a study of mechanisms might be undertaken. Most of this is thoroughly reviewed by Lockhart (1965).

Mohr (1972) was especially clear in his discussion of what *does not* constitute an interaction. Say two factors influence the same steady-state rate of some process such as stem growth. There are only two kinds of results in such an experiment that indicate no interaction (Figure 6):

1. *Additive responses.* If the two factors act upon different causal sequences or compartments leading to a response, then the effects of either one are simply added onto the other. An analysis of variance indicates no interaction, since it shows that the two curves describing the responses are statistically parallel to each other. Say, for example, that ascorbic acid is produced in two parts of the cell, and that its production is influenced independently by different factors. It is easy to imagine that the sum of the responses to changes in the factors

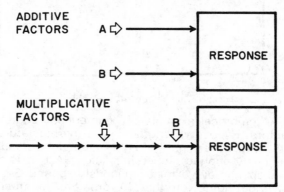

Figure 6 An illustration of additive and multiplicative factors according to the analysis of Mohr (1972). See discussion in the text.

applied separately is equal to the response to changes in the factors applied simultaneously. An example is stem growth in white mustard in response to gibberellic acid and red light. These responses are perfectly additive (Figure 7). The dose–response curves for growth as a function of gibberellic acid have the identical form with and without red light (which inhibits); the curves are parallel in the statistical sense. The conclusion of this particular study is that light does not act upon stem growth by an effect upon gibberellic acid—an important conclusion, indeed.

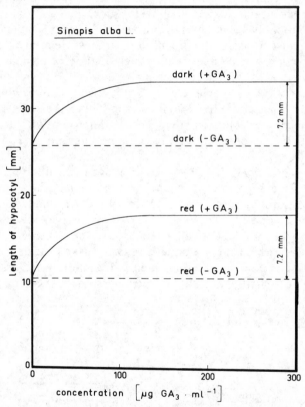

Figure 7 An empirical example of "numerically additive behavior" of two factors. Hypocotyl lengthening in the mustard seedling was investigated under the control of light (continuous standard red light) and exogenously applied gibberellic acid (GA_3). It is apparent that the dose–response curve for exogenously applied GA_3 is the same with and without light. Note that GA_3 promotes lengthening whereas red light inhibits lengthening of the hypocotyl. Hypocotyl length was measured 72 hr after sowing. After Mohr (1972).

2. *Multiplicative responses.* If two factors influence different steps in the same reaction sequence, then the effect of one is always some fraction of the effect of the other. If the fraction is greater than one, both factors act in the same direction; if less than one, they act against each other (one may inhibit, the other promote). As Lockhart (1965) points out, this form of no interaction is indicated by analysis of variance when the response data are first converted to logarithms. After such a conversion, curves of responses will appear parallel (in a statistical sense) just as in the additive case. Lockhart states that this is a common result in analysis of factor interactions in plants — more common than the additive responses.

In any case, it is important to remember that these two cases indicate no interaction, while any other kind of response indicates interaction. Lockhart summarizes additive and multiplicative responses in a simple table (Table 3).

Lockhart's (1965) analysis of multiple factor interactions is penetrating and impressive. Space will allow only a brief summary here. First it will be well to review a few of his definitions:

Growth: an irreversible increase in weight, volume, area or length of a plant or plant part.

Growth factor: a set of substances (interchangeable) that support growth when all other growth factor sets are provided. Growth factors vary for different organisms and are minimal for autotropic organisms. The simplest growth factor set contains only water. The various possible nitrogen sources available to a plant provide a more complex example of a growth factor set.

Growth factor flux: the flow of growth factors, which is proportional to their concentration differences and inversely proportional to the resistance encountered by the flow.

Modifying factors: such factors as temperature and light that exert

Table 3 Lockhart's (1965) Illustration of Additive and Multiplicative Responses to Two Factors, A and B, Applied in Combinations of High and Low Levels

	Multiplicative response			
	A_{low}	A_{high}	A_{low}	A_{high}
B_{low}	1	2	1	2
B_{high}	3	4	3	6
	$V = A + B$			$V = AB$	

their effects by influencing the concentration or flux of growth factors. (Light in photosynthesis is a growth factor rather than a modifying factor.)

Saturation: when a further increase in growth factor concentration has no effect upon response (unless other growth factors change). Effects of growth factors applied at supraoptimal concentrations should be considered in an analysis such as this, but we will not take the time to do so here.

Interaction: a measure of the influence of one variable upon the magnitude of the response to another variable—with additive and multiplicative responses constituting no interaction as discussed above. Actually, the term interaction can be used in various ways, but Lockhart suggests that we should restrict its usage to the statistical sense (Fisher's analysis of variance). A correlation between the responses of two dependent variables to one experimental variable is not an interaction, for example.

Lockhart considers how factors might interact in their effects upon growth of a plant. He emphasizes that the possible kinds of interaction are completely analogous to the interactions observed in enzymology. An interaction with a growth factor (e.g., increasing the growth factor increases the response as in the nutrition experiments of Figures 1–5) is perhaps the simplest interaction and is analogous to increasing the substrate concentration (at levels below saturation) in an enzymatically controlled reaction. No interaction of growth factors (independence in an analysis of variance) is analogous to noncompetitive effects on an enzyme. Complete interaction of growth factors is analogous to competitive enzyme interactions, in which an antimetabolite competes with the substrate for the active site on an enzyme. Finally, an incomplete interaction of growth factors is analogous to uncompetitive enzymatic inhibition or promotion, as when the inhibitor or promoter acts allosterically on an enzyme.

Mathematical Formulations for Growth

Numerous attempts have been made to formulate mathematical models of growth. Usually yield is expressed as a function of one or more growth factors. At least two criteria must be met by any such formulation: at zero concentration of growth factor, no growth occurs; and as the growth factor approaches infinity, growth approaches a limit. The three following systems have been rather widely applied (Lockhart, 1965).

Mitscherlich (1930):
$$y = V_{max}(1 - e^{-cx}) \simeq v$$
Balmukand (1928):
$$1/y = (c/x) + a$$
$$y = x/c + ax \simeq v$$
Michaelis and Menton (1913):

$$v = V_{max}x/(K + x) = x/(K/V_{max} + x/V_{max})$$

where: y = yield, V_{max} = maximum growth rate, e = base of natural logarithms, c = constant, x = concentration of growth factor, v = growth rate, a = constant, and K = Michaelis constant.

All three of these formulations produce saturation-type curves such as those in Figures 1–5. If time had permitted, it would have been instructive to attempt curve fitting with the data of these figures.

Several years ago, I was intrigued with the question of limiting factors; i.e., on what theoretical grounds might we expect only one growth factor at a time to limit growth? Or conversely, on what grounds might we expect two growth factors to be simultaneously limiting? When would we expect the "Blackman curves," and when would we expect the curves to diverge from each other as soon as they leave the origin?

At that time, I thought of a rather simpleminded approach that seemed to help me think about these questions. Assume that two interacting growth factors combine in some reaction, the product of which produces growth. The extent to which the two factors might be individually or simultaneously limiting will depend upon the extent to which the reaction goes to completion. Ignoring such sophistications as reaction rates, limitations due to diffusion, etc., we can simply think of two reactants, A and B, forming C:

$$A + B \rightleftharpoons C$$

The equilibrium constant for this reaction is indicated by $K = [A][B]/[C]$. If C is plotted as a function of A at various levels of B, typical saturation curves are produced (Figure 8). If the equilibrium constant K is very small, then A is completely limiting when B is not. This produces perfect "Blackman curves" and expresses exactly the concept of limiting factors in the restricted sense as originally envisioned by Liebig. This is the law of the minimum. That is, if the reaction goes virtually to completion, then any one of the reactants will be totally limiting when the other is not.

On the other hand, if K is large, indicating that the reaction goes only partially to completion, then A and B will both promote when increased

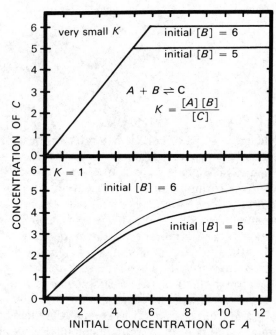

Figure 8 An illustration of the principle of limiting factors as it might be observed in a chemical equilibrium reaction. Concentration of hypothetical product is plotted as a function of initial concentration of one reactant (A) in the presence of two initial concentrations of the other reactant (B). (top) With a very small equilibrium constant, virtually all of the available A enters into the formation of C until B becomes limiting at its two concentrations. This is the ideal limiting factor response. If K is as large as 1 (bottom), then even at low concentrations, both A and B limit the amount of product formed. After Salisbury and Ross (1969).

in concentration. The sharp-breaking "Blackman curves" do not appear. Both A and B can be limiting factors at the same time, indicating a more general sense for the concept of limiting factors. Of course the more complex formulations above would provide the same analysis, but this approach seems to get at the heart of the matter rather directly. It suffers from the important deficiency that it seems to imply that an infinite increase in such reactants as A and B would lead to infinite growth. (We could solve this by adding the stipulation that the reaction is catalyzed by an enzyme that occurs in a finite amount. But including this in the equation destroys the "simpleminded" approach.)

I had hoped, in performing my mineral nutrition experiments, to see whether a true law of the minimum might be expressed or whether two factors could be simultaneously limiting. Examination of Figures 2, 4, and 5 reveals that the law of the minimum is indeed rather closely approached—closely enough to justify it as a valid and important generalization. It is obvious, however, that phosphate, for example, can limit growth somewhat even while nitrogen is strongly limiting. Thus the law of the minimum, as we might well expect, is at best an approximation of the truth, but a valuable one because of the insights it provides. Incidentally, it is not difficult to find other situations where the curves diverge

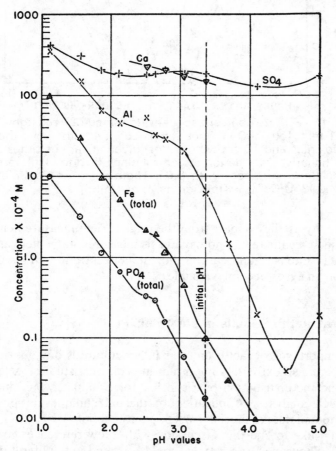

Figure 9 Concentrations of five ions as a function of pH of an equilibrium soil solution of hydrothermally altered material from the Big Rock Candy Mountain. Samples of soil were treated with various amounts of acid or base and a standard quantity of distilled water. After equilibrium had been achieved (over night), filtrates were analyzed. After Salisbury (1954).

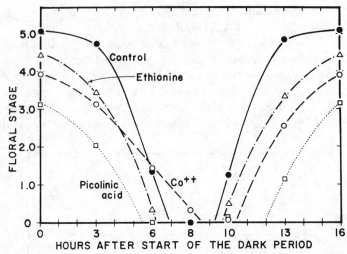

Figure 10 Effects upon subsequent flowering of a red light interruption (1 min, four 300 W flood lamps about 40 cm above the plants; red Plexiglas and 10 cm water filter) given at various times during a 16-hr inductive dark period to control plants and to plants previously treated (leaves dipped) with 0.01 M ethionine or picolinic acid or with 0.003 M CoCl$_2$. After Collins *et al.* (1963).

rather rapidly as they depart from the origin. Field measurements often provide such results (e.g., photosynthesis measured in the field as a function of light intensity and carbon dioxide concentration). This is where regression analyses become valuable.

Incorporating the Results in our Thinking

The importance of factor analysis in agriculture is obvious, and such analyses are also extremely important in ecological studies. Attempts to understand the distribution of a species, for example, would inevitably utilize such analyses. Application of these techniques in physiology helps us to understand mechanisms of plant function.

I would like to end this discussion with a few references to specific examples. Thousands of examples could be found in the literature, but I thumbed through my own reprints to come up with the following five examples:

1. Salisbury (1954, 1964). The Big Rock Candy Mountain in southcentral Utah is an exposed cross section of an ancient hot spring. It

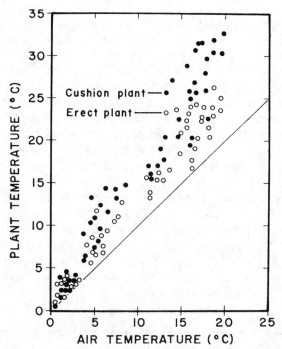

Figure 11 Plant temperature data obtained at about 3800 m (12500 ft) near The Trail Ridge Road of Rocky Mountain National Park in Colorado shown as a function of air temperature. The data are representative of those obtained on three occasions. The line shows equal plant and air temperatures. After Salisbury and Spomer (1964).

supports a few species, notably *Pinus ponderosa,* but *Artemisia tridentata* and other species of the region do not grow on the brightly colored, highly acidic (pH 3.4) material. Analysis (Figure 9) showed that nitrogen was extremely low in this material and that other elements such as phosphorus, iron, and aluminum were strongly influenced in their concentration by pH. The many observable interactions could be used to explain why certain vegetation could not grow on the material, but survival of the existing vegetation remains a mystery.

2. Collins *et al.* (1963). Numerous interactions have appeared over the years in our studies of the physiology of flowering. For example, a brief light interruption given at various times during a single 16-hr inductive dark period inhibits flowering of *Xanthium strumarium* (cocklebur) in a highly characteristic way (Figure 10). Two chemicals, ethionine and picolinic acid, applied to the plants just before the dark period also inhibit flowering, and their inhibition is essentially

additive to the inhibition due to light—indicating no interaction. Cobaltous ion, however, interacts strongly with the light inhibition, changing the time of maximum inhibition.

3. Salisbury and Spomer (1964). During one summer, George G. Spomer made hundreds of measurements of leaf temperatures in the alpine tundra of Colorado. Many environmental variables such as wind velocity, radiation, humidity, temperature, etc., were measured simultaneously (within the time limitations imposed by the necessity to record the data). Figure 11 shows some of the results. Several regression analyses were run, indicating a number of correlations and interactions. My conclusion from the study, however, was that effects on leaf temperature were simply too complex to be completely understood. It was obvious that several correlations existed, but there was always an extensive and unexplained scatter in the data.

4. Drake *et al.* (1970). In laboratory studies, Bert G. Drake measured leaf temperatures as a function of wind velocity, air temperature, and humidity at constant radiant input. It became apparent (Figure 12) that the difference between leaf and air temperature decreased as air temperature increased, up to about 35°C. These interactions imply

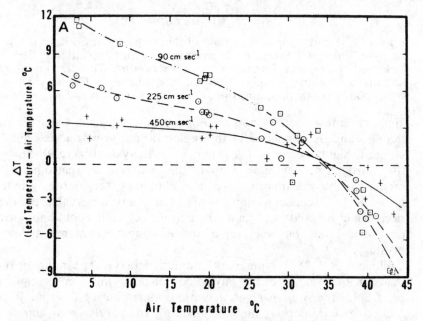

Figure 12 The difference between leaf and air temperature at three wind velocities plotted as a function of air temperature. Note that air and leaf temperature are about equal at 35°C. After Drake *et al.* (1970).

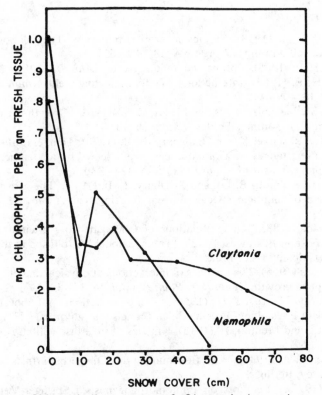

Figure 13 Chlorophyll contents of *Claytonia lanceolata* and *Nemophila breviflora* as a function of the depth of snow covering the plants. The dip in the *Nemophila* curve at 10 cm was correlated with the presence of a tree that produced heavy shade. In general, chlorophyll content appears to be proportional to the intensity of light penetrating the snow. After Kimball *et al.* (1973).

that, as the air temperature varies, the plants have a mechanism for controlling leaf temperature via control of transpiration.

5. Kimball *et al.* (1973). In recent years, we have been studying growth of certain spring ephemerals under the snow. Among other things, these plants apparently synthesize chlorophyll in response to the light penetrating the snow, as indicated by Figure 13.

Although statistics were used in two of the above studies, most of the analyses were carried out by plotting of the data and inspection of these plots. This is probably quite adequate in the majority of cases, but we should not overlook the powerful tools afforded to us by statistical treatments.

References

Balmukand, B. H. (1928). Studies in crop variation V. The relation between yield and soil nutrients. *J. Agr. Sci.* **18**, 602–627.

Blackman, F. F. (1905). Optima and limiting factors. *Ann. Bot.,* 281–295.

Clements, H. F. (1964). Interaction of factors affecting yield. *Annu. Rev. Plant Physiol.* **15**, 409–442.

Collins, W. T., Salisbury, F. B., and Ross, C. W. (1963). Growth regulators and flowering. III. Antimetabolites. *Planta* **60**, 131–144.

Drake, B. G., Raschke, K., and Salisbury, F. B. (1970). Temperatures and transpiration resistances of *Xanthium* leaves as affected by air temperature, humidity, and wind speed. *Plant Physiol.* **46**, 324–330.

Kimball, S. L., Bennett, B. D., and Salisbury, F. B. (1973). The growth and development of montane species at near freezing temperatures. *Ecology* **54**, 168–173.

Liebig, J. Von. (1885). "The Relations of Chemistry to Agricultural Experiments of Mr. J. B. Lawes," p. 23. (Trans. Samuel W. Johnson at the author's request.) Albany, New York.

Lockhart, J. A. (1965). The analysis of interactions of physical and chemical factors on plant growth. *Annu. Rev. Plant Physiol.* **16**, 37–52.

Machlis, L., and Torrey, J. G. (1956). "Plants in Action – A Laboratory Manual of Plant Physiology. Freeman, San Francisco, California.

Michaelis, L., and Menton, L. (1913). Kinetics of invertase action. *Biochem. Z.* **49**, 333–369.

Mitscherlich, E. A. (1930). "Die Bestimmung des Düngerbedürfnisses des Bodens." Parey, Berlin.

Mohr, H. (1972). "Lectures on Photomorphogenesis." Springer-Verlag, New York.

Salisbury, F. B. (1954). Some chemical and biological investigations of materials derived from hydrothermally altered rock in Utah. *Soil Sci.* **78**, 277–294.

Salisbury, F. B. (1964). Soil formation and vegetation on hydrothermally altered rock material in Utah. *Ecology* **45**, 1–9.

Salisbury, F. B., and Ross, C. (1969). "Plant Physiology." Wadsworth, Belmont, California.

Salisbury, F. B., and Spomer, G. G. (1964). Leaf temperatures of alpine plants in the field. *Planta* **60**, 497–505.

Multiple Factor Effects on Animals

W. B. Vernberg

University of South Carolina
Columbia, South Carolina

The environment is the sum of many abiotic and biotic factors acting constantly, and organisms are a part of this dynamic fluctuating complex. Although biologists have long recognized that capacity and resistance adaptations of animals are a function of the interaction of many environmental stimuli, by far the majority of studies have dealt with the influence of only one factor on an organism, with other variables held as nearly constant as possible. In view of the complex nature of environment, however, it is difficult to know which variables are significant, for physical forces may interact to kill an organism at intensity levels, which, if taken separately, would not be lethal.

When measured individually, the tolerances of some organisms to a number of environmental factors typically is much greater than the animal will normally experience in its habitat. If various combinations of these factors are studied simultaneously, the resultant tolerance limits more nearly approximate the concomitant fluctuations in environmental parameters experienced by the organism in the field. Recent and extensive reviews of multiple factor interaction can be found in Kinne (1970) and Alderdice (1972). These reviews demonstrate that multiple factor interactions influence many facets in the life of an organism including lethal limits, reproduction, larval development, osmoregulation, respiration, and behavior. Rather than duplicating these reviews, this paper will be directed primarily to recent papers that relate results of studies on multiple factor interaction to the physiological adaptations of animals to their environment.

It has long been recognized that salinity can modify thermal responses (for review, see Kinne 1970). Whether an organism can tolerate thermal stress best in combination with high or low salinity depends in large part on the temperature–salinity regime it encounters in nature. A good example can be found in the work of Kenny (1969) on the tube-dwelling polychaete *Clymenella torquata*. At 37°C the upper thermal limits of this worm is markedly reduced at lowered salinities; at low temperatures, however, *C. torquata* can withstand low salinities for long periods of time. This increased tolerance to low salinities in combination with low temperature can be correlated with the normal environmental regimes *C. torquata* encounters in nature, since the Newport River estuary in North Carolina, where this study was done, is a winter low salinity system. Periods of low salinity, therefore, usually coincide with periods of low temperature.

In some animals tolerance to thermal-salinity stress can be linked to osmoregulatory performance. During the winter the southern flounder *Paralichthys lethostigma* migrates from estuaries and low salinity coastal waters to a fully marine habitat on the continental shelf. This species shows seasonal differences in renal performance. The glomerular filtration rate, which is important in volume regulation, is low under a winter temperature–salinity regime when temperatures are low and salinity is high. In the warmer months when the fish returns to warmer and low salinity inshore waters, it has a high rate of glomerular filtration (Hickman, 1968).

Whether developing organisms tolerate low salinity best at high or low temperatures is also a function of the environmental parameters of their habitat. The mollusk *Adulus californiensis* lives in estuaries where salinity varies seasonally, but temperatures do not. Spawning occurs along the Oregon coast during the summer months when high salinity waters are carried into the estuary. During the first 3 days of development, tolerances are limited to temperatures ranging from 9° to 16°C and salinities from 28 to 33 o/oo (Lough and Gonor, 1971). These conditions are essentially oceanic, and would be favorable to those larvae swept out of the bay into the oceans. Metabolic measurements confirm the suitability of the oceanic environment for development of these mollusks (Lough and Gonor, 1973). Low salinity is particularly stressful at higher temperatures, and the relatively low salinity, high temperature conditions farther up in the estuary would result in high mortality rates. However, as the larvae age, they develop the necessary tolerances en-

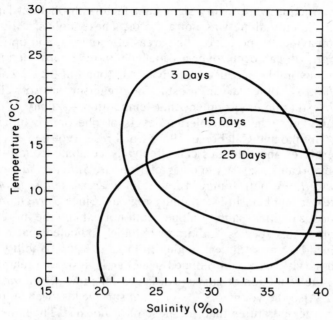

Figure 1 Comparison of 60% survival contours for 3-, 15-, and 25-day-old *Adula californiensis* larvae (from Lough and Gonor, 1973).

abling the mollusks to survive and reproduce under estuarine conditions (Figure 1).

In contrast to the low salinity, high temperature sensitivity of *A. californiensis,* larvae of species reproducing in high temperature water tend to be especially sensitive to low temperature and low salinity. Highest survival rates of *Menippe mercenaria* were obtained under a 30°C, 30 – 35 o/oo regime; low temperature in combination with low salinity was especially stressful (Ong and Costlow, 1970). Zoeae of the fiddler crab *Uca pugilator* also survived best under high temperature, high salinity (25°C, 30 o/oo) conditions (Vernberg *et al.,* 1974). Both *M. mercenaria* and *U. pugilator* spawn during the warmer months of the year when temperatures and salinity are most favorable for development, i.e., high temperature and high salinity. The thermal tolerance of larvae may be different from that of the adult stage. For example, first stage zoeae of the tropical fiddler crab, *Uca rapax,* can withstand lower temperatures than adults, but the opposite responses are found for the temperate zone species *Uca pugilator* and *U. pugnax* (Vernberg, 1969). Cain (1973) reported that larvae of *Rangia cuneata* become more tolerant to temperature and salinity as they age. However, temperature and temperature –

salinity interaction were highly significant factors throughout larval development. Salinity alone was not a factor. These mollusks live in low salinity embayments and oligohaline areas of estuaries, and optimal survival and growth can occur over a wide salinity range provided the temperature is favorable. Reduced survival was found at 32°C, 2 o/oo and 8°C, 20 o/oo. Yet other larvae of estuarine organisms are so well adapted to their estuarine environment that temperature–salinity interaction is important only when the tolerant levels of one or the other is approached (Brenko and Calabrese, 1969; Calabrese, 1969).

Temperatures and salinities can effectively combine to limit the distribution of organisms. Two species of isopods, *Sphaeroma rugicauda* and *S. hookeri*, are both found in low salinity areas, but *S. hookeri* occurs in greater numbers in low salinity regions. Since *S. rugicauda* survives in most salinities, salinity alone could not explain the more limited distribution of this species. Laboratory studies indicated that both species survived best at salinities ranging from 15 to 30 o/oo; ability of both species to survive was also reduced at either high or low temperature. However, the reduction of survival was greater in *S. rugicauda* than in *S. hookeri*. Also the young of *S. rugicauda* survive less well at lower salinities at all temperatures than do those of *S. hookeri*. Thus, the greater sensitivity of all stages in the life cycle of *S. rugicauda* to temperature–salinity interaction appears to limit distribution of this species (Jansen, 1970).

A good example of how the response of an organism can be linked with the ranges of environmental fluctuations it encounters in nature can be found in a recent study by Bayne (1973) on the responses of three species of mollusks to declining oxygen tensions and reduced salinity. Two of the species, *Gelonia ceylonica* and *Anadara granosa*, are tropical species; the third is *Mytilus edulis*, a boreal species. *Gelonia* can be characterized as an euryhaline organism that is tolerant of low oxygen tensions. It occurs intertidally and is out of water much of the time; oxygen tensions of the water that does cover it are low. *Anadara* occurs in shallow burrows in muddy sand; it is subjected to a wide range of oxygen tensions and is relatively stenohaline. *Mytilus* is euryhaline, and is also subject to low oxygen tensions from time to time. The two euryhaline species, *Mytilus* and *Gelonia* were better able to maintain a high metabolic rate in declining oxygen tensions than was *Anadara* over a salinity range of 20–30 o/oo. At a higher salinity (32.5 o/oo), however, *Gelonia* regulated better than *Anadara*, but *Anadara* regulated better than *Mytilus*.

Interaction of multiple factors also occurs in the deep sea, where there seems to be some correlation between resistance to pressure and eurythermy. A good example can be found in the study by Schlieper *et al.* (1967) on excised gill tissue from tropical and temperate zone mollusks. In the tropical zone species *Chama corrucopia* and *Modiolus auriculatus*, cellular gill activity decreased at 300 atm, reaching zero activity at 350–400 atm. Cellular activity in gill tissue of the eurythermal temperate zone *Mytilus edulis* and *Ostrea edulis* decreased at 400 atm pressure, ceasing completely between 700 and 800 atm. When the cellular resistance of gill tissue from the cold water stenotherm, *Cyprina islandica*, were compared with that of *M. edulis*, the latter was more resistant to pressure than the stenothermal species. Pressure resistance of tissues of the boreal species, *Modiolus modiolus*, which is found at the 15–50 m level, was much more resistant than the tropical shallow water species, *M. auriculatus*.

In another study (Menzies and George, 1972) investigated the pressure response of eight intertidal species found in tropical waters in comparison to eurythermal temperate zone species. These authors found that the pressure required to achieve the LD_{50} increased with decreasing temperature. Their data suggest that the survival of invertebrates under hydrostatic pressures should be better among cold water species than for tropical species or species living at high temperatures. These findings are in agreement with the zoogeographic and ecological implications of deep water communities which indicate that cold water species tend to be more eurybaric than warm water species.

Although vast regions of the sea are as yet unexploited, patches of oil and detectable quantities of DDT have been reported in some of the most remote parts of the ocean. Coastal and estuarine areas, on the other hand, tend to be heavily populated and industrialized, and the great majority of estuarine systems today are polluted to some extent with a wide variety of toxicants. Scientists should be aware of possible interaction between these pollutants and multiple factors in the environment.

Low dissolved oxygen content is not a pollutant in itself, but it is symptomatic of polluted waters, and can markedly influence survival of a species. In a study on the sand shrimp *Crangon septemspinosa* under different temperature–salinity conditions, Haefner (1969) found that 100% survival occurred over a relatively wide temperature–salinity range. Ovigerous shrimp, for example, could survive within the ranges of 4°–22°C and 20–40o/oo (Figure 2a). In comparable mortality studies but under low dissolved oxygen concentrations, temperature–salinity tolerances were greatly narrowed (Figure 2b). None had 100% survival and the tolerance zones were shifted toward lowered temperatures and higher salinities. From these data Haefner (1970) concluded that sand

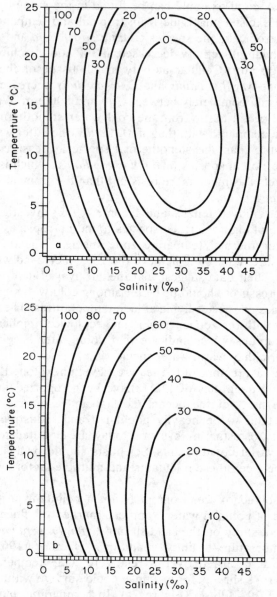

Figure 2   a, Estimation of percentage mortality of ovigerous *Crangon septemspinosa,* based on response surface fitted to observed mortality under 12 combinations of salinity and temperature in aerated water (from Haefner, 1970). b, Estimation of percentage mortality of ovigerous *Crangon septemspinosa,* based on response surface fitted to observed mortality under 12 combinations of salinity and temperature at low concentrations of dissolved oxygen (from Haefner, 1970).

shrimp populations could experience high mortalities and even decimation when dissolved oxygen levels remained at 2–3 ppm for extended periods of time.

Radioactivity is another potential hazard in the marine environment. Ecological aspects of radioactivity in the marine environment have been reviewed by Rice and Baptist (1970), who point out that the principal source of manmade radioactivity in the environment has been fallout from atomic test explosions, but unless extensive testing is resumed or there is a nuclear war, the contribution from this activity will continue to diminish. The amount of radioactive wastes will increase, however, from the use of nuclear reactors in electric power plants and ships.

It has been found that cesium-137 from fallout was more concentrated in the brackish water clam *Rangia cuneata* than in those clams from higher salinities in the same estuary (Wolfe and Schelske, 1969). It has also been noted that the cesium-137 content of *Rangia* fluctuated seasonally with an inverse relation to salinity of the water (Wolfe, 1967). These observations were confirmed in laboratory experiments by Wolfe and Coburn (1970), who found that concentration factors decreased with increasing salinity but increased with temperature (Table 1).

In another study on the interaction of environmental factors and radionuclides, it was found that the euryhaline fish *Fundulus heteroclitus* had a markedly increased LD_{50} when exposed to the combined effects of ionizing radiation, temperature and salinity (Angelovic et al., 1969). Mortalities of the fish were markedly affected with ^{22}Na efflux in combination with temperature-salinity stress. At temperatures above 20°C, mortality increased, but in lower salinities mortality was reduced in temperatures below 20°C. This may be linked to a limited osmoregulatory capability at the higher temperature since an irradiated fish generally lost ^{22}Na more rapidly than unirradiated fish (White et al., 1967).

Generally, larvae are much more sensitive to toxicants than are adults (Connor, 1972; DeCoursey and Vernberg, 1972), and very low concentrations of a toxicant can interact with environmental factors to

Table 1 Predicted Concentration Factors for Cesium-137 in Soft Tissues of *Rangia cuneata* at Different Temperatures and Salinities[a]

Salinity (o/oo)	Predicted concentration factor at different temperatures				
	5°C	10°	15°	20°	25°
1	7.33	11.6	14.5	16.6	18.4
5	5.04	7.15	8.55	9.64	10.5
10	4.11	5.68	6.73	7.54	8.22
20	3.31	4.47	5.26	5.87	6.38

[a]From Wolfe and Coburn, 1970.

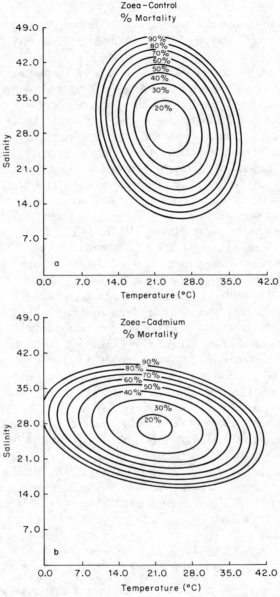

Figure 3 a, Estimation of percentage mortality of *Uca pugilator* zoeae based on response surface fitted to observed mortality under 13 combinations of salinity and temperature (from Vernberg *et al.*, 1974). b, Estimation of percentage mortality of *Uca pugilator* zoeae based on response surface fitted to observed mortality under 13 combinations of salinity and temperature (from Vernberg *et al.*, 1974).

cause increased mortalities among larvae. When zoeae of *Uca pugilator* were reared under different thermal–salinity regimes with and without the addition of 1 ppm cadmium, the tolerance levels of the cadmium-exposed zoeae were narrowed (Figure 3a, b). After 96 hr, 80% of the control larvae survived temperatures of 21°–28°C and salinities of 23–34o/oo. In experimental larvae, these ranges were 18°–23°C and 24–29o/oo. In the predictive equation where temperature and salinity were used as predictors of mortality, temperature (T_1, T_2) was the most important cause of death among control zoeae, but salinity (S_1, S_2) was the most important factor among the experimental ones (Vernberg *et al.*, 1974). Larvae exposed to very low levels of Hg (1.8 ppb) in combination with suboptimal thermal–salinity regimes also showed increased mortalities in comparison to control zoeae (Vernberg *et al.*, 1974). Unlike cadmium-exposed larvae, however, the interaction between Hg and temperature was the most important cause of death. These studies point up the fact that responses of the weakest link in a life cycle must be taken into account when assessing the effects of low level pollution.

That concentration of a pollutant which is sublethal under optimum thermal–salinity regimes can be lethal under a suboptimal regime is illustrated by the study of Vernberg and Vernberg (1972) and O'Hara and Vernberg (unpublished) on adult *U. pugilator*. Concentrations of 0.18 ppm Hg (as $HgCl_2$) and 1.0 ppm Cd (as $CdCl_2$) were sublethal under optimum conditions of temperature and salinity (25°C, 30o/oo) for 2–3 months (Vernberg and Vernberg, 1972; O'Hara and Vernberg, unpublished). When placed under suboptimal temperature–salinity regimes, however, survival was markedly affected. Although increased mortalities were noted under both high and low thermal–salinity stress, generally mercury-exposed crabs withstood high temperature and low salinity better than low temperature and low salinity, while cadmium-exposed crabs could better tolerate low temperature and low salinities. Such studies reinforce the comment of Sprague (1970) that "no assumption should be made about temperature effects on toxicity."

These results suggested that perhaps cause of death could be related to a greater accumulation of metals under the suboptimal regimes. It was established that most of the body burden was found in two tissues, the gill and hepatopancreas (Vernberg and Vernberg, 1972; O'Hara, 1973), and the total amount of metals in the gills and hepatopancreas was considered as total body burden. When crabs were exposed to a number of environmental regimes in combination with Hg, the total amount of mercury remained relatively unchanged under all temperature–salinity regimes. In contrast it became evident that the total body burden of cadmium was dependent on the thermal and, to a lesser extent, the salinity regime. After a 72-hr exposure to 1 ppm Cd, the amount of cadmium increased markedly with temperature, particularly in combination with low salinity. Not only was the uptake of cadmium dependent upon temperature–salinity conditions, but also the lethal concentration of cadmium can be corrrelated with these factors. O'Hara (1973) determined the cadmium concentration lethal to 50% of the test organisms in 240 hr (TLm-240 hr) under different thermal and salinity regimes (Figure 1). At 10°, 10o/oo, a concentration of 2.9 ppm Cd was fatal, whereas at 10°, 30o/oo, the concentration level was 47.0 ppm (Figure 4). Values generally were more influenced by temperature than by salinity within a given thermal regime. Thus, even within the usual ecological range experienced by these crabs, the tolerance level to cadmium was markedly altered.

Although the total amount of Hg does not change with shifts in temperature and salinity, the experimental regime did influence the distribu-

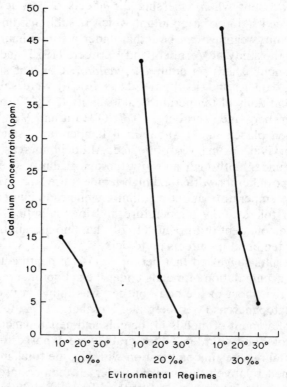

Figure 4 Cadmium concentration lethal to 50% of adult *Uca pugilator* after 240 hr under different temperature–salinity regimes (based on data from O'Hara, 1973).

tion of the mercury in the gill and hepatopancreas. After a 24-hr exposure to 0.18 ppm Hg, the amount of mercury in the gill increased with decreasing temperature. Conversely, the amount of mercury in the hepatopancreas decreased with increasing temperature (Vernberg and O'Hara, 1972). These results suggest that the inability to transfer mercury from the gill tissue to the hepatopancreas at low temperature could be a factor in the toxicity of mercury to fiddler crabs at low temperature.

The distribution of cadmium in the gills and hepatopancreas of crabs proved to be very different from that of mercury. The amount of cadmium in both the gills and hepatopancreas tended to increase with temperature, especially in combination with low salinity. At each temperature, crabs in low-salinity accumulated more than those in high-salinity water. The increased amount of cadmium at low salinities is probably a function of osmoregulation. In several brachyuran crabs osmotic regulation is controlled by salt exchange in addition to water regulation. Thus, the increased uptake of Cd is probably the result of active uptake of salts necessary to maintain the hyperosmotic condition of the internal medium.

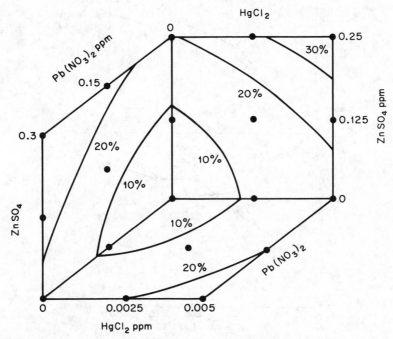

Figure 5 Effects of interactions of two heavy metals on *Cristigera* growth rate, showing mercury × zinc, mercury × lead, lead × zinc interactions (from Gray, 1974).

If an estuary is polluted, it is highly probable that more than one toxicant would be present. In such a situation, what would the effect be on uptake rates of each of the metals? When fiddler crabs were exposed to sublethal concentrations of mercury and cadmium, the general trend was to increase the amount of each metal in the gills when compared to exposure to a single metal and to decrease the amount in the hepatopancreas (O'Hara and Vernberg, unpublished). Mercury uptake in the gills was more influenced by the presence of cadmium, particularly at high salinities, than was cadmium uptake by the addition of mercury. It is unclear why high salinity should have this effect. The concomitant decrease in the hepatopancreas would suggest that the movement of the Hg from the gills to the hepatopancreas is being blocked.

Two or more metals present in the environment also can interact to significantly alter growth rates as illustrated in the studies by Gray and Ventilla (1973) and Gray (1974) on the ciliate *Cristigera*. Low level con-

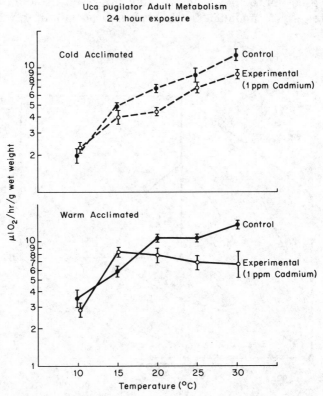

Figure 6 Metabolic-temperature curves of cold- and warm-acclimated *Uca pugilator*. Experimental animals have been exposed to 1 ppm cadmium for 24 hr.

centrations and mixtures of $HgCl_2$, $Pb(NO_3)_2$, $ZnSO_4$ were added to ex-potentially growing cultures of *Cristigera*. Mercury (5 ppb) alone re-duced growth rates 9.5% lead (300 ppb) reduced growth rates by 11.7%, and zinc (250 ppb) by 13.7%. If viewed from an additive basis, then, mix-ing of the chemicals should reduce growth rate by 37.4%. Instead, growth rate was reduced 67.2%, indicating supplemental synergistic effects. A graphic presentation is shown in Figure 5 of the effects of interactions of two heavy metals on *Cristigera* growth rate, showing mercury × zinc, mercury × lead, lead × zinc interactions.

Interactions of environmental factors with a pollutant are also appar-ent in other aspects of the biology of the animals. Studies on thermal-metabolic acclimation patterns indicate that patterns are modified in the presence of cadmium. Respiration rates were determined on cold- and warm-acclimated crabs that had been exposed to a sublethal concentra-tion of $CdCl_2$ (1 ppm Cd) for 24 hr or 14 days. Rates were measured at

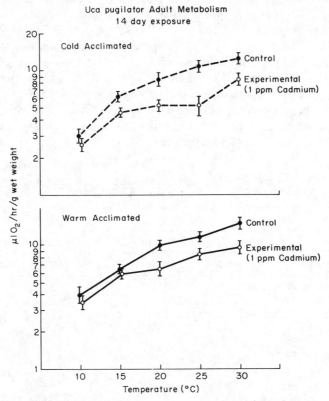

Figure 7 Metabolic-temperature curves of cold- and warm-acclimat-ed *Uca pugilator*. Experimental animals have been exposed to 1 ppm cadmium for 14 days.

temperatures ranging from 10° to 30°C at 5° intervals; the salinity was maintained at 30 o/oo. After a 24-hr exposure to cadmium, the pattern of response of the experimental crabs had been markedly modified, especially in the warm-acclimated crabs (Figure 6). In these crabs the oxygen consumption appeared to be independent of temperature increase above 15°C. In both cold- and warm-acclimated animals, 24-hr exposure to cadmium tended to significantly decrease oxygen uptake rates. Following exposure to cadmium for 14 days, the pattern of response of cold-acclimated animals was altered to greater extent than the patterns of warm-acclimated animals (Figure 7). Rates of the experimental crabs were significantly depressed over those of controls at all temperatures above 10°C and, again, there was a period of temperature insensitivity. Significantly decreased rates in the warm-acclimated experimental crabs were also noted at the higher temperature. Differences in Q_{10} patterns also point up the effect of Cd on these crabs (Table 2).

Other modifying effects of pollutants on temperature response have been noted. Temperature preference of salmonids changed after exposure to DDT (Ogilvie and Anderson, 1965), and Anderson (1968) found that the lateral line nerves of DDT-exposed salmonids showed increased and uncontrolled firing upon stimulation at 5°C and below. In goldfish an increase in water temperature from 21.1° to 21.5°C in the presence of $CuCl_2$ increased the attractiveness of the water (Kleerekoper et al., 1973). Another behavioral response, phototactic response, can be significantly altered by a temperature–salinity–mercury interaction. Mercury generally increases photopositive responses, but the interaction effects

Table 2 Q_{10} Values of Cold- and Warm-acclimated *Uca pugilator* following 1- and 14-Day Exposure to 1 ppm Cadmium

Temperature range (°C)	Q_{10}			
	Warm acclimated		Cold acclimated	
	Control	Experimental	Control	Experimental
After 1-day exposure				
10–15	2.7	1.2	2.8	1.1
15–20	4.8	2.4	2.0	3.2
20–25	1.0	1.1	1.6	1.3
25–30	1.0	3.3	1.7	1.5
After 14-day exposure				
10–15	2.7	3.5	4.2	3.4
15–20	2.0	1.0	1.8	1.2
20–25	1.6	1.4	1.7	1.0
25–30	1.6	1.5	1.3	3.1

are not the same for all stages. Analysis of variance data indicates that T × Hg and S Hg were significant at the 5% level in stage I zoeae while only the T × Hg interaction was significant in stage III larvae (Vernberg *et al.*, 1974).

Studies aimed at determining the effects of a pollutant on a particular organism obviously must take into account thermal history and temperature and salinity responses. It also must be recognized that man-induced environmental changes are now a part of what classically has been called a "normal environment." In the present-day concept of physiological adaptation to the environment, the interaction of pollutants with other parameters must be included.

References

Alderdice, D. F. (1972). Factor combinations—responses of marine poikilotherms to environmental factors acting in concert. In ' Marine Ecology," (O. Kinne, ed.), Vol. 1, part 3, pp. 1659–1722, Wiley (Interscience.), New York.

Anderson, J. M. (1968), Effect of sublethal DDT on the lateral line of brook trout, *Salvelinus fontinalis. J. Fish, Res. Bd. Can.* **25**, 2677–2682.

Angelovic, J. W., White, J. C., Jr., and Davis, E. M. (1969). Interactions of ionizing radiation, salinity and temperature on the estuarine fish, *Fundulus heteroclitus, Proc. 2nd Symp. Radioecol.* (D. J. Nelson, and F. C. Evans, ed.), pp. 131–141. Oak Ridge, Tenn. USAEC Conf-670503.

Bayne, B. (1973). The responses of three species of bivalve mollusc to declining oxygen tension at reduced salinity. *Comp. Biochem. Physiol.* **45A**, 793–806.

Brenko, M. H., and Calabrese, A. (1969). The combined effects of salinity and temperature on larvae of the mussel *Mytilus edulis. Mar. Biol.* **4**, 224–226.

Cain, T. D. (1973). The combined effects of temperature and salinity on embryos and larvae of the clam *Rangia cuneata. Mar. Biol.* **21**, 1–6.

Calabrese, A. (1969). Individual and combined effects of salinity and temperature on embryos and larvae of the coot clam *Mulinia lateralis* (Say). *Biol. Bull. Mar. Biol. Lab Woods Hole, Mass.* **137**, 417–428.

Connor, P. M. (1972). Acute toxicity of heavy metals to some marine larvae. *Mar. Poll. Bull.* **3**, 190–192.

DeCoursey, P. J., and Vernberg, W. B. (1972). Effect of mercury on survival, metabolism, and behaviour of larval *Uca pugilator* (Brachyura). *Oikos* **23**, 241–247.

Gray, J. S. (1974). Synergistic effects of three heavy metals on growth rates of a marine ciliate protozoan. *In* "Pollution and the Physiological Ecology of Estuarine and Coastal Water Organisms," (F. J. Vernberg and W. B. Vernberg, eds.); pp. 465–486. Academic Press, New York.

Gray, J. S., and Ventilla, R. J. (1973). Growth rates of sediment-living protozoan as a toxicity indicator for heavy metals. *Ambio* **2,** 118–121.

Haefner, P. A., Jr. (1969). Temperature and salinity tolerance of the sand shrimp, *Crangon septemspinosa* Say. *Physiol. Zool.* **42,** 388–397.

Haefner, P. A., Jr. (1970). The effect of low dissolved oxygen concentrations on temperature–salinity tolerance of the sand shrimp. *Crangon septemspinosa* Say. *Physiol. Zool.* **43,** 30–37.

Hickman, C. P. (1968). Glomerular filtration and urine flow in the euryhaline southern flounder, *Paralichthys lethostigma,* in sea water. *Can. J. Zool.* **46,** 427–437.

Jansen, K. P. (1970). Effect of temperature and salinity on survival and reproduction in Baltic populations of *Sphaeroma hookeri* Leach, 1814 and *S. rugicauda* Leach, 1814 (Isopoda). *Ophelia* **7,** 177–184.

Kenny, R. (1969). Effects of temperature, salinity and substrate on distribution of *Clymenella torquata* (Leidy), Polychaeta. *Ecology* **50,** 624–631.

Kinne, O. (ed.) (1970). Temperature. Animals. Invertebrates. *In* "Marine Ecology," Vol. 1, Part 1, pp. 407–514. Wiley (Interscience), New York.

Kleerekoper, H., Waxman, J. B., and Matis, J. (1973). Interaction of temperature and copper ions as orienting stimuli in the locomotor behavior of the goldfish *(Carassius auratus). J. Fish. Res. Bd. Can.* **30,** 725–728.

Lough, R. G., and Gonor, J. J. (1971). Early embryonic stages of *Adula californiensis* (Pelecypoda: Mytilidae) and the effect of temperature and salinity on developmental rate. *Mar. Biol.* **8,** 118–125.

Lough, R. G., and Gonor, J. J. (1973). A response-surface approach to the combined effects of temperature and salinity on the larval development of *Adula californiensis* (Pelecypodo: Mytilidae). I. Survival and Growth of three and fifteen-day old larvae. *Mar. Biol.* **22,** 224–250.

Menzies, R. J., and George, R. Y. (1972). Temperature effects on behavior and survival of marine invertebrates exposed to variations in hydrostatic pressure. *Mar. Biol.* **13,** 155–159.

Ogilvie, D. M., and Anderson, J. M. (1965). Effect of DDT on temperature selection by young Atlantic salmon, *Salmo salar. J. Fish. Res. Bd. Can.* **22,** 503–512.

O'Hara, J. (1973). The influence of temperature and salinity on the toxicity of cadmium to the fiddler crab, *Uca pugilator. Fish. Bull.* **71,** 149–153.

Ong, K. S., and Costlow, J. D., Jr. (1970). The effect of salinity and temperature on the larval development of the stone crab, *Menippe mercenaria* (Say), reared in the laboratory. *Chesapeake Sci* **11,** 16–29.

Rice, T. R., and Baptist, J. P. (1970). Ecological aspects of radioactivity in the marine environment. *In* "Environmental Radioactivity Symposium," (J. C. Clopton, ed.), pp. 107–180. The Johns Hopkins Univ. Dep. of Geogr. and Environmental Engineering, Baltimore, Maryland.

Schlieper, C., Flügel, H., and Theede, H. (1967). Experimental investigations of the cellular resistance ranges of marine temperate and tropical bivalves: Results of the Indian Ocean expedition of the German Research Association. *Physiol. Zool.* **40,** 354–360.

Sprague, J. B. (1970). Measurement of pollutant toxicity to fish. II. Utilizing and applying bioassay results. *Water Res.* **4**, 3–32.

Vernberg, F. J. (1969). Acclimation of intertidal crabs. *Amer. Zool.* **9**, 331–341.

Vernberg, W. B., and O'Hara, J. (1972). Temperature–salinity stress and mercury uptake in the fiddler crab, *Uca pugilator. J. Fish. Res. Bd. Can.* **29**, 1491–1494.

Vernberg, W. B., and Vernberg, F. J. (1972). The synergistic effects of temperature, salinity and mercury on survival and metabolism of the adult fiddler crab, *Uca pugilator. Fish. Bull.* **70**, 415–420.

Vernberg, W. B., DeCoursey, P. J., and O'Hara, J. (1974). Multiple environmental factor effects on physiology and behavior of the fiddler crab, *Uca pugilator. In* "Pollution and the Physiological Ecology of Estuarine and Coastal Water Organisms," (F. J. Vernberg and W. B. Vernberg, eds.) pp. 381–426. Academic Press, New York.

White, J. C. Jr., Angelovic, J. W., Engel, D. W., and Davis, E. M. (1967). Interactions of radiation, salinity and temperature on estuarine organisms. *U. S. Fish Wildl. Serv. Circ.* (270), 29–35.

Wolfe, D. A. (1967). Seasonal variation of Caesium-137 from fallout in a clam, *Rangia cuneata*, Tray. *Nature London* **215**, 1270.

Wolfe, D. A., and Coburn, C. B. Jr. (1970). Influence of salinity and temperature on the accumulation of Cesium-137 by an estuarine clam under laboratory conditions. *Health Physics* **18**, 499–505.

Wolfe, D. A., and Schelske, C. L. (1969). Accumulation of fallout radioisotopes by bivalve molluscs from the lower Trent and Neuse Rivers. *Proc. 2nd Symp. Radioecol.* ed. by (D. J. Nelson and F. C. Evans, ed.), pp. 493–504. Oak Ridge, Tenn. USAEC Conf-670503.

On the Mathematical Modeling of Biological Systems: A Qualified "Pro"

F. Eugene Yates

Department of Biomedical Engineering
University of Southern California
Los Angeles, California

If our brains had infinite capacity for recording experience and could note and instantaneously recall all past associations of causes and effects, then, perhaps, modeling of reality and carrying out internal simulations would not be the outstanding human characteristics that they obviously are (Monod, 1971). If we had observed every case of forces *(F)*, masses *(m)* and accelerations *(a)*, and could recall their exact values, then we would not need to use a compact, abstracted relationship,

$$F = ma$$

to codify these relationships. But in fact, internal simulation, the formulation of some kind of model of the past (history), present (orientation), and future (planning), is the chief occupation of the conscious mind of man. We are designed to be modelers, and our models often take the form of external simulations of aspects of reality, which simulations are transmittible to other human beings.

When we create an external simulation, we usually make a point of using explicit, mathematical models. Models are usually of the equivalent network type, that is, they describe connections among specified functional components. The mathematical formulations serve at least eight related purposes which seem appreciated by engineers more than

539

by biologists. The eight purposes of simulation by means of such mathematical models are shown in Table 1 (Yates, 1971a).

The practitioners of the biological scientific art sometimes obscure the real issues behind modeling by assuming in advance that living systems are too complex to model mathematically. Can this view also mean, too complex to understand? If so, then what are the skeptics doing when they write their own nonmathematical papers?

Since modeling is a universal manifestation of the psychology of science, it is presumptuous for any one person to tell others how or why to do it. Nevertheless, by chance and inclination, I have been reflecting upon mathematical models in biology over a 10-year period. My views are developed in detail in 13 references that range from specific examples to general philosophy (Brown-Grant et al., 1970; Yates, 1967, 1969, 1971a,b, 1973; Yates and Brennan, 1967, 1969; Yates and Iberall, 1975; Yates and Urquhart, 1962; Yates et al., 1968, 1969, 1972).

To illustrate the problems I have encountered with mathematical models in biology, I wish to consider in a somewhat whimsical way, the relationships among the three processes of description, explanation and understanding. I assume, without defining the term, that what we wish to achieve by modeling is "understanding." Understanding, in turn, is a function of the interactions of descriptions (observational data, requiring money to accumulate) and explanation. Explanation can be considered as a framework we use to interpret data, and may be of several kinds, as indicated below.

The Scale of Explanation

Explanation in its most primitive form is purely verbal (and mere words, of course, can be used to mean almost anything, regardless of their assigned meanings). In the next most advanced form, explanation consists of diagrams. In biology these are usually arrow diagrams asserting dynamic relations by means of static pictures. It is very easy to be a professor, if students will accept as explanation such schemes as:

$$DNA \rightarrow mRNA \rightarrow protein$$

What dynamic mysteries lurk uncaptured by that (static) sequence written on a blackboard!

In still more advanced forms, explanation consists of empirical equations "fitting" (and here the criteria of agreement or fit are seldom presented) a specified set of data, but without proven capacity to predict any other set. At the next more advanced level, explanation consists of a logical structure expressed by either of two types of mathematical formalisms. The first is in the form of Boolean algebra which captures functional relations (Gann *et al.*, 1973). The second is in the form of homomorphic sets of algebraic and differential equations which, in the ideal, map dynamic properties of solutions of equations onto dynamic processes in a real system on a one-to-one basis. The correspondence between equation structure and system structure begins to be high at this stage of explanation.

Finally, at the highest level with which I am familiar, explanation invokes powerful, general physical concepts for the illumination of dynamic system properties. This approach attempts to find a nearly universal set of physical principles to explain properties of all viable systems. The principles may be found, for example, in statistical and irreversible process thermodynamics combined with nonlinear mechanics (Iberall, 1972). Out of extensive observation (description) and most advanced explanation comes the highest understanding.

Figure 1 illustrates the relationship among description, explanation, and understanding and shows a peculiarity of the resulting terrain of knowledge, the surface of understanding upon which the scientist attempts to climb upward for a better view. The peculiarity is seen in the Hill of Illusion. As we obtain more data, and extend the richness of our explanations from words toward homomorphic or isomorphic equation sets, and create a simulator, we increase our understanding to a point

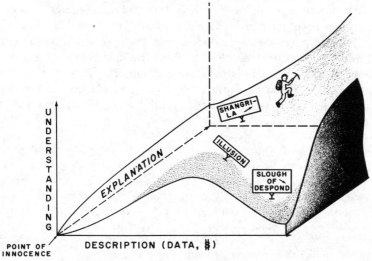

Figure 1 Whimsical relationships among description, explanation, and understanding. The axes are defined in the text.

shown at the top of the hill in the foreground of the figure. But then we find, to our consternation and disappointment, that every way from there is down. As we gather more data our model fails in predictive power. The unpredicted actually occurs. If we then try to extend our model, we become confronted with an overwhelmingly large set of new parameters or relations to identify, beyond the reach of our experimental methods. Thus we can't easily defend our model by extending the data base upon which it rests. The data remain always too limited to validate the extended model. At this point we have achieved a limited, though useful simulation of a special case of a living system or one of its components. Generality eludes us, and we have not discovered or expressed a theory of the living state with our model. Perhaps it is not too cynical to say that when we reach this point, what we actually understand is our limited model.

Uses of Limited Models (Simulators)

Limited, special-case models (simulators), can be very valuable to an investigator because they may provide him with one or more of the eight features listed in Table 1. If the modeler keeps in mind the importance of knowing what question it is that he or she is trying to answer through the act of modeling, he or she is unlikely to be either too grandiose in his claims or hopes, or defeated by the limited results he obtains. We must be content in choosing as our purpose in modeling, some goal that modeling is capable of reaching. Otherwise, we may end up concluding merely that computers are versatile, or that the essence of biological systems cannot be captured mathematically. The first conclusion is correct but trivial, and the latter is false. I wish to emphasize again that each of the eight features listed in Table 1 as possible yields from mathematical modelling is in fact realizeable and useful. Claude Levi-Strauss (1966) put it as follows in "The Savage Mind":

> And when we do finally succeed in understanding life as a function of inert matter, it will be to discover that the latter has properties very different from those previously attributed to it. Levels of reduction cannot therefore be classed as superior and inferior, for the level taken as superior must, through reduction, be expected to communicate retroactively some of its richness to the inferior level to which it will have been assimilated. Scientific explanation consists not in moving from the complex to the simple but in the replacement of a less intelligible complexity by one which is more so.

Table 1 Uses of Mathematical Models of the Equivalent Network Type (Simulators).

1. Codification of current facts and beliefs about a system of interest (bookkeeping).
2. Exposure of contradictions in the data sets or beliefs.
3. Explorations of the major implications of the beliefs about the system (which implications may be strongly counterintuitive).
4. Exposure of incompletness in the data sets.
5. Prediction of system performance under new conditions.
6. Prediction of values of experimentally inaccessible variables or parameters.
7. Identification of the essentials of system structure.
8. Representation of the current "understanding" of the system of interest.

At least to the creator of a model, the model represents a more intelligible complexity than does the raw set of data upon which it operates.

Models of Exceedingly Complex Biological Systems

For each model there is an appropriate level of structure and function, and the degree of complexity within models tends to approach the same extent whether the model deals with subcellular processes or human population dynamics. It is not required, useful, or possible to go from molecular events to political systems with a model continuous through all levels in the hierarchy. Instead, perhaps we should look down and up only one level in each direction from the predominant level at which the model is structured. In any event, living systems are probably only piecewise continuous themselves (Yates and Iberall, 1975).

Probably most people would agree that human political and economic systems represent the most complex living systems. As pointed out by Arthur Iberall (personal communication) only three different approaches have been used in the formulation of models of such systems: (1) casual, conversational constructs; (2) the social inventory approach, which consists of gathering data and tabulating relationships; and (3) the equivalent network approach, which consists of establishing feedback circuits of relations among levels and rates, as exemplified in the work of Forrester (1969a,b; 1971), and elaborated most recently by Meadows *et al.* (1972) in aa extension of Forrester's earlier work "World Dynamics" (1971). In the equivalent network approach, functional relationships are established on an empirical basis, if there is no theoretical basis for their formulation (as usually there is not), and feedback effects are noted and incorporated into the connections within the model. Multiple loop models result which are usually nonlinear and these can be strikingly counterintuitive in their performance. Objections to the equivalent network approach, which I do not share, have been vigorously expresssed in an article by Passell *et al.* (1972) in which they deal simultaneously with "The Limits to Growth," "World Dynamics," and "Urban Dynamics." To give a sample of the flavor of their review, I have selected one of their pungent paragraphs:

> The *Limits to Growth,* in our view, is an empty and misleading work. Its imposing apparatus of computer technology and systems jargon conceals a kind of intellectual Rube Goldberg device—one which takes arbitrary assumptions, shakes them up, and comes out with arbitrary conclusions that have the ring of science. "Limits" pretends to a degree of certainty so exaggerated as to obscure the few modest (and unoriginal) insights that it genuinely contains. Less than pseudo-science and little more than polemical fiction, the *Limits to Growth* is best summarized not as a rediscovery of the laws of nature, but as a rediscovery of the oldest maxim of computer science: Garbage In, Garbage Out.

Even though I do not share this disparaging viewpoint with respect to the equivalent network approach to the modeling of complex systems, I believe, along with A. S. Iberall, that the most satisfying understanding of these systems will come from a fourth approach, that of nonequilibrium thermodynamics, combined with nonlinear mechanics. In this approach, there is hope for a general systems theory (Iberall, 1972; Yates *et al.*, 1972; Yates and Iberall, 1975) and the means to leave the Hill of Illusion and ascend the higher slopes of understanding, shown in the right, rear region in Figure 1.

Obviously, part of the difficulty in discussing or appreciating mathematical modeling applied in the life sciences has to do with the uncertain and incomplete nature of the act of mathematical modeling. As an art, it has room for many different tastes; as an expression of logical relations, it is as vulnerable as the assumptions made at the outset. It has been my experience that among able scientists, both those who have attempted mathematical modeling of systems of interest, and those who take the view that biological systems have some innate properties that remove them from the domains accessible by mathematical modeling, can achieve coherence of thought. But let us not be deceived—this congenial result is obtained because the human brain is a remarkably capable, compulsive, internal simulator and modeler, even in those persons who disdain such external, overt acts of modeling as writing a differential, algebraic, or Boolean equation. In the end, if we seek understanding, models are the only truths we ever find. So far, the most powerful, predictive, compact, and unambiguous models we have achieved have been of the Model that he might have perceived and cast down.

I must carefully define the sort of model that I have in mind "the ill and unfit choice of words wonderfully obstructs the nding" (N.O. 43). My object is not to construct a windmill by a class of model that is easily and profitlessly attacked. Rather, define and consider a class of model that is as unexceptionable le, thus making my criticisms more substantial than the jousting mill that I built to destroy.

ubject is the mathematical class of model because calculation is cific than prose. It deals in cause and effect rather than the in-ut of a black box and thus makes good use of fundamental ge. It calculates change, for example, as the growth of plant uring a week from a knowledge of a causal change such as the thesis per hour that has a characteristic time perhaps a hun-ut not a billionth of the characteristic time of the calculated growth. Finally, the simulated causes must mimic the real nd the calculated outcome must mimic the real outcome.

is the most unexceptionable class of model that I can define, if it can be criticized, all models can be criticized and have idols casting down.

revity, I shall refer to this class of model as the "simulator." criticisms will apply to the problems that arise when the fore-teria for simulators are not followed. Then, I shall relate the s that may occur even with these simulators.

s of Models That Are Not Simulators

fining the class of model to be discussed here I said that the change would be calculated from knowledge of a causal pro-was nearby in a scale of characteristic times. Thus if one tried g the change in weight of a plant from the much shorter times h faster rates of molecular reactions, he or she would not be simulator as I have specified it.

nderstanding must not . . . be allowed to jump and fly from particu-remote axioms . . . and taking stand upon them as truths that cannot ken, proceed to prove and frame the middle axioms by reference to . . . Then only, may we hope well of the sciences, when in a just f ascent, and by successive steps not interrupted or broken, we rise articulars to lesser axioms; and then to middle axioms, one above the and last of all to the most general [N.O. 104].

mathematical. The burden of proof lies heavily upon those who would insist, for whatever (vitalistic?) reasons, that in biology it should be different. But the question is open. Let us work.

References

Brown-Grant, K., Brennan, R. D., and Yates, F. E. (1970). Simulation of the thyroid hormone-binding protein interactions in human plasma. *J. Clin. Endocrinol. Metab.*, **30**, 733–751.

Forrester, J. W. (1969a). "Principles of Systems." Wright-Allen Press, Cambridge, Massachusetts.

Forrester, J. W. (1969b). "Urban Dynamics." M.I.T. Press, Cambridge, Massachusetts.

Forrester, J. W. (1971). "World Dynamics." Wright-Allen Press, Cambridge, Massachusetts.

Gann, D. S., Cryer, G. L., and Schoeffler, J. D. (1973). Finite level models of biological systems. *Ann. Biomed. Eng.* **1**, 385–445.

Iberall, A. S. (1972). "Toward a General Science of Viable Systems." McGraw-Hill, New York.

Levi-Strauss, C. (1966). "The Savage Mind," pp. 247–248. Univ. of Chicago Press, Chicago, Illinois.

Meadows, D. H., Meadows, D. L., Randers, J., and Behrens W. W. III, (1972). "The Limits to Growth." Universe Books, New York.

Monod, J. (1971). "Chance and Necessity." Knopf, New York.

Passell, P., Roberts, M., and Ross, L. (1972). *N.Y. Times Book Rev.* April 2, 1972.

Yates, F. E. (1967). Physiological control of adrenal cortical hormone secretion. *In* "The Adrenal Cortex," (A. Eisenstein, ed.), Chap. 4, pp. 133–183. Little, Brown and Co., Boston, Massachusetts.

Yates, F. E. (1969). The adrenal glucocorticoid endocrine system: simulation of a biological controller. *J. Basic Eng., Trans. ASME* **92**, 305–312.

Yates, F. E. (1971a). A physical view of endocrine and metabolic systems. *Acta Cient. Venez.* **22** (Suppl. 2), 46–50.

Yates, F. E. (1971b). Systems analysis in biology. *In* "Biomedical Engineering," (J. H. U. Brown, J. Jacobs, and L. Stark, eds.), pp. 3–19. Davis, Philadelphia, Pennsylvania.

Yates, F. E. (1973). Systems Biology as a Concept. *In* "Engineering Principles in Physiology," (J. H. U. Brown and D. S. Gann, eds.), Vol. I, pp. 3–12. Academic Press, New York.

Yates, F. E., and Brennan, R. D. (1967). Study of the mammalian adrenal glucocorticoid system by computer simulation. *IBM Tech. Rep.* #320-3228, December 1967, IBM Data Processing Division, Palo Alto Scientific Center.

Yates, F. E., and Brennan, R. D. (1969). Digital simulation of a biochemical control system. *Proc. IBM Sci. Computing Symp. Computers Chem.* IBM Data Processing Division Form 320-1954-0, White Plains, New York.

Yates, F. E., and Iberall, A. S. (1975). Temporal and hierarchical organization in biosystems. *In* Temporal Aspects of Therapeutics," (J. Urquhart and F. E. Yates, eds.). *Proc. 2nd Alza Conf.,* Plenum Press (in press).

Yates, F. E., and Urquhart, J. (1962). Control of plasma concentrations of adrenal cortical hormones. *Physiol. Rev.* **42**, 359–443.

Yates, F. E., Brennan, R. D., Urquhart, J., Dallman, M. F., Li, C. C., and Halpern, W. (1968). A continuous system model of adrenocortical function. *In* "Systems Theory and Biology," (M. Mesarovic, ed.), pp. 141–184. Springer-Verlag, New York.

Yates, F. E., Brennan, R. D., and Urquhart, J. (1969). The adrenal glucocorticoid control system. *Fed. Proc.* (Symp. issue) **28**, 71–83.

Yates, F. E., Marsh, D. J., and Iberall, A. S. (1972). Integration of the whole organism: a foundation for a theoretical biology. *In* "Challenging Biological Problems: Directions Towards Their Solution," (J. A. Behnke, ed.). AIBS 25 year celebration volume, Oxford Press, pp. 110–132.

are Ido

Firs
becaus
underst
definin
I want
as poss
at a wi

My
more s
put-out
knowle
weight
photos
dredth
weekly
causes

Thi
and thu
that ne

For
First, r
going
difficul

Idols of the Model or Bringir

Paul E. Waggoner

The Connecticu

Introduction

In 1620 Pilgrims stepped off the Mayflo
in the Commonwealth of Massachusetts, v
lawyer and politician, Francis Bacon, publi
casting down the Idols of the Tribe, the C
Theater that beset men's minds and constr
empty controversies and idle fancies" (N.
modern science, devised the mixture of e
that broke the Idols and with them broke
sy, starting the straighter trajectory of sc
three and a half centuries to a still imperfe
standing of nature. It was Bacon who sho
gate between high-flown generalizations a
stead "from works and experiments to ex
again from these causes and axioms, new
legitimate interpreter of nature" (N.O. 11
ing, I can do no better than bring Bacon ho

Proble

In
simulat
cess th
calcula
and m
making

The
lars
be s
then
scal
from
othe

*N.O. 43 refers to the 43d aphorism of Bacon's "Great Instauration."

mathematical. The burden of proof lies heavily upon those who would insist, for whatever (vitalistic?) reasons, that in biology it should be different. But the question is open. Let us work.

References

Brown-Grant, K., Brennan, R. D., and Yates, F. E. (1970). Simulation of the thyroid hormone-binding protein interactions in human plasma. *J. Clin. Endocrinol. Metab.*, **30**, 733–751.

Forrester, J. W. (1969a). "Principles of Systems." Wright-Allen Press, Cambridge, Massachusetts.

Forrester, J. W. (1969b). "Urban Dynamics." M.I.T. Press, Cambridge, Massachusetts.

Forrester, J. W. (1971). "World Dynamics." Wright-Allen Press, Cambridge, Massachusetts.

Gann, D. S., Cryer, G. L., and Schoeffler, J. D. (1973). Finite level models of biological systems. *Ann. Biomed. Eng.* **1**, 385–445.

Iberall, A. S. (1972). "Toward a General Science of Viable Systems." McGraw-Hill, New York.

Levi-Strauss, C. (1966). "The Savage Mind," pp. 247–248. Univ. of Chicago Press, Chicago, Illinois.

Meadows, D. H., Meadows, D. L., Randers, J., and Behrens W. W. III, (1972). "The Limits to Growth." Universe Books, New York.

Monod, J. (1971). "Chance and Necessity." Knopf, New York.

Passell, P., Roberts, M., and Ross, L. (1972). *N.Y. Times Book Rev.* April 2, 1972.

Yates, F. E. (1967). Physiological control of adrenal cortical hormone secretion. *In* "The Adrenal Cortex," (A. Eisenstein, ed.), Chap. 4, pp. 133–183. Little, Brown and Co., Boston, Massachusetts.

Yates, F. E. (1969). The adrenal glucocorticoid endocrine system: simulation of a biological controller. *J. Basic Eng., Trans. ASME* **92**, 305–312.

Yates, F. E. (1971a). A physical view of endocrine and metabolic systems. *Acta Cient. Venez.* **22** (Suppl. 2), 46–50.

Yates, F. E. (1971b). Systems analysis in biology. *In* "Biomedical Engineering," (J. H. U. Brown, J. Jacobs, and L. Stark, eds.), pp. 3–19. Davis, Philadelphia, Pennsylvania.

Yates, F. E. (1973). Systems Biology as a Concept. *In* "Engineering Principles in Physiology," (J. H. U. Brown and D. S. Gann, eds.), Vol. I, pp. 3–12. Academic Press, New York.

Yates, F. E., and Brennan, R. D. (1967). Study of the mammalian adrenal glucocorticoid system by computer simulation. *IBM Tech. Rep.* #320-3228, December 1967, IBM Data Processing Division, Palo Alto Scientific Center.

Yates, F. E., and Brennan, R. D. (1969). Digital simulation of a biochemical control system. *Proc. IBM Sci. Computing Symp. Computers Chem.* IBM Data Processing Division Form 320-1954-0, White Plains, New York.

Yates, F. E., and Iberall, A. S. (1975). Temporal and hierarchical organization in biosystems. *In* Temporal Aspects of Therapeutics," (J. Urquhart and F. E. Yates, eds.). *Proc. 2nd Alza Conf.*, Plenum Press (in press).

Yates, F. E., and Urquhart, J. (1962). Control of plasma concentrations of adrenal cortical hormones. *Physiol. Rev.* **42,** 359–443.

Yates, F. E., Brennan, R. D., Urquhart, J., Dallman, M. F., Li, C. C., and Halpern, W. (1968). A continuous system model of adrenocortical function. *In* "Systems Theory and Biology," (M. Mesarovic, ed.), pp. 141–184. Springer-Verlag, New York.

Yates, F. E., Brennan, R. D., and Urquhart, J. (1969). The adrenal glucocorticoid control system. *Fed. Proc.* (Symp. issue) **28,** 71–83.

Yates, F. E., Marsh, D. J., and Iberall, A. S. (1972). Integration of the whole organism: a foundation for a theoretical biology. *In* "Challenging Biological Problems: Directions Towards Their Solution," (J. A. Behnke, ed.). AIBS 25 year celebration volume, Oxford Press, pp. 110–132.

Idols of the Model or Bringing Home the Bacon

Paul E. Waggoner

The Connecticut Agricultural Experiment Station
New Haven, Connecticut

Introduction

In 1620 Pilgrims stepped off the Mayflower and onto Plymouth Rock in the Commonwealth of Massachusetts, while back home in England a lawyer and politician, Francis Bacon, published the "Novum Organum," casting down the Idols of the Tribe, the Cave, the Marketplace, and the Theater that beset men's minds and constrained science to "numberless empty controversies and idle fancies" (N.O. 43).* Bacon, the herald of modern science, devised the mixture of experimentation and reasoning that broke the Idols and with them broke the circle of empty controversy, starting the straighter trajectory of science that has brought us in three and a half centuries to a still imperfect but certainly clearer understanding of nature. It was Bacon who showed how science could navigate between high-flown generalizations and dumb cataloguing and instead "from works and experiments to extract causes and axioms and again from these causes and axioms, new works and experiments as a legitimate interpreter of nature" (N.O. 117). As I criticize model building, I can do no better than bring Bacon home to the task, seeing if there

---

*N.O. 43 refers to the 43d aphorism of Bacon's "Novum Organum" and G.I. to his "Great Instauration."

are Idols of the Model that he might have perceived and cast down.

First, I must carefully define the sort of model that I have in mind because "the ill and unfit choice of words wonderfully obstructs the understanding" (N.O. 43). My object is not to construct a windmill by defining a class of model that is easily and profitlessly attacked. Rather, I want to define and consider a class of model that is as unexceptionable as possible, thus making my criticisms more substantial than the jousting at a windmill that I built to destroy.

My subject is the mathematical class of model because calculation is more specific than prose. It deals in cause and effect rather than the input-output of a black box and thus makes good use of fundamental knowledge. It calculates change, for example, as the growth of plant weight during a week from a knowledge of a causal change such as the photosynthesis per hour that has a characteristic time perhaps a hundredth but not a billionth of the characteristic time of the calculated weekly growth. Finally, the simulated causes must mimic the real causes, and the calculated outcome must mimic the real outcome.

This is the most unexceptionable class of model that I can define, and thus if it can be criticized, all models can be criticized and have idols that need casting down.

For brevity, I shall refer to this class of model as the "simulator." First, my criticisms will apply to the problems that arise when the foregoing criteria for simulators are not followed. Then, I shall relate the difficulties that may occur even with these simulators.

Problems of Models That Are Not Simulators

In defining the class of model to be discussed here I said that the simulated change would be calculated from knowledge of a causal process that was nearby in a scale of characteristic times. Thus if one tried calculating the change in weight of a plant from the much shorter times and much faster rates of molecular reactions, he or she would not be making a simulator as I have specified it.

> The understanding must not . . . be allowed to jump and fly from particulars to remote axioms . . . and taking stand upon them as truths that cannot be shaken, proceed to prove and frame the middle axioms by reference to them . . . . Then only, may we hope well of the sciences, when in a just scale of ascent, and by successive steps not interrupted or broken, we rise from particulars to lesser axioms; and then to middle axioms, one above the other; and last of all to the most general [N.O. 104].